D1611227

LYMPH NODES

Cambridge Illustrated Surgical Pathology

This text-atlas is a practical, integrated, and modern approach to lymph node pathology. Intended for both practicing pathologists and pathologists in training, it provides a personal view of lymph node diagnosis by one of the international leaders in the field.

Illustrated with more than 250 full-color photographs, this book covers the entire range of disease that may be encountered in lymph node pathology. It features extensive coverage of nonneoplastic lymphoid lesions and non-lymphoid lesions, and discusses all malignant lymphomas and other neoplasms that may involve lymph nodes in both adult and pediatric populations. The orientation is unique, as the text not only showcases various disease entities but also portrays the progression of disease states from incipient to advanced. Finally, the author emphasizes differential diagnosis, covering all of the methods used in distinguishing different easily confused entities.

Dr. Lawrence M. Weiss is a Board-certified anatomic pathologist and the current chairman of pathology at the City of Hope National Medical Center in Duarte, California. He has published more than 300 papers on varied topics in surgical pathology and hematopathology. He is also the editor of four books on hematologic malignancies and surgical pathology. In 2000, he was honored by the United States and Canadian Academy of Pathology as its Young Investigator of the Year.

LYMPH NODES

Cambridge Illustrated Surgical Pathology

Lawrence M. Weiss

City of Hope National Medical Center

WH
17
· W431i
2008

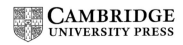
CAMBRIDGE
UNIVERSITY PRESS

CAMBRIDGE UNIVERSITY PRESS
Cambridge, New York, Melbourne, Madrid, Cape Town, Singapore, São Paulo, Delhi

Cambridge University Press
32 Avenue of the Americas, New York, NY 10013-2473, USA

www.cambridge.org
Information on this title: www.cambridge.org/9780521871617

© Lawrence M. Weiss 2008

This publication is in copyright. Subject to statutory exception
and to the provisions of relevant collective licensing agreements,
no reproduction of any part may take place without the
written permission of Cambridge University Press.

First published 2008

Printed in Hong Kong by Golden Cup

A catalog record for this publication is available from the British Library.

Library of Congress Cataloging in Publication Data

Weiss, Lawrence M.

  Lymph nodes / Lawrence Weiss.
    p. ; cm.
  Includes bibliographical references and index.
  ISBN 978-0-521-87161-7 (hardback)
  1. Lymph nodes–Diseases. 2. Histology, Surgical. I. Title.
  [DNLM: 1. Lymph Nodes–pathology–Atlases. 2. Pathology,
Surgical–Atlases. WH 17 W431i 2008]
RC646.W45 2008
616.4'2075–dc22   2007034894

ISBN 978-0-521-87161-7 hardback

Every effort has been made in preparing this publication to provide accurate and up-to-date information
that is in accord with accepted standards and practice at the time of publication.
Nevertheless, the authors, editors, and publisher can make no warranties that the information
contained herein is totally free from error, not least because clinical standards are
constantly changing through research and regulation. The authors, editors, and publisher
therefore disclaim all liability for direct or consequential damages resulting from the use of material
contained in this book. Readers are strongly advised to pay careful attention to information
provided by the manufacturer of any drugs or equipment that they plan to use.

Cambridge University Press has no responsibility for the persistence or accuracy of URLs for external
or third-party Internet Web sites referred to in this publication and does not guarantee that any
content on such Web sites is, or will remain, accurate or appropriate.

CONTENTS

Preface   ix

1   Specimens and Studies   1

2   Normal Lymph Node   5
    Structure and Cells   5
    Trafficking and the Immune Response   10

3   Benign Lymphadenopathies   13
    Reactive Follicular Hyperplasia   15
        Autoimmune Disease   18
        Kimura Disease   19
        Syphilis   22
        Toxoplasmosis   22
        Castleman Disease   25
        HIV-Related Benign Lymphadenopathy   32
        Progressive Transformation of Germinal Centers   36
    Reactive Paracortical Hyperplasia   38
        Acute Infectious Mononucleosis   39
        CMV Lymphadenitis   42
        Herpes Simplex Lymphadenitis   43
        Postvaccinial Reactive Paracortical Hyperplasia   44
        Drug-Induced Reactive Paracortical Hyperplasia   44
        Dermatopathic Lymphadenitis   45
    Sinus Hyperplasia   48
        Nonspecific Sinus Histiocytosis   48
        Monocytoid B-Cell Hyperplasia   48
        Whipple Lymphadenopathy   51
        Lymphadenopathy Due to Deposition of Exogenous Material   51
        Lymphadenopathy Due to Deposition of Endogenous Lipid Material   53
        Rosai-Dorfman Disease   53
        Hemophagocytic Lymphohistiocytosis   58
    Benign Lymphadenopathy with Extensive Necrosis   59
        Complete Necrosis   59
        Kikuchi Histiocytic Necrotizing Lymphadenitis   61
        Systemic Lupus Erythematosus   64
        Kawasaki Disease   65

Reactive Lymphadenopathies with a Primary Granulomatous
    Pattern: Noninfectious   66
    Granulomatous Inflammation in Malignant Neoplasms   67
    Sarcoidosis   67
Reactive Lymphadenopathies with a Primary Granulomatous
    Pattern: Infectious   67
    Tuberculosis   69
    Atypical Mycobacterial Infection   69
    Lepromatous Lymphadenitis   69
    Fungal Lymphadenitis   70
    Cat Scratch Lymphadenitis   71
    Lymphogranuloma Venereum   73
    Yersinial Lymphadenitis   73
Lymphadenopathy Due to Alteration of the Connective Tissue
    Framework   73
    Inflammatory Pseudotumor of Lymph Nodes   75
    Vascular Transformation of Lymph Node Sinuses   76
    Bacillary Angiomatosis   78
Deposition of Interstitial Substance   79
    Proteinaceous Lymphadenopathy   79
    Immunoglobulin Deposition Lymphadenopathy   80
    Pneumocytis Lymphadenitis   81

4 Epithelial and Nevomelanocytic Lesions of Lymph Nodes   **82**
Epithelial Lesions   82
    Benign Epithelial Inclusions   82
    Carcinoma   84
Nevomelanocytic Lesions   87

5 Stromal Tumors and Tumorlike Lesions of Lymph Nodes   **89**
Lipomatosis   89
Palisaded Myofibroblastoma   90
Smooth Muscle Neoplasms   90
Vascular Tumors and Tumorlike Lesions   93
    Angiomyomatous Hamartoma   93
    Epithelioid Hemangioma   95
    Vascular Lesion Arising in Castleman Disease   96
    Hemangioendothelioma   97
    Kaposi Sarcoma   98
    High-Grade Angiosarcoma   100

6 Hodgkin Lymphoma   **101**
Classical Hodgkin Lymphoma   101
Nodular Lymphocyte–Predominant Hodgkin Lymphoma   115

7 Non-Hodgkin Lymphoma   **122**
Chronic Lymphocytic Leukemia/Small Lymphocytic Lymphoma   125

Lymphoplasmacytic Lymphoma 130

Plasmacytoma 133

Hairy Cell Leukemia 135

Nodal Marginal Zone B-Cell Lymphoma 138

Extranodal Marginal Zone B-Cell Lymphoma of Mucosa-Associated
Lymphoid Tissue (MALT) Involving Lymph Nodes 142

Splenic Marginal Zone Lymphoma Involving Lymph Nodes and
Primary Nodal Marginal Zone Lymphoma of Splenic Type 143

Follicular Lymphoma 145

Mantle Cell Lymphoma 156

Diffuse Large B-Cell Lymphoma 161

Burkitt Lymphoma 175

Precursor B-Lymphoblastic Lymphoma/Leukemia 181

Precursor T-Lymphoblastic Lymphoma/Leukemia 183

Mature T-Cell and NK-Cell Neoplasms 187

Angioimmunoblastic T-Cell Lymphoma 187

Peripheral T-Cell Lymphoma, Unspecified 190

Anaplastic Large-Cell Lymphoma, ALK-Negative Type 197

Anaplastic Large-Cell Lymphoma, ALK-Positive Type 200

Mycosis Fungoides/Sezary Syndrome 205

Adult T-Cell Leukemia/Lymphoma 208

T-Cell Prolymphocytic Leukemia 209

Other Mature T- and NK-Cell Neoplasms 210

    T-Cell Large Granular Lymphocytic Leukemia 211

    Aggressive NK-Cell Leukemia 211

    Extranodal NK/T-Cell Lymphoma, Nasal Type 212

    Enteropathy-Associated T-Cell Lymphoma 213

    Hepatosplenic T-Cell Lymphoma 213

    Subcutaneous Panniculitis-Like T-Cell Lymphoma 215

8 Composite Lymphomas and Interface Between Classical Hodgkin and Non-Hodgkin Lymphoma **216**

Composite Classical Hodgkin and B-Cell Non-Hodgkin
Lymphoma 216

Sequential Hodgkin Lymphoma and B-Cell Lymphoma 217

B-Cell Lymphoma with Features Intermediate Between Diffuse
Large B-Cell Lymphoma and Classical Hodgkin Lymphoma
(Gray-Zone Lymphoma) 217

Hodgkin Lymphoma and T-Cell Lymphoma 219

9 Immunodeficiency-Associated Lymphoproliferative Disorders **220**

Primary Immunodeficiency Syndromes 220

HIV-Associated Malignant Lymphomas 224

Posttransplantation Lymphoproliferative Disorders 228

Immunosuppression Associated with Treatment of Other Diseases 231

Methotrexate-Associated Lymphoproliferative Disorders   231

Fludarabine-Associated Lymphoproliferative Disorders   231

Immunosuppression Associated with Aging   231

10   **Histiocytic and Dendritic Cell Neoplasms**   **234**

Histiocytic Sarcoma   234

Langerhans Cell Histiocytosis   237

Langerhans Cell Sarcoma   241

Interdigitating Dendritic Cell Sarcoma   241

Follicular Dendritic Cell Sarcoma   244

Fibroblastic Reticulum Cell Neoplasm   247

Precursor Plasmacytoid Dendritic Cell Neoplasm   248

11   **Myeloid and Mast Cell Neoplasms**   **250**

Extramedullary Hematopoiesis   250

Myeloid Sarcoma   251

Mast Cell Neoplasia   253

Reference List   257

Index   285

PREFACE

Although there are many well-trained hematopathologists, I have found that most diagnostic lymph node biopsies are still signed out by general surgical pathologists. This book is written for the general surgical pathologist in pathology. This book is not a comprehensive textbook of hematopathology. It does not discuss every paper in the literature. It is a single-authored book by intent, with my goal being to impart my personal approach to lymph node diagnosis. In this age of Internet access, I have used references sparingly – not to prove a statement – but selecting those that contribute to diagnostic acumen, with an emphasis on review articles. I have not completely ignored extranodal lymphomas, but that is not the focus of this book. This book hopefully covers all that one may encounter in a lymph node biopsy. I am hoping that this book can take the place of a sign-out session with me and guide the surgical pathologist to the correct diagnosis on his or her own.

I would like to thank my two mentors in hematopathology, Dr. Ronald Dorfman, the consummate master of the hematoxylin and eosin slide, and Dr. Roger Warnke, the consummate master of the immunostain. I also thank my colleague of many years, Dr. Karen Chang, as well as my colleagues in hematopathology, particularly the members of the International Lymphoma Study Group, who have brought the field (and my knowledge of hematopathology) to the state we find it in today. Finally, I thank Gina Lewis for her terrific secretarial assistance.

Lawrence M. Weiss, M.D.

1 SPECIMENS AND STUDIES

Lymph node specimens may include fine-needle aspiration biopsies, needle core biopsies, excisional lymph node biopsies, including sentinel lymph node biopsies, and lymph node dissections.[1-6] The first three types of specimens are typically used for lymphoma diagnosis, while sentinel lymph node biopsies and lymph node dissections are performed in the assessment and treatment of metastatic neoplasm and are discussed later. Fine-needle aspiration biopsies may be very useful but in general should be interpreted by only those with adequate training in their interpretation. They are most useful in ruling out neoplastic disease or in staging or determining recurrence of disease. Nonetheless, in conjunction with ancillary studies, they may be used by experienced practitioners to establish an initial diagnosis of malignant lymphoma. These ancillary studies commonly include flow cytometry, immunohistochemical studies performed on cytospin preparations, fluorescence in situ hybridization (FISH) studies performed on the smears, and/or microbiologic culture, as appropriate. Needle core biopsies are fast replacing excision biopsies as the primary means of lymphoma diagnosis. Multiple cores may be obtained, with some cores fixed in formalin or other fixatives for light microscopic examination and paraffin section immunohistochemical studies; snap-frozen for possible molecular studies, immunohistochemical studies (rare antibodies), or microbiologic studies, as appropriate; and touch preparations saved for possible FISH studies.

Excisional lymph node biopsies still provide the best material for primary lymphoma diagnosis. Optimally, the largest abnormal lymph node should be excised. The specimen should be received fresh if possible, in a capped empty container, but should be placed in a small amount of sterile saline if greater than 1 hour between excision and processing is expected. Specimens should not be placed on sponge, gauze, or any material that can desiccate or introduce other artifacts into the tissue. The specimen should be bread-loafed into thin slices, with the first slices removed sterile for possible cytogenetic and/or microbiologic studies, as appropriate. Touch or preferably scrape preparations should be made for assessment of cytologic detail and possible FISH studies. A portion of the specimen should be sent for flow cytometry studies, and another portion should be snap-frozen for possible molecular studies or rare immunohistochemical studies that do not work well in paraffin sections. The remainder of the tissue should be fixed and paraffin embedded. Most laboratories prefer formalin fixation, which is sufficient if the tissue is sliced thin and adequate time for fixation is allowed. Some laboratories also employ a second fixative; although governmental regulations generally do not permit the use of metal-based fixatives any more, reasonable surrogate commercial alternatives are available. I do not recommend fixation in glutaraldehyde for cases of suspected lymphoma, as there is no good role for electron microscopy in the diagnosis and classification.

The Association of the Directors of Anatomic and Surgical Pathology (ADASP) has made a series of recommendations for the handling of lymph node specimens with possible metastatic disease. They recommend that, in the absence of gross tumor, a lymph node biopsy be cut into 3- to 4-mm slides and entirely submitted, processing different surfaces for microscopic examination. Furthermore, they recommend the examination of several levels with hematoxylin and eosin (H&E). For lymph node dissections, they recommend fresh processing. They do not believe that clearing of adipose tissue is necessary, although others have found that this technique may be necessary for finding the smallest lymph nodes. Every lymph node should be submitted for microscopic examination, again submitting each node in its entirety, unless it shows grossly evident tumor. Levels are not recommended for lymph node dissections. For sentinel lymph node biopsies, they recommend levels on each block, if tumor is not seen grossly or at the time of frozen section. They provide no recommendations on the performance of immunostains, although it is my laboratory's practice to routinely perform keratin and S-100 stains for carcinoma and malignant melanoma, respectively.

Ancillary studies are as important for lymphoma diagnosis as routine light microscopic evaluation. A list of paraffin section immunohistochemical markers useful in the workup of cases of suspected malignant lymphoma is given in Table 1. Flow cytometry studies can supplement immunohistochemical analysis, particularly in several areas: determination of specific kappa:lambda ratios and determination of surface marker antigen expression that may be weak or not detected in paraffin sections due to sensitivity issues (Table 2). Nonetheless, there are potential pitfalls to the interpretation of flow cytometry studies, including gating on the wrong population, the obvious inability to assess antigen expression in an architectural context, the relative inability to detect nuclear antibodies, the inability to determine kappa:lambda ratios when the neoplastic population lacks surface immunoglobulin expression, and the inability to detect abnormal antigen expression in rare cell populations. Detection of antigen receptor gene rearrangement studies is most often determined using polymerase chain reaction (PCR) studies as opposed to the older (and much slower) Southern blot studies. While the detection of clonal gene rearrangements is not synonymous with malignancy, and their absence is not synonymous with benignity, their detection or lack of detection may be very helpful, when interpreted in the proper context and in conjunction with the results of other studies. Finally, a variety of specific recurring chromosomal translocations have been associated with various subtypes of malignant lymphoma and may be helpful in both diagnosis and classification of lymphoma.

Table 1. Commonly Used Major Leukocyte Antigens Detectable in Paraffin Sections

Antibody	Predominant Hematolymphoid Cell Expression
ALK	Anaplastic large-cell lymphomas with ALK translocation
Bcl-2	Non–germinal center B-cells, most T-cells, most follicular lymphomas, many low-grade and some higher grade B-cell lymphomas
Bcl-6	Germinal center B-cells, lymphomas of follicular origin
BOB.1	B-cells and B-cell lymphomas, nodular lymphocyte-predominant Hodgkin lymphoma
Cyclin D1 (Bcl-1)	Mantle cell lymphoma, hairy cell leukemia
DBA.44	Hairy cells, B-cells
Elastase	Myeloid tumors, leukemia
Epithelial membrane antigen	Plasma cells and plasma cell neoplasms, many cases of nodular lymphocyte predominance, anaplastic large-cell lymphoma, and T-cell–rich B-cell lymphoma
EBV latent membrane protein	Some EBV-infected cells, including EBV+ Hodgkin cells, posttransplantation lymphoproliferative disorders, and EBV-associated infectious mononucleosis
Fascin	Dendritic cells, Reed-Sternberg cells
Granzyme B	NK-cells and cytotoxic T-cells
Hemoglobin A	Nucleated erythroid cells (benign and neoplastic)
HLA-DR	B-cells, interdigitating cells, Langerhans cells, immature granulocytes, and erythroid cells
Immunoglobulin light and heavy chains	Plasma cells, plasma cell and plasmacytoid neoplasms, some follicular and marginal zone lymphomas
Ki-67 (MIB-1)	Proliferating cells
Langerin	Langerhans cells
Lysozyme	Histiocytes–monocytes and myeloid cells (benign and neoplastic)
Myeloperoxidase	Myeloid cells (benign and neoplastic)
MUM-1/IRF	Plasma cells, classical Hodgkin lymphoma, subset of diffuse large B-cell lymphomas
OCT-2	B-cells and B-cell lymphomas and nodular lymphocyte-predominant Hodgkin lymphoma
PAX-5	B-cells and neoplasms
Perforin	Cytotoxic T-cells and NK-cells
Tartrate-resistant acid phosphatase	Hairy cell leukemia
TdT	Thymic lymphoid cells, lymphoblastic neoplasms, and some myeloid neoplasms
TIA-1	Cytotoxic T-cells and NK-cells
Tryptase	Mast cells
ZAP-70	Subset of small lymphocyte leukemia/small lymphocytic lymphoma
CD1a	Thymocytes, some T-lymphoblastic lymphomas, and Langerhans cells
CD2	T-cells and T-cell lymphomas
CD3	T-cells and many T-cell lymphomas
CD4	Histiocytes and histiocytic neoplasms, T-helper cells, and many T-cell lymphomas
CD5	T-cells and many T-cell lymphomas, B chronic lymphocytic leukemia/small lymphocytic lymphoma, mantle cell lymphoma
CD7	T-cells, some T-cell neoplasms, some myeloid leukemias
CD8	T-cytotoxic suppressor cells, some T-cell lymphomas
CD10 (CALLA)	Precursor B-cells and B-lymphoblastic neoplasms, lymphomas of follicular origin, Burkitt lymphoma
CD15	Myeloid cells, Hodgkin lymphoma, rare non-Hodgkin lymphomas

continued on next page

Table 1. *continued*

CD16	NK-cells and neoplasms, some myeloid cells
CD20	B-cells and B-cell lymphomas, nodular lymphocyte-predominant Hodgkin lymphoma
CD21	Follicular dendritic cells and neoplasms, mantle and marginal zone B-cells
CD23	Follicular dendritic cells, mantle zone B-cells, and most B chronic lymphocytic leukemia/small lymphocytic lymphoma
CD25	Cells expressing IL-2R, classical Hodgkin lymphoma, human T-cell leukemia/lymphoma, subset of other T-cell lymphomas
CD30	Activated lymphoid cells, classical Hodgkin lymphoma, anaplastic large-cell lymphoma
CD34	Progenitor cells, some myeloid and lymphoblastic neoplasms
CD35	Follicular dendritic cells and neoplasms
CD43	T-cells, myeloid cells, mast cells, T-cell lymphomas, some B-cell lymphomas, myeloid leukemia, mast cell neoplasms
CD45/CD45RB	All hematolymphoid cells, nodular lymphocyte-predominant Hodgkin lymphoma; relatively low expression in anaplastic large-cell lymphoma and lymphoblastic neoplasms; not on Reed-Sternberg cells
CD45RA	B-cells and subset of T-cells, B-cell lymphomas, nodular lymphocyte-predominant Hodgkin lymphoma
CD45RO	Most T-cells, histiocytes, myeloid cells, T-cell lymphomas
CD56	NK-cells and subset of T-cell lymphomas
CD57	Subset of T-cells and NK-cells, subset of T-cell lymphomas
CD61	Megakaryocytes (including dysplastic and neoplastic forms)
CD68	Histiocytes, myeloid cells, mast cells and neoplasms, some non–Hodgkin lymphomas
CD79a	Immature and mature B-cells and lymphomas, plasma cells and plasma cell neoplasms
CD99	Lymphoblastic lymphoma/leukemia
CD117	Immature myeloid cells
CD138	Plasma cells, plasma cell lesions
CD163	Histiocytes

Table 2. Flow Cytometry Markers Not Typically Performed in Paraffin Sections

FMC-7	Conformational epitope on CD20; expressed in most B-cell lymphomas except chronic lymphocytic leukemia/small lymphocytic lymphoma
CD11c	Hairy cell leukemia, acute myeloid leukemia, some chronic lymphocytic leukemia/small lymphocytic lymphoma
CD14	Macrophages
CD19	B-cells and B-cell lymphomas
CD22	B-cells and B-cell lymphomas
CD33	Cells of monocytic/myeloid lineage
CD38	Activated lymphocytes, subset of cases of chronic lymphocytic leukemia/small lymphocytic lymphoma
CD52	Mature lymphocytes (protein targeted by alemtuzumab)
CD103	Mucosal intraepithelial lymphocytes, enteropathy-associated T-cell lymphoma, hairy cell leukemia

2 NORMAL LYMPH NODE

Structure and Cells	5
Trafficking and the Immune Response	10

STRUCTURE AND CELLS[7,8]

Since the lymph nodes participate in immune reactions, there is no fixed or archetypical normal lymph node architecture; the specific histologic appearance of each lymph node reflects its level of stimulation by antigens. Nonetheless, one can discern major features that are shared by most lymph nodes. Lymph nodes are composed of a cortex, paracortical region, medullary cords, and sinuses, covered by a capsule. Afferent lymphatic and a few afferent blood vessels enter the lymph node at multiple points through the capsule, while most afferent blood vessels and all efferent blood vessels and lymphatics enter and leave through a depressed central area of the capsule called the hilum. Trabeculae composed of fibrosis tissue branch off the capsule to partially penetrate the lymph node parenchyma. The lymph node structure is further supported by a network of fibroblastic reticulum cells. These cells represent a heterogeneous mixture of spindled cells that may express vimentin, desmin, myosin, the isoform of alpha-actin specific for smooth muscle, desmoplakin I, desmoglein, or keratin.

The cortex essentially consists of primary and secondary follicles. Primary follicles are composed predominantly of naive and memory B-lymphocytes expressing a high density of surface immunoglobulin composed of mu and delta heavy chains combined with polytypic light chains (Figure 1). They express bcl-2 protein, but lack CD10 and bcl-6 protein (Figure 2). Secondary follicles contain germinal centers and a mantle zone. The mantle zone is composed of the same B-cells that comprise the primary follicle and may be thick or thin; thin or seemingly absent mantle cells may be particularly common in children. The germinal center consists of a mixture of B-cells, T-cells, antigen-processing cells, and tingible-body macrophages (Figure 3). The B-cells usually predominate and are a mixture of small cleaved and large cleaved cells (centrocytes) as well as large noncleaved cells (centroblasts). They are bcl-2 protein negative and express both CD10 and bcl-6 protein. They have low levels of surface immunoglobulin, but have cytoplasmic immunoglobulin, usually of mu–heavy chain type. The T-cells

Figure 1. Primary follicle. The follicle consists of a round collection of small mature lymphocytes. No germinal center is seen and small and large cleaved cells are absent.

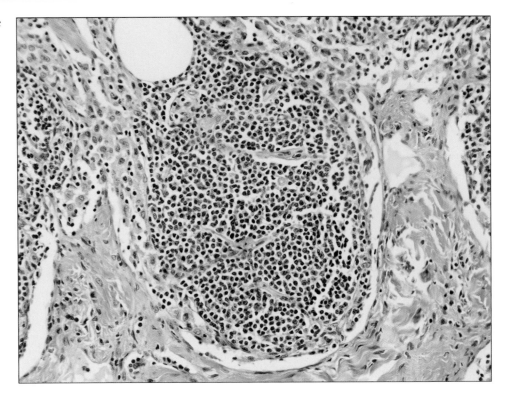

Figure 2. Primary follicle, bcl-2 stain. The cells are bcl-2 positive. This bcl-2 staining of follicles cannot be presumed to be evidence of follicular lymphoma, until the possibility of primary follicles has been eliminated. Primary follicles lack the cleaved cells characteristic of follicular lymphoma.

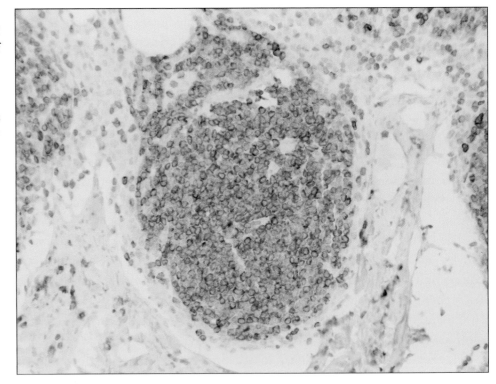

are CD4-positive/CD8-negative helper/inducer cells, and a subset is CD57 positive. The antigen-processing cells are mostly follicular dendritic cells. These cells express an array of antigens, suggesting that they are a specialized form of myofibroblasts and may derive from bone marrow stromal cell progenitors. They are usually histologically inapparent, although one can identify them by

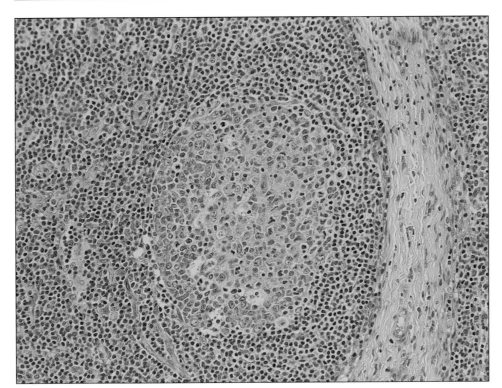

Figure 3. Secondary follicle with germinal center. Notice the polarization, with *light* zone adjacent to the capsule and a *dark* zone with a higher mitotic rate adjacent to the interior of the lymph node. The larger cells predominate in the light zone.

their frequent multinucleation with a relatively fine chromatin pattern with small evident nucleoli and inconspicuous cytoplasm. When highly multinucleated, they have been called polykaryocytes or Warthin-Finkeldey cells (Figure 4). Immunohistochemical studies show expression of CD21, CD35, CD23, and clusterin. In highly stimulated lymph nodes, the germinal centers consist of a light zone (facing the capsule) composed of centrocytes and T-helper/inducer cells and an opposing dark zone (facing the medulla), composed of highly proliferative centroblasts and tingible-body macrophages, so-called polarization. Occasionally, one also sees a marginal zone external to the mantle zone, often best developed in mesenteric lymph nodes. These areas are composed of marginal zone B-cells, cells with nuclear irregularities, and relatively abundant pale cytoplasm.

The paracortical zone varies markedly depending on the degree of immune stimulation. In the unstimulated state, it consists of small mature T-lymphocytes, predominantly of CD4-positive phenotype (Figure 5). It usually comprises the largest area of a stimulated lymph node, consisting of a mixture of T-lymphocytes of both CD4-positive/CD8-negative and CD4-negative/CD8-positive type in widely varying ratios, B-cells, particularly B-immunoblasts, dendritic cells, macrophages, plasma cells, and, depending on the stimulus, eosinophils and plasmacytoid monocyte/dendritic cells (Figure 6). B-immunoblasts are large lymphoid cells, generally with a pale chromatin pattern with a prominent nucleolus and abundant basophilic cytoplasm. The dendritic cells are usually interdigitating dendritic cells (CD1 negative, S-100 protein positive), but may be Langerhans cells (CD1 positive, S-100 protein positive). Plasmacytoid monocytic/dendritic cells are dendritic cells that are slightly larger than resting

Figure 4. Warthin-Finkeldey cells. The cells have multiple nuclei with a fine chromatin pattern and thin nuclear membranes arranged in a grapelike cluster. The cytoplasm is not discernible.

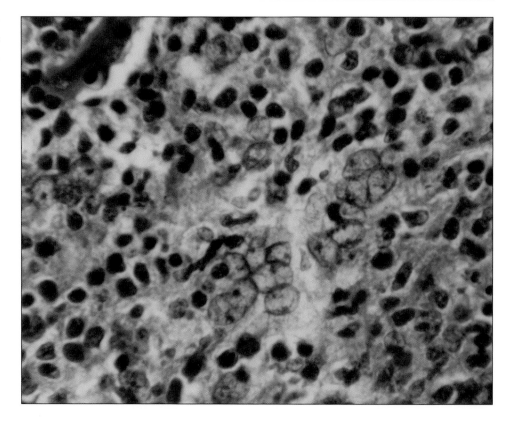

Figure 5. Paracortical region. The paracortical in a typical lymph node consists of a predominance of small mature lymphoid cells, with scattered histiocytes, plasma cells, and large lymphoid cells, with the number depending on the degree of immune stimulation. A germinal center is seen at the right.

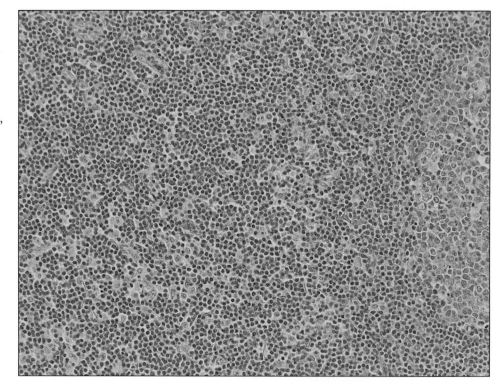

lymphocytes, with moderately abundant and well-demarcated eosinophilic to faintly basophilic cytoplasm. The nucleus is round, oval, or slightly indented, with finely dispersed chromatin and one or two small nucleoli. They may be identified on light microscopy when they form clusters or may be identified by

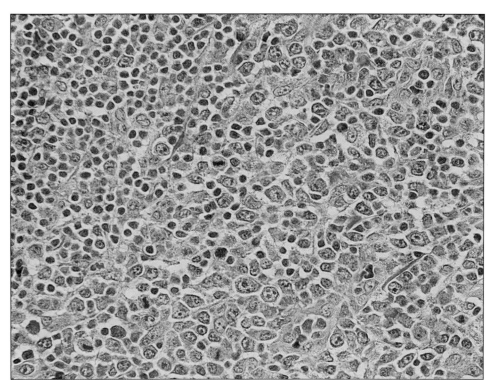

Figure 6. Reactive paracortical hyperplasia. A mottled appearance is imparted by the mixture of small and large cells. There is a mixture of immunoblasts, small lymphocytes, plasma cells, histiocytes, and rare eosinophils in this field. The blood vessels are hard to see, since the nuclei of the high endothelial venules are somewhat vesicular and blend in with the lymphoid cells.

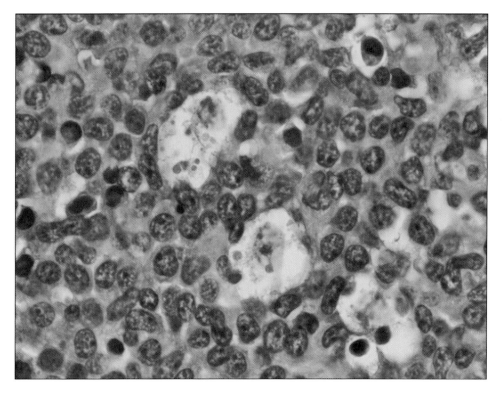

Figure 7. Plasmacytoid dendritic cells. These cells are most easily identified when they are found in clusters. Frequent apoptosis, as seen here, is typical and aids in their identification.

virtue of expression of CD123 (Figure 7). They are probably derived from the lymphoid system and upon stimulation with interleukin (IL)-3 mature into a subset of interdigitating cells in the paracortex. Another feature of the para-cortical zone is the presence of high endothelial venules. These are venules lined by cuboidal rather than the typically flattened endothelial cells and have fairly

9

Figure 8. Medullary sinus, with adjacent medullary cords. The sinuses contain loose collections of histiocytes, small lymphocytes, and plasma cells. The cords contain small lymphocytes and plasma cells.

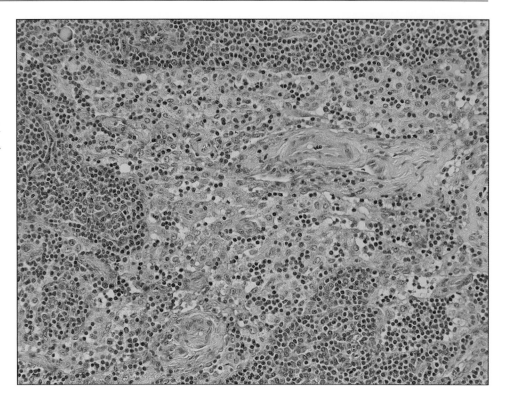

large nuclei. They possess an unusually abundant amount of cytoplasm that appears to almost completely obliterate the vessel lumen.

The sinuses of a lymph node include the subcapsular sinuses, which receive lymph from afferent vessels, and the medullary sinuses, which deliver lymph to the efferent lymphatics (Figure 8). The most frequent cellular component of the sinuses is the sinus histiocyte. Occasionally, the sinuses are filled with collections of monocytoid B-cells. These cells are B-lineage cells that are bcl-2 negative and have nuclear irregularities and a more abundant cytoplasm than naive B-cells (and even more than marginal zone B-cells); there are often admixed neutrophils (Figure 9). The medullary cords are thin to thick cords of lymphoid cells, often with admixed plasma cells, present between the medullary sinuses.

TRAFFICKING AND THE IMMUNE RESPONSE[9]

T-lymphocytes and, to a lesser extent, B-lymphocytes enter the lymph node via the high endothelial venules, utilizing L-selectin (CD62L) receptors concentrated on lymphocyte microvilli. B-cells may also enter via the subcapsular sinuses, as monocytoid B-cells. Many of the B-cells migrate to primary follicles and the mantle zones of secondary follicles. Antigen enters the lymph node via the afferent lymphatics. Although most antigens are ingested by macrophages within the sinuses, some enter the paracortical and cortical regions and become retained on the cell processes of interdigitating and follicular dendritic cells, respectively. Interdigitating and follicular dendritic cells present these antigens to T-cells and B-cells (in association with class I and II major histocompatibility

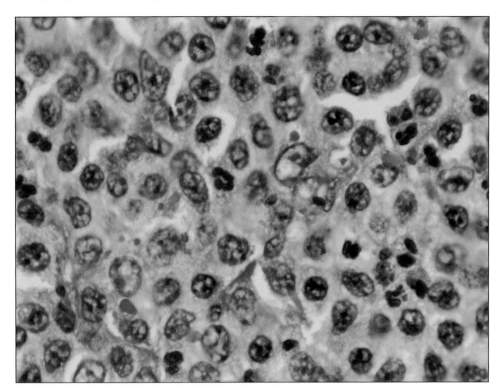

Figure 9. Reactive monocytoid B-cell hyperplasia. The cells have medium-sized nuclei, with abundant pale cytoplasm. Note the admixed neutrophils.

[MHC] antigens). The B-cell response starts in the paracortical region, with increased migration to primary follicles and the mantle zones of secondary follicles, as well as the generation of B-immunoblasts, which develop into short-lived plasma cells producing predominantly IgM heavy chain antibodies. The T-cell response results in T-cell activation and helper/inducer T-cell migration to follicles.

Although the B-cell response starts in the paracortical region, most of the action occurs within the follicles. First, correlating with loss of bcl-2 protein, gain of bcl-6 protein, gain of CD10, and the morphologic transformation to centroblasts, there is intense proliferation of the centroblasts (with a generation time of about 6 hours), leading to the formation of germinal centers. Each germinal center is the product of about three to ten founder B-cells and may generate over 10,000 B-cells during its life. During this intense proliferative activity, the naive B-cells undergo somatic hypermutation at the immunoglobulin gene V region. Eventually, the centroblasts are transformed into centrocytes, which are nonproliferating cells. Those germinal center B-cells in which the hypermutation process has led to loss of affinity for their immunoglobulin with antigen undergo apoptosis and phagocytosis by tingible-body macrophages, while those germinal center B-cells in which the hypermutation process has led to increased affinity with immunoglobulin take up the antigen via their surface immunoglobulin, process it, and present it to the T-helper/inducer cells in conjunction with class II antigens. As a result of this interaction, T-cells express CD40 ligand, which is in turn recognized by the CD40 present on the centrocytes, leading to loss of bcl-6 protein and CD10, reexpression of bcl-2 protein, and the morphologic transformation to memory (marginal zone) B-cells or plasma cells. The plasma cell pathway is regulated by expression of the transcription factor IRF4 (MUM-1) and the transcriptional repressor Blimp-1. Plasma cells accumulate in the medullary sinuses in transit to other locations, including the bone marrow and other extranodal sites. Plasma cells lack CD45 and CD20 and express CD138 and cytoplasmic immunoglobulin.

As mentioned above, naive T-cells interact with antigen presented on the surface of antigen-presenting dendritic cells in the paracortical region. Helper/inducer cells expressing CD4 bind to MHC class II molecules on the dendritic cells, while suppressor cells expressing CD8 bind to MHC class I molecules. These interactions lead to transformation to T-immunoblasts, and ultimately to effector T-cells, which are morphologically indistinguishable from small non-proliferating lymphocytes. In addition to helper/inducer and suppressor functions, which modulate other immune reactions via cytokines, CD8-positive, and to a lesser extent, CD4-positive cells, can have direct cytotoxic effects to cells harboring antigens. These cytotoxic cells contain cytotoxic granules, which may contain granzyme B, perforin, and/or TIA-1. Natural killer (NK) cells are another cell type that may show cytotoxic effects. NK-cells do not rearrange their antigen receptor genes and possess surface CD16, CD56, and/or CD57 and cytoplasmic CD3. Morphologically, they correspond to large granular lymphocytes. NK-cells kill cells that lack class I MHC or express allogenic MHC. Their cytotoxic granules are similar in composition to those of T-cells.

3   BENIGN LYMPHADENOPATHIES

Reactive Follicular Hyperplasia   **15**
  Autoimmune Disease   18
  Kimura Disease   19
  Syphilis   22
  Toxoplasmosis   22
  Castleman Disease   25
  HIV-Related Benign Lymphadenopathy   32
  Progressive Transformation of Germinal Centers   36
Reactive Paracortical Hyperplasia   **38**
  Acute Infectious Mononucleosis   39
  CMV Lymphadenitis   42
  Herpes Simplex Lymphadenitis   43
  Postvaccinial Reactive Paracortical Hyperplasia   44
  Drug-Induced Reactive Paracortical Hyperplasia   44
  Dermatopathic Lymphadenitis   45
Sinus Hyperplasia   **48**
  Nonspecific Sinus Histiocytosis   48
  Monocytoid B-Cell Hyperplasia   48
  Whipple Lymphadenopathy   51
  Lymphadenopathy Due to Deposition of Exogenous Material   51
  Lymphadenopathy Due to Deposition of Endogenous
       Lipid Material   53
  Rosai-Dorfman Disease   53
  Hemophagocytic Lymphohistiocytosis   58
Benign Lymphadenopathy with Extensive Necrosis   **59**
  Complete Necrosis   59
  Kikuchi Histiocytic Necrotizing Lymphadenitis   61
  Systemic Lupus Erythematosus   64
  Kawasaki Disease   65
Reactive Lymphadenopathies with a Primary Granulomatous
       Pattern: Noninfectious   **66**
  Granulomatous Inflammation in Malignant Neoplasms   67
  Sarcoidosis   67

continued on next page

Reactive Lymphadenopathies with a Primary Granulomatous Pattern: Infectious	67
Tuberculosis	69
Atypical Mycobacterial Infection	69
Lepromatous Lymphadenitis	69
Fungal Lymphadenitis	70
Cat Scratch Lymphadenitis	71
Lymphogranuloma Venereum	73
Yersinial Lymphadenitis	73
Lymphadenopathy Due to Alteration of the Connective Tissue Framework	73
Inflammatory Pseudotumor of Lymph Nodes	75
Vascular Transformation of Lymph Node Sinuses	76
Bacillary Angiomatosis	78
Deposition of Interstitial Substance	79
Proteinaceous Lymphadenopathy	79
Immunoglobulin Deposition Lymphadenopathy	80
Pneumocytis Lymphadenitis	81

All lymph nodes (unless an individual without any autoimmune or genetic disease, including cancer, lives under sterile conditions) are exposed to varying concentrations of different types of antigens.[10–12] Thus, all nonneoplastic lymph nodes show varying degrees of reactive changes. The most important consideration in assessing the reactive lymph node is in its distinction from a neoplasm, mainly the various types of malignant lymphoma. In a minority of circumstances, the specific pattern of reaction may strongly suggest a specific etiology. For these two reasons, I try to characterize reactive lymphadenopathies by patterns of reaction. Each pattern suggests specific types of malignant lymphoma, which should be considered in the differential diagnosis, and each pattern suggests a general type of immune response, which raises certain disease classes in the differential diagnosis.

I like to characterize benign lymphadenopathies into the following seven categories:

1. Follicular
2. Paracortical
3. Sinus
4. Extensive necrosis
5. Granulomatous
6. Connective tissue framework
7. Deposition of interstitial substance.

One should also keep in mind that these patterns are never pure. Thus, reactive follicular hyperplasia usually has a component of paracortical hyperplasia, and sometimes one cannot even determine the dominant process. Nonetheless, from a differential diagnostic standpoint, it is useful to try to assess the dominant process, for the reasons given above.

REACTIVE FOLLICULAR HYPERPLASIA[13–20]

Follicular hyperplasia is the most common pattern of reactive lymphadenopathy. It is usually associated with varying degrees of paracortical and/or sinus hyperplasia. It is particularly commonly seen in children and young adults, but may be encountered in all ages, including the very elderly. Clinically, the lymphadenopathy is usually localized, but may be generalized. The cervical and axillary areas are most frequently involved, corresponding with the lymph node groups most likely to drain antigens. Table 3 lists the most common diseases that give rise to histologic findings that may suggest the specific etiology of the follicular hyperplasia.

Table 4 lists the main histologic differential diagnostic features between reactive follicular hyperplasia and follicular lymphoma. Please note that there is no one pathognomonic histologic feature. Therefore, one should rather rely upon a constellation of characteristics. At the outset, even the history can be helpful. The older the patient, the more likely the diagnosis is follicular lymphoma. Generalized lymphadenopathy is also more commonly seen with follicular lymphoma than reactive follicular hyperplasia. The one single most useful histologic feature is the density of follicles (cortical:paracortical ratio) on low magnification. The more the follicles and the less the paracortical areas, the more likely is the diagnosis of malignant lymphoma. In fact, a complete back-to-back arrangement of the follicles is seen in over 75% of cases of follicular lymphoma, while it is seen only in the most florid cases of reactive follicular hyperplasia. The greatest exception to this rule is when there are areas of nodal effacement, another feature favoring follicular lymphoma. These areas are usually focal, but mass-forming, and not distributed evenly around individual follicles. Floridly reactive follicles may also occasionally show one or more of the following features: extension of the process outside the capsule, the presence of follicles throughout the node, predominance of centroblasts, and absent or greatly diminished mantle zones (Figures 10 and 11). These latter two features are particularly common in florid reactive follicular hyperplasia occurring in childhood.

Immunohistochemical and other special studies may be very helpful in distinguishing reactive follicular hyperplasia and follicular lymphoma. These studies are summarized in Table 5. Determination of bcl-2 expression in paraffin sections is the single most useful ancillary study, being consistently negative in reactive follicular hyperplasia, but positive in about 90% of cases of follicular lymphoma. One can occasionally see large numbers of bcl-2-positive T-helper/inducer cells in cases of reactive follicular hyperplasia. Comparison with CD3 stains and the observation that the bcl-2–positive cells are not centroblasts can help with this pitfall (Figure 12). The types of follicular lymphoma that are most likely to be bcl-2 negative include grade 3 follicular lymphoma and follicular

Table 3. Reactive Lymphadenopathies with a Primary Follicular Pattern

- Autoimmune disease
- Kimura disease
- Toxoplasmosis
- Syphilis
- Castleman disease
- HIV-associated lymphadenopathy
- Progressive transformation of germinal centers

Table 4. Follicular Hyperplasia vs. Lymphoma

Reactive Follicular Hyperplasia	*Follicular Lymphoma*
Low density of follicles	High density of follicles
Follicles usually limited to subcortical region	Follicles distributed evenly throughout nodal parenchyma
Follicles rarely extend beyond capsule	Follicles often extend beyond capsule
Follicles of uneven size and shape	Follicles usually of similar size and shape
Mixture of cell types in germinal center	Monomorphic or polymorphic population
Tingible-body macrophages present	Tingible-body macrophages rarely seen
Usually moderate to high mitotic rate	Usually low to moderate mitotic rate
Mantle zone usually distinct	Mantle zone usually indistinct or absent
Cell polarization sometimes seen	Cell polarization absent
Large interfollicular areas evident	Compressed interfollicular areas
Areas of nodal effacement seen	May contain areas of nodal effacement

Figure 10. Reactive follicular hyperplasia. This case featured follicles with diminished or absent mantle zones and had a predominance of large noncleaved cells in the germinal centers. All special studies supported a benign diagnosis.

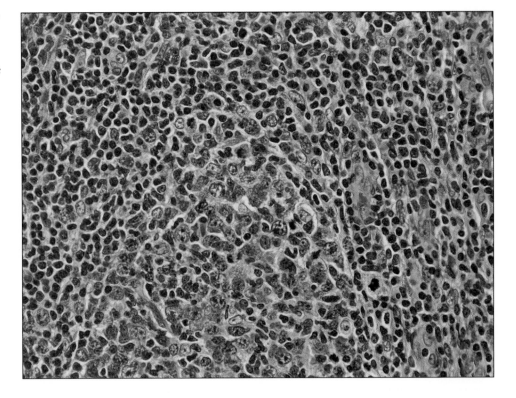

lymphoma arising in children. In situ colonization by follicular lymphoma may show only scattered bcl-2–positive cells, but the bcl-2 expression in this process is usually much stronger than the adjacent bcl-2 staining of either T-helper/inducer cells or adjacent B-mantle cells. Ki-67 stains may also be useful. Not only are higher numbers of germinal center cells usually positive in reactive follicular hyperplasia than follicular lymphoma but also the stain may demonstrate a pattern of polarity that may not have been evident on routine light microscopy (Figure 13).[21] Immunoglobulin protein studies are helpful in only a minority of cases, as is also the case for in situ hybridization studies for mRNA expression.

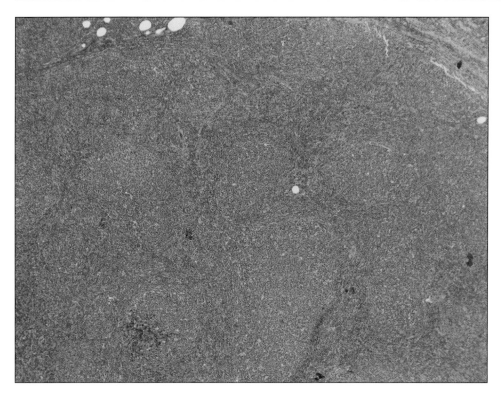

Figure 11. Reactive follicular hyperplasia. The follicles are densely packed and are relatively uniform in size. Despite these two features, this turned out to be a case of florid reactive follicular hyperplasia.

Table 5. Follicular Hyperplasia vs. Lymphoma: Special Studies

Reactive Follicular Hyperplasia	Follicular Lymphoma
Bcl-2 negative in B-cells of germinal centers	Bcl-2 positive in B-cells in germinal enters (90%)
No light chain restriction on immunos	Light chain restriction (20% in paraffin)
No light chain restriction on flow cytometry	Light chain restriction or absence, when gated correctly (100%)
Ig rearrangements absent	Ig rearrangements usually detected (80%)
t(14;18) absent (99%)	t(14;18) usually present (90%)

Rarely, highly reactive follicular hyperplasia, particularly in children, may show light chain restriction, often of lambda–light chain type. These cases are extraordinarily rare and, although monotypic, are polyclonal.

Gene rearrangement studies may be helpful in the distinction of reactive vs. neoplastic follicular proliferations, although one must keep in mind that PCR studies for immunoglobulin heavy and light chains may be false negative in up to 20% of cases of follicular lymphoma due to the process of somatic hypermutation and that *pseudoclonal* immunoglobulin gene rearrangements may be rarely seen in reactive follicular hyperplasia when small aliquots (less than 50 ng) are analyzed. Similarly, although the detection of a t(14;18) (bcl-2 gene rearrangement) usually provides strong support for a diagnosis of lymphoma, up to 10% of cases of follicular lymphoma (usually grade 3) may be negative and the t(14;18) may be rarely truly observed in reactive follicular hyperplasia.

Figure 12. Follicle in reactive follicular hyperplasia, CD3 stain. There may be many CD3-positive cells in reactive follicles, all of which will be bcl-2 positive. Although they are often seen toward the peripheral of the germinal center, this may not be evident in every follicle. Note the negatively stained large germinal center cells.

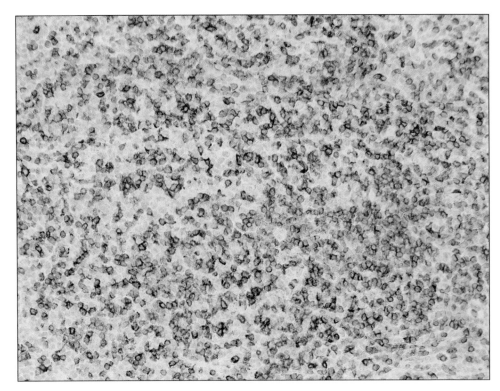

Figure 13. Reactive follicular hyperplasia, Ki-67 stain. Polarization of the germinal center is often best appreciated on a Ki-67 stain.

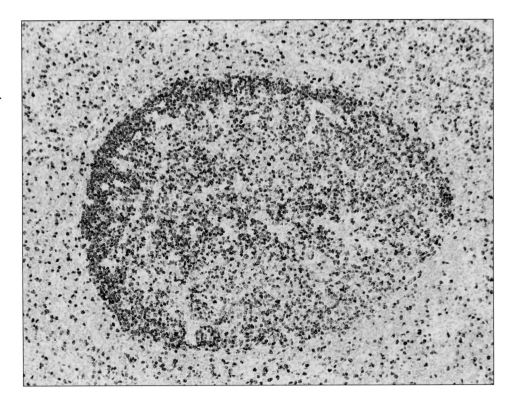

Autoimmune Disease[22–25]

Autoimmune disease may give rise to a striking reactive follicular hyperplasia. This is usually associated with a marked paracortical and medullary sinus polytypic plasma cell proliferation, and plasmacytoid features may be evident within the

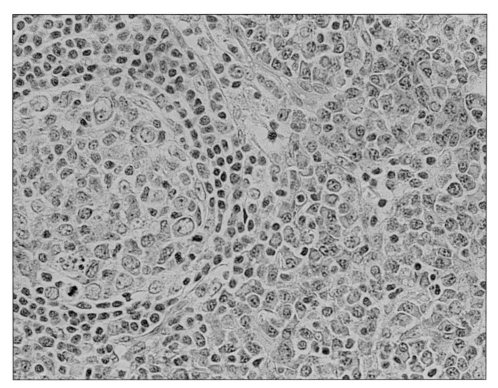

Figure 14. Collagen vascular disease. This case shows reactive follicular hyperplasia with paracortical plasmacytosis, the most common pattern seen. Several plasma cells show cytoplasmic Russell bodies.

follicles as well (Figure 14). The third part of the triad, neutrophils in the sinuses, sometimes with the formation of neutrophilic microabscesses, is commonly mentioned in textbooks, but infrequently actually seen, in my experience. Occasionally, the follicles in rheumatoid lymphadenopathy may show a predominance of small centrocytes, with a relatively low proliferative rate and few tingible-body macrophages, simulating a follicular lymphoma. One should also look for histologic findings of lymph proliferations that may develop in patients with rheumatoid arthritis who have been treated with methotrexate or other immunosuppressive regimens. Patients with rheumatoid arthritis who have been treated with gold may show nonbirebringent crystalline structures scattered throughout the lymph node parenchyma, either lying free in spaces or within histiocytes. Diagnosis may be made by x-ray microanalysis. In Sjogren syndrome, one may see a sinusoidal or paracortical monocytoid B-cell proliferation in addition to the reactive follicular hyperplasia. These proliferations must be distinguished from a marginal zone B-cell lymphoma, which may complicate cases of Sjogren syndrome.

Kimura Disease[26–29]

Kimura disease is an idiopathic chronic inflammatory disease, which predominantly affects young to middle-aged men. It is infrequent in the United States, but is endemic throughout Asia. Its etiology is unknown, but an aberrant immune reaction to an unknown antigenic stimulus has been suggested. The pathogenesis may involve mast cells via secretion of IL-4, IL-5, and RANTES. Patients present with one or more subcutaneous masses of the head and neck, accompanied by involvement of local lymph nodes and salivary glands. Patients

Figure 15. Kimura disease. This reactive germinal center has infiltration by eosinophils, as well as deposition of a proteinaceous substance.

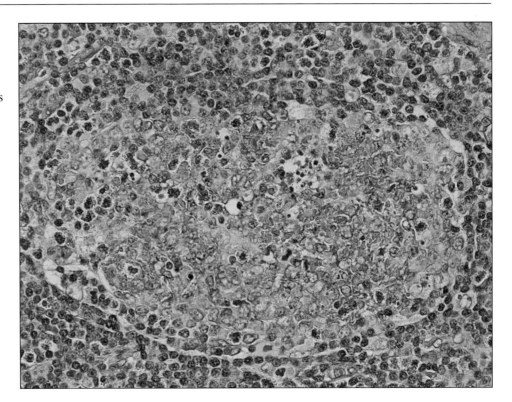

have eosinophilia in the peripheral blood accompanied by elevated serum levels of IgE. The disease is usually stable and self-limiting, with slow regression frequent. Surgery is employed for diagnosis and to treat disfiguring mass effects; however, recurrences occur in 25% of cases. Patients may have nephrotic syndrome due to circulating IgE immunocomplex deposition. Steroids have been used to treat recurrences or for nephrotic syndrome, with localized radiotherapy used for relapses after steroid withdrawal.

Histologically, Kimura disease shows a reactive follicular hyperplasia characterized by highly vascularized germinal centers. The border with the mantle zone may show frequent invagination of mantle B-lymphocytes. They often contain an eosinophilic proteinaceous material (which includes IgE), numerous eosinophils, and polykaryocytes (Figure 15). There may be partial necrosis of the germinal center (follicle lysis), occasionally with the formation of intrafollicular eosinophilic abscesses. The paracortex is also hypervascular and may similarly show numerous eosinophils, eosinophilic microabscesses, and polykaryocytes (Figures 16 and 17). There is often patchy sclerosis, particularly in association with blood vessels. The sinuses also may show eosinophilia.

The triad of florid reactive hyperplasia, cortical and paracortical eosinophilia, and cortical and paracortical hypervascularity is characteristic of Kimura disease. Kimura disease should be distinguished from a completely different entity with a name that provides the confusion: angiofollicular hyperplasia with eosinophilia. This disease has a completely different epidemiology (middle-aged women in Western populations), pathogenesis (vascular neoplasm), histologic appearance (epithelioid hemangioma with eosinophils), and behavior (completely benign not requiring treatment beyond excision). Several other

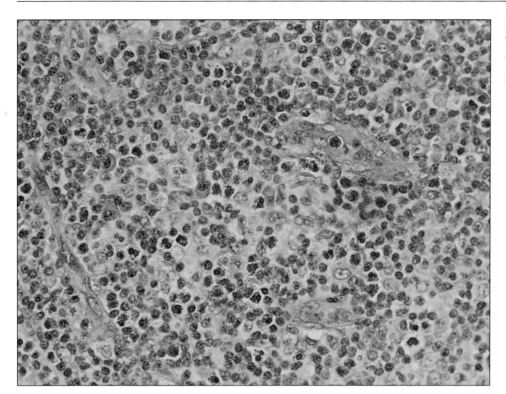

Figure 16. Kimura disease. The interfollicular areas are very vascular and contain numerous eosinophils.

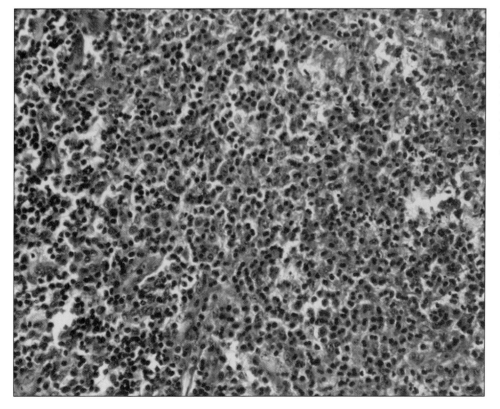

Figure 17. Kimura disease. An eosinophilic microabscess is seen. The differential diagnosis of eosinophilic microabscesses includes Hodgkin lymphoma, Langerhans cell histiocytosis, fungal infection, and allergic disorders.

lymphadenopathies feature numerous eosinophils, including allergic responses such as drug reaction and parasitic infestation. The clinical setting (Asian individual with neck localization) can be very helpful, although the combination of features seen in Kimura disease is usually not encountered in these other diseases.

Figure 18. Syphilis. Reactive follicular hyperplasia is seen in the lymph node parenchyma, while the capsule shows fibrosis and infiltration with plasma cells and lymphocytes.

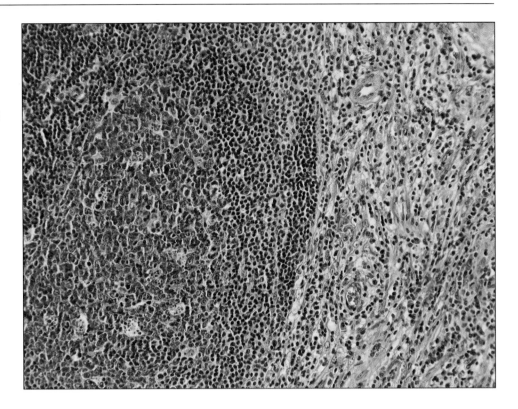

Syphilis[22]

Syphilis is rarely seen in lymph node biopsies, since patients are usually identified by VDRL and RPR screening tests. Patients usually present with primary or secondary syphilis. They are mainly young adults and often have evidence of human immunodeficiency virus (HIV) or other venereal diseases. Patients who come to biopsy usually present with inguinal lymphadenopathy, which is usually bilateral, or generalized lymphadenopathy. There is often a history of a prior skin or mucosal lesion, and the patient may have general malaise, fever, and weight loss.

Histologically, syphilis usually shows a prominent reactive follicular hyperplasia. The most distinctive finding is a prominent perilymphadenitis, with thickening of the capsule, infiltration by plasma cells, and frequent endarteritis and phlebitis. Trabeculae coming off the capsule may also show thickening and plasma cell infiltration (Figure 18). The paracortical area often shows an intense plasmacytosis, particularly in a perivenular distribution, and may also show an endarteritis, phlebitis, epithelioid granulomas with multinucleated giant cells, and, occasionally, frank abscesses. Warthin-Starry stains or specific immunostains may provide confirmation of the diagnosis, with the demonstration of spirochetes, particularly within and around the walls of venules and sometimes even within germinal centers.

Toxoplasmosis[30–32]

Toxoplasmosis is a disease due to infection by the protozoal parasite *Toxoplasma gondii*. This organism has a worldwide distribution and is present in

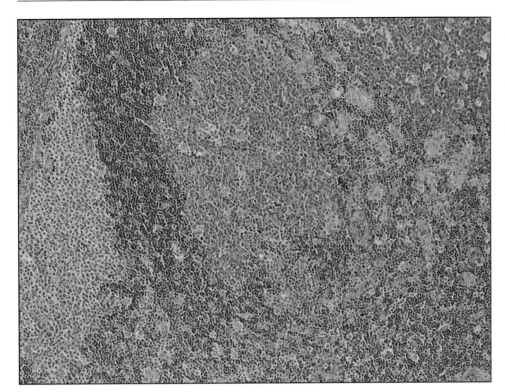

Figure 19. Toxoplasmosis. The characteristic triad of reactive follicular hyperplasia, clusters of epithelioid histiocytes, and reactive monocytoid B-cell hyperplasia is seen.

approximately 50% of adults in the United States. Most individuals have asymptomatic infection, although a subset may present with an acute febrile disease, which may mimic influenza or infectious mononucleosis. Lymphadenopathy may occur in the late stages of acute infection, following defervescence, typically in children or young adults. Lymphadenopathy most often occurs in the posterior cervical region, although other lymph nodes may be affected, and even generalized lymphadenopathy may occur.

Histologically, toxoplasmosis shows a characteristic triad of reactive follicular hyperplasia, a reactive monocytoid B-cell proliferation, and a proliferation of epithelioid histiocytes. This triad is typically seen in proximity of each other, often within one low-magnification field (Figure 19). The epithelioid histiocytes may be present as single cells or small clusters, both within the paracortical region as well as encroaching upon or frankly involving the germinal centers (Figure 20). However, they do not form well-formed granulomas with multinucleated giant cells, and they do not show necrosis. Toxoplasmic cysts and/or intracellular organisms are only rarely found, identified in less than 1% of cases. Once the diagnosis is suspected, serologic studies can confirm the diagnosis. Immunohistochemical or PCR studies do not have a high sensitivity in the analysis of involved lymph nodes.

Only rarely will the characteristic triad of histologic findings be seen outside of the setting of toxoplasmosis. The most common exception is HIV lymphadenopathy. In these cases, there are often other histologic findings that may suggest that diagnosis. Another rare exception is leishmaniasis, which may be a closer mimic of toxoplasmosis. However, in leishmaniasis, discrete granulomas may be seen, foci of necrosis may be present, and one may see intracellular organisms within the histiocytes (Figures 21 and 22).

Figure 20. Toxoplasmosis. The epithelioid histiocytes are present as single cells and small clusters and do not aggregate into well-formed granulomas with giant cells.

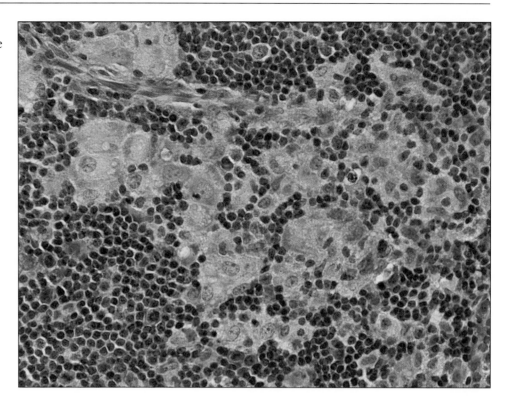

Figure 21. Leishmaniasis. There is a superficial resemblance to toxoplasmosis, but discrete granulomas with giant cells are seen.

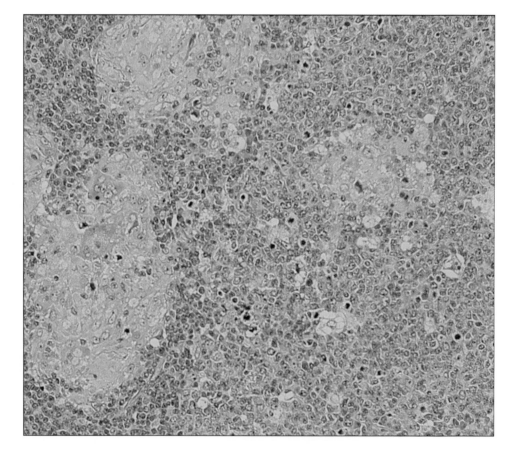

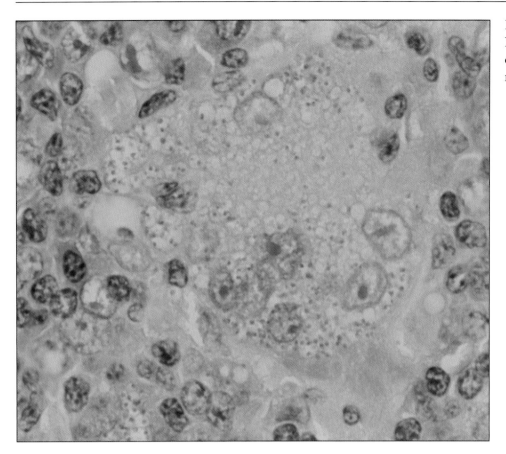

Figure 22. Leishmaniasis. Numerous intracellular organisms are seen in this multinucleated giant cells.

Table 6. Castleman Disease

Type	Unicentric Hyaline-Vascular	Unicentric Plasma Cell	Multicentric
Demographics	M = F median in 20s; 80% of cases	M = F median in 20s; 10% of cases	M = F median in 50s; 10% of cases
Site	Single lymph node, most often mediastinum	Single lymph chain, most often abdomen	Multiple lymph node sites
Symptoms	Rarely any symptoms	Systemic symptoms	Systemic symptoms; POEMS syndrome (15%)
Pathogenesis	Unknown	↑ IL-6	↑ IL-6, often due to HHV-8, often in the setting of HIV

Castleman Disease[25,33–51]

Castleman disease has classically been thought of to consist of at least two separate entities, and possibly three (Table 6), including a localized (unicentric) hyaline-vascular type, a localized plasma cell type, and a multicentric plasma cell type. The hyaline-vascular type is the best characterized. It occurs in a wide age distribution, with a median in young adults. There is no sex predilection. Patients are usually asymptomatic and present with a solitary mass, with a mean diameter of about 6 cm. The mass is most often found in the mediastinum, although cervical, abdominal, and axillary lymph nodes may also be sites of involvement. Some patients may present with unusual findings, such as anemia,

Figure 23. Castleman disease, hyaline-vascular type. This follicle shows three germinal centers, typical for this disease. Note the fibrosis in the interfollicular area.

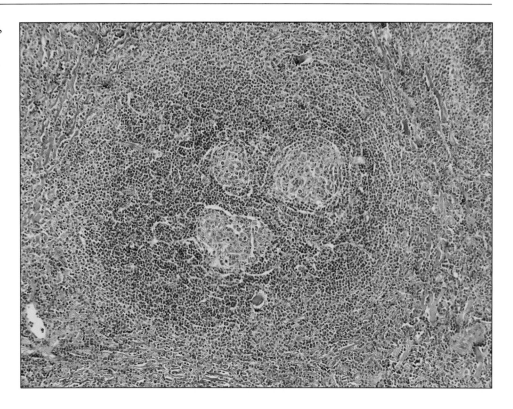

paraneoplastic pemphigus, or thrombotic thrombocytopenic purpura. Surgical excision is almost always curative.

Histologically, the hyaline-vascular type of Castleman disease shows capsular thickening, with thick trabeculae extending from the capsule and into the lymph node parenchyma. Sinuses are usually diminished and are absent in extranodal locations. The follicles are highly distinctive. They show expanded mantle zones, often arranged in concentric rings, occasionally enclosing two or more germinal centers (Figures 23 and 24). The germinal centers are usually atrophic and highly vascularized (regressed germinal centers) (Figure 25). Follicular dendritic cells are often prominent and may show nuclear atypia, including enlarged hyperchromatic or bizarre nuclei. They are usually seen within regressed germinal centers, but may also be present in the mantle areas. The paracortical region is also highly vascularized and may show hyalinization, particularly around vessels (Figure 26). It consists of a mix of cells, sometimes with increased numbers of plasmacytoid monocytic/dendritic cells, with formation of clusters (Figure 27). Plasma cells are variable in number and range from absent to abundant. The latter has been referred to as the mixed or transitional type of localized Castleman disease. Some cases show diffuse areas of dendritic, myoid, or reticular cells; these cases have been termed the *stromal-rich* variant. Immunohistochemical studies show aberrant networks of follicular dendritic cells (Figure 28). Many follicles have a contracted tight network of follicular dendritic cells, and expanded networks may be seen in other follicles. The B-cells and plasma cells are polytypic and polyclonal. One case has been reported to show clonal chromosomal abnormalities, including a t(1;16) and deletions involving the long arms of chromosomes 7 and 8. Hyaline-vascular Castleman

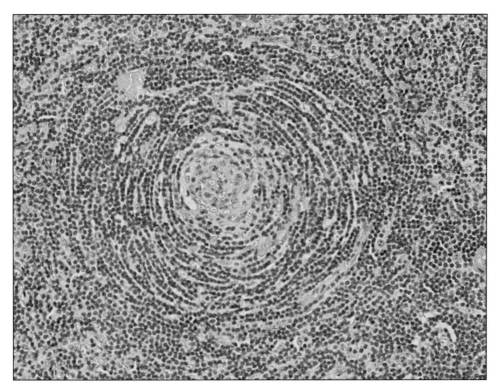

Figure 24. Castleman disease. This follicle shows marked regression, with *onion-skinning* of mantle zone lymphocytes.

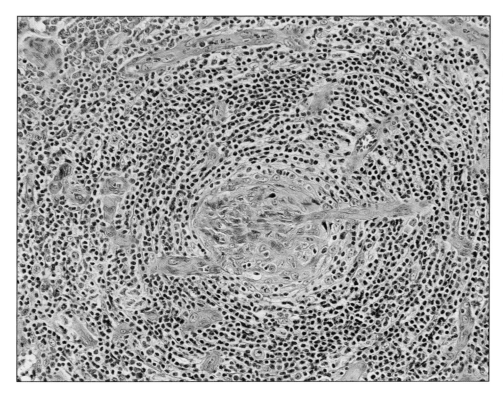

Figure 25. Castleman disease, hyaline-vascular type. A regressed germinal center is seen, with a lollypop appearance imparted by hypervascularity.

disease may be complicated or accompanied by vascular neoplasms, including angiomyoid proliferations, and follicular dendritic cell neoplasms. Regressed germinal centers can be found in a number of diseases, most notably HIV infection and angioimmunoblastic lymphadenopathy–like peripheral T-cell lymphoma.

Figure 26. Castleman disease, hyaline-vascular variant. The interfollicular areas show intense hypervascularization, with hyalinization present around individual vessels.

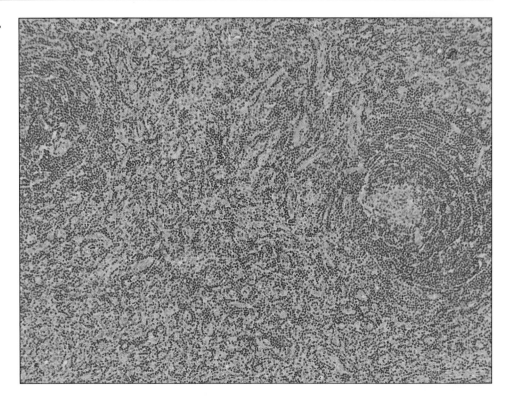

Figure 27. Castleman disease, hyaline-vascular type. A cluster of plasmacytoid dendritic cells is seen at left, in comparison to the reactive germinal center seen at right. Both areas may have tingible-body macrophages, which can lead to confusion between the two.

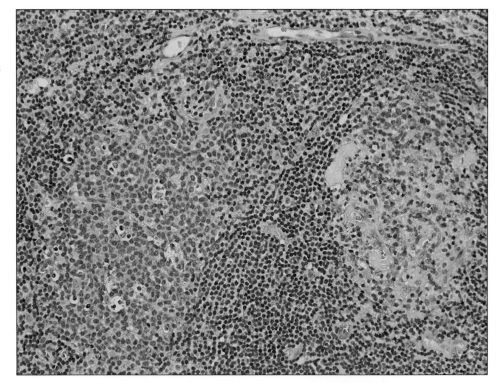

The plasma cell type of localized Castleman disease is the poorest characterized of the three subtypes and may be closely related to multicentric Castleman disease. Many of the cases reported in the early literature probably correspond to multicentric Castleman disease, but when these cases are removed, there is an equal sex distribution, with a median age in young adulthood.

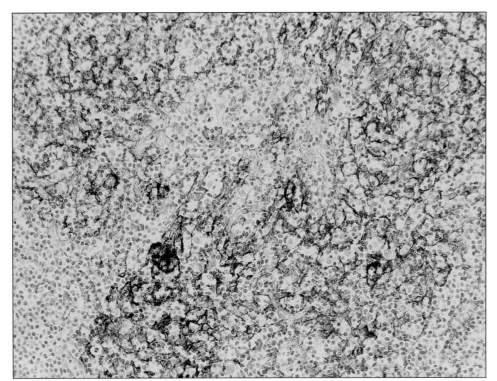

Figure 28. Castleman disease, hyaline-vascular type, CD21. A markedly disordered dendritic pattern is seen. The germinal center is at the area of the tight cluster of CD21-positive cells.

This subtype is at least ten times less frequent than the hyaline-vascular subtype. Patients often present with malaise, fevers, and night sweats. Laboratory studies show frequent cytopenias (mostly anemia and thrombocytopenia), polyclonal hypergammaglobulinemia, and plasmacytosis in the bone marrow. In addition, there are consistently elevated IL-6 levels, a finding that may have pathogenetic significance. There is also an association with amyloidosis and renal insufficiency. This subtype usually presents in abdominal lymph nodes. Surgical excision is usually curative, although some patients continue to have systemic symptoms.

Histologically, the localized plasma cell form of Castleman disease shows retained lymph node architecture. The germinal centers may be hyperplastic or normal, show regression, and show a proteinaceous precipitate. The paracortical region shows marked plasmacytosis, often with plasmacytoid immunoblasts (Figure 29). The paracortical areas may be focally hypervascular. Immunohistochemical studies show normal networks of follicular dendritic cells, although the plasma cells may show monotypic lambda–light chain restriction in up to one-half of cases. This finding does not correlate with aggressive behavior. Large numbers of truly unicentric cases have not been studied for human herpesvirus (HHV)-8, so the association with this virus is not yet firmly established, although it has been hypothesized that many of the cases showing monotypic lambda–light chain restriction may be HHV-8 associated. The histologic findings are not pathognomonic, and a variety of other disease may show similar histologic features, including autoimmune disease, HIV-associated lymphadenopathy, immunosuppression, Hodgkin lymphoma (as an area adjacent to the Hodgkin), or even lymph nodes draining a site of carcinoma. The finding of

Figure 29. Castleman disease, plasma cell type. The germinal center shows some Castleman-like features, and the interfollicular region shows a plasma cell infiltrate.

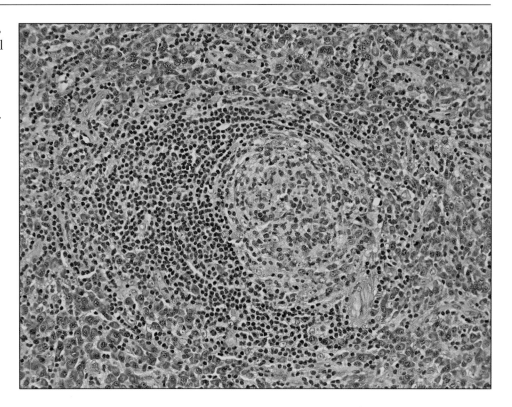

elevated serum levels of IL-6 would provide strong support for the localized plasma cell form of Castleman disease.

Multicentric Castleman disease also has an equal sex predilection, but occurs in an older age group than the localized subtypes, with a median age in the 50s. Those patients with HIV infection may have a younger age at presentation. By definition, multiple lymph node groups are affected, and there is usually splenomegaly or hepatosplenomegaly as well. Patients often have systemic symptoms, including malaise, fever, and night sweats. Abnormal laboratory studies include pancytopenia (usually anemia and thrombocytopenia), hypoalbuminemia, and hypergammaglobulinemia. Many patients with multicentric Castleman disease have HIV infection, and about 15% have the POEMS syndrome (Crow-Fukase disease), consisting of polyneuropathy, organomegaly, endocrinopathy, monoclonal gammopathy, and skin changes. Virtually all of the patients with HIV infection have identifiable HHV-8/Kaposi sarcoma herpesvirus (KSHV) in lesional tissue, while about 40% of non–HIV-infected patients also have identifiable HHV-8 in lesional tissue. Since the copy number of HHV-8 in blood correlates with symptoms and HHV-8 is known to produce a viral homologue of IL-6, it is thought that the HHV-8 plays an important role in pathogenesis. Patients with multicentric Castleman disease have been treated by splenectomy (to treat hematologic complications), chemotherapy, antiherpesvirus therapy, highly active antiretroviral therapy (HAART) in acquired immunodeficiency syndrome (AIDS)–infected patients, and monoclonal antibodies for IL-6 and CD20. Optimal therapy has not been achieved, and patients generally have a poor prognosis. Many of these patients progress to malignant lymphoma, particularly those who are HIV infected.

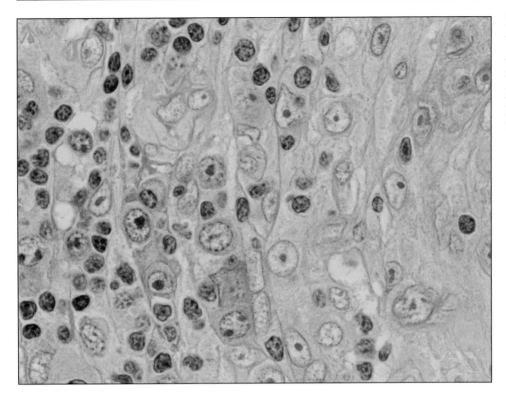

Figure 30. Plasmablastic variant of Castleman disease. A regressed germinal center is seen, with scattered atypical plasma cells and plasmablasts present at the interface with the mantle zone.

Involved lymph nodes in multicentric Castleman disease show similar histologic features to that seen in the localized plasma cell variant. Those cases associated with HHV-8 preferentially show follicular dissolution resulting from blurring of the mantle zone boundary, the presence of atypical plasma cells and plasmablasts in these areas, and more prominent paracortical vascular proliferation than in HHV-8–negative cases, designated the plasmablastic variant of Castleman disease (Figure 30). There is also associated dilation of the intranodal sinuses. Immunostains demonstrate positivity using antibodies against the ORF73/latency-associated nuclear antigen-1 of HHV-8. Specifically, there is homogeneous or stippled nuclear staining within predominantly small lymphocytes and immunoblasts of HHV-8–associated cases, largely restricted to the mantle zones of the most disrupted and regressed follicles. Alternatively, HHV-8 positivity may be demonstrated using appropriate PCR studies. In the HHV-8–positive cases, the atypical plasma cells and plasmablasts in the mantle zones are monotypic for lambda light chain, while the mature plasma cells in the paracortical areas show a polytypic pattern of staining. In fact, it has been shown that these cells are polyclonal naive (nonmutated) B-cells expressing IgM heavy chain and exclusively lambda light chain. In contrast, an exclusively polytypic pattern of light chain staining is seen in the HHV-8–negative cases. Epstein–Barr virus (EBV) studies may show scattered positive cells, but this is not of diagnostic or pathogenetic significance. The differential diagnosis of multicentric Castleman disease is similar to that discussed under the unicentric plasma cell variant. These patients are at risk of further (or concurrent) development of non-Hodgkin lymphoma, Kaposi sarcoma, plasmacytoma, Hodgkin lymphoma, and glomeruloid hemangioma. The most important lymphoma to

Figure 31. Plasmablastic lymphoma, arising in multisystemic Castleman disease in an HIV-positive patient. A proliferation of plasmablasts is seen in the germinal center and extends to efface areas of the internodal region.

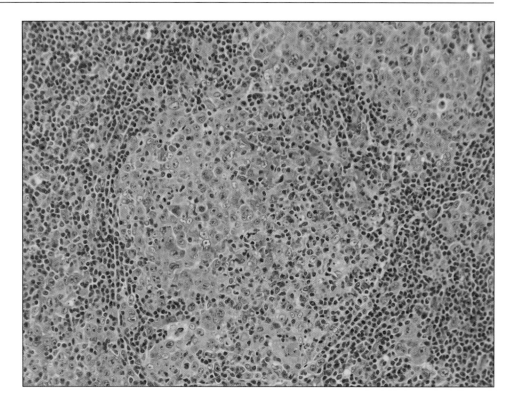

Table 7. Castleman Disease – Modern Classification

Non–HHV-8 associated

Unicentric hyaline-vascular

Unicentric plasma cell

Multicentric plasma cell

HHV-8 associated (plasmablastic)

Without associated plasmablastic lymphoma

With associated plasmablastic lymphoma

distinguish from the plasmablastic variant of Castleman disease is HHV-8–associated plasmablastic lymphoma. These lymphomas show a proliferation of plasmablasts that are HHV-8 positive, EBV negative, and show exclusively IgM immunoglobulin heavy chain and lambda light chain. Some cases arise in association with the plasmablastic variant of multicentric Castleman disease, showing micronodules either adjacent to or replacing some follicles, probably representing an early stage of lymphoma and strongly suggesting that this lymphoma probably arises out of progression from the plasmablastic variant (Figure 31). The prognosis of these lymphomas is poor, with death usually within 1 year.

Since the pathogenesis, histologic findings, and clinical implications of HHV-8–associated Castleman disease are different than those of HHV-8–negative Castleman disease, a proposal has been made to classify the disease along these lines (Table 7). The first category includes cases of hyaline-vascular Castleman disease that are segregated, since these seem to be its own unique disease, easily curable by surgical excision. The second category includes all HHV-8–associated cases – the plasmablastic variant. The remaining cases probably represent a mixture of cases, some representing nonspecific histologic findings, while others probably represent a further distinct form of plasma cell Castleman disease in which increased endogenous IL-6 production is of pathogenetic significance.

HIV-Related Benign Lymphadenopathy[52–58]

Patients with HIV infection may develop enlarged lymph nodes due to a wide variety of causes, including malignant lymphoma (non-Hodgkin and Hodgkin lymphoma), Kaposi sarcoma, multicentric Castleman disease, or numerous types of infection. However, the most frequent cause of isolated or generalized lymphadenopathy in this patient population is a lymph node reaction that develops in relation to response to the HIV itself. Persistent generalized lymphadenopathy was a term coined for lymphadenopathy that occurred in homosexual men in which there was lymph node enlargement of at least 3 months, absence of any illness or drug use known to cause lymph node enlargement, and histologic evidence of hyperplasia on biopsy. Although several discrete categories of lymph node pathology were characterized, including florid follicular hyperplasia, mixed follicular hyperplasia and involution, follicular involution, and lymphocyte depletion, it is now widely recognized that the changes form a continuum that correlate with other features of disease progression, such as CD4 T-cell counts and levels of virus. This section will discuss all of the stages of HIV-related benign lymphadenopathy, with emphasis on the forms that most commonly pose problems in differential diagnosis, particularly at the early stages of presentation with HIV infection.

Florid follicular hyperplasia is the histology seen in about 90% of patients who meet the criteria for persistent generalized lymphadenopathy as well as in about 20% of those patients who have lymph node enlargement in the context of AIDS. HIV-associated florid follicular hyperplasia has several characteristic features, none of which alone, or even together, is pathognomonic for this condition. Nonetheless, the constellation of findings in the appropriate clinical setting should raise consideration of HIV infection. First, there are numerous large, irregular germinal centers, often taking up much of the lymph node parenchyma (Figure 32). The centers usually have an extremely high proliferative rate and a high complement of large noncleaved cells and tingible-body macrophages, giving a prominent starry-sky appearance. They may contain hemorrhage and polykaryocytes are prominent in about one-quarter of cases. The mantle zones are often disrupted, thin, or completely absent and often invaginate into the germinal center, sometimes isolating clusters of germinal center cells, a phenomenon known as follicle lysis (Figure 33). The paracortical region often contains a mixed population of cells including plasma cells, immunoblasts, histiocytes, eosinophils, and neutrophils, with prominent high endothelial venules. Additional features include a focal to extensive monocytoid B-cell proliferation, focal dermatopathic changes, and clusters of or well-formed granulomas composed of epithelioid histiocytes. The differential diagnosis of HIV-associated florid follicular hyperplasia is any other reactive follicular hyperplasia, as well as follicular lymphoma, particularly given the high density of follicles, the often large number of large, noncleaved cells, and the frequently attenuated or absent mantle zones.

With progression of disease, florid follicular hyperplasia persists; however, other follicles show evidence of follicular regression, with small, atrophic, and hyalinized, follicles, and attenuated or absent mantle zones. The paracortical area is often expanded in area, with an increase in histiocytes and plasma cells and a corresponding decrease in the number of small lymphocytes. The

Figure 32. Reactive follicular hyperplasia. The follicle is enormous in size, wrapping around the blood vessel at the right. The mantle zone is diminished in size.

Figure 33. Follicular lysis. There is extensive hemorrhage in the follicle with separation of the germinal center cells into small clusters.

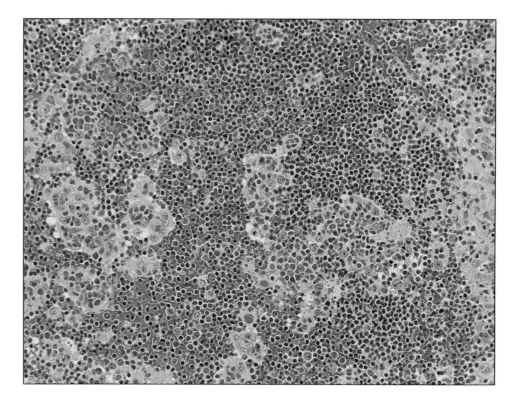

vasculature is increased in prominence, with numerous high endothelial venules. The lymph node capsule often shows areas of fibrosis, which may lead to obliteration of the underlying sinuses. The constellation of histologic features may raise consideration of Castleman disease. Eventually, the florid follicular hyperplasia is lost, and all the follicles show involution (Figure 34). The

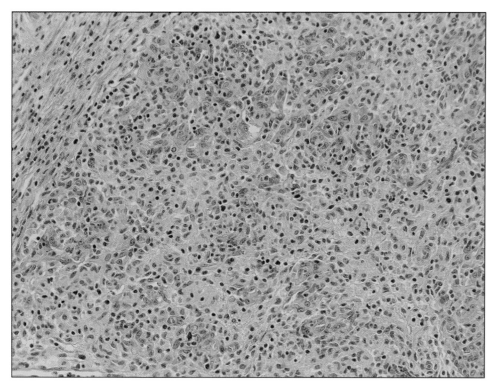

Figure 34. AIDS, lymphocyte depletion. This lymph node shows severe lymphocyte depletion, with an absence of follicles or appreciable numbers of paracortical lymphocytes. Instead, numerous histiocytes and small blood vessels are present.

majority of these patients have AIDS clinically. The paracortical areas may show a deposition of an eosinophilic material, and there may be a fine fibrosis. At this stage of disease, the histologic appearance of angioimmunoblastic lymphaden-opathy–like T-cell lymphoma may be mimicked. The areas of hypocellularity and fibrosis should raise consideration of Kaposi sarcoma, which should be ruled out by careful histologic examination of these areas. Eventually (often seen at autopsy), there is a complete loss of germinal centers with replacement by fibrous scars and an almost complete loss of small lymphocytes from the para-cortical region. The lymph nodes are small and dominated by medullary cords and dilated sinuses. Histiocytes are common and may show phagocytosis of hematopoietic cells. One should rule out *Mycobacterium avium intracellulare* infection.

Immunostains are not necessary for diagnosis, but do show interesting findings. The germinal centers of florid follicular hyperplasia show increased number of CD8-positive T-cells, often bearing cytotoxic markers. The lysis of the follicles is reflected in a disruption of the follicular dendritic cell network as shown by stains for follicular dendritic cells. The paracortex shows a decrease in the CD4:CD8 ratio, although not to the extent seen in the per-ipheral blood. Involuting follicles show a low proliferative rate as revealed by Ki-67 staining, with a loss of CD10 expression. The paracortical regions of later stage lymph nodes show an increase in interdigitating cells as revealed by S-100 protein and CD1 stains. Lymph nodes showing lymphocyte depletion show clusters of B-cells and CD8-positive T-cells, with a virtual absence of CD4-positive T-cells. Stains for follicular dendritic cells show a virtual absence of these cells.

Figure 35. Progressive transformation of germinal centers. A normal-sized germinal center is seen in the corner, while the central follicle is greatly enlarged and is segmented by invaginated small lymphocytes.

Progressive Transformation of Germinal Centers[59–68]

Progressive transformation of germinal centers is often seen as an isolated incidental finding in a lymph node that otherwise shows nonspecific reactive follicular hyperplasia. Rarely, it may be a dominant finding resulting in localized lymph node enlargement, most commonly occurring in the cervical region. It may occur in all ages, but favors children and young adults, with a male predominance. Excision is usually curative, although the disease may recur, usually in the same site. Beside its potential for confusion with malignant lymphoma, its importance lies in the fact that it may precede, coexist, or follow a biopsy showing lymphocyte-predominant Hodgkin lymphoma; it has been reported that the risk of developing nodular lymphocyte–predominant Hodgkin lymphoma after a diagnosis of progressive transformation of germinal centers is approximately 1–5%.

Excised lymph nodes are usually large and show a distinct nodular appearance on low magnification. A key finding is that progressively transformed germinal centers always occur in the context of nonspecific reactive follicular hyperplasia in a lymph node that has retained its overall architecture. The progressively transformed germinal centers stand out as well-circumscribed nodules from three to ten times in size as the adjacent follicles (Figure 35). When multiple progressively transformed germinal centers are present in one lymph node, they show varying sizes, reflecting their appearance at different stages of evolution. At high magnification, the dominant finding in the nodules is an expansion of mantle zone B-cells. The mantle cells not only form a large cuff but also more importantly they extensively infiltrate the germinal centers, isolating clusters of residual germinal center cells and dendritic cells. Ultimately, the germinal center cells become lost in a large round nodule seemingly entirely composed of mantle zone B-cells. Occasional cases may show a wreath of epithelioid histiocytes around the nodules, although this phenomenon is much more common in lymphocyte-predominant Hodgkin lymphoma. Most importantly, the lymphocytic and histiocytic (L&H) cells of lymphocyte-predominant Hodgkin lymphoma are not found in progressive transformation of germinal centers.

Immunohistochemical studies demonstrate that the majority of lymphocytes in the nodules show features of mantle cells, with IgM and IgD expression. The number of CD57-positive cells in the follicles is often increased, but there is no rosetting around large B-cells. Stains for follicular dendritic cells show distorted and disrupted networks of follicular dendritic cells. The bcl-2 staining shows the areas of residual germinal center cells. Importantly, CD20 stains do not identify L&H cells in, around, or outside the nodules, although there is staining of the residual large noncleaved cells of the reactive germinal center. Similar to this, epithelial membrane antigen, an inconsistent marker of L&H cells, is negative in large cells. Flow cytometry studies have shown the presence of population of CD4-positive and CD8-positive cells in about one-third of cases.

The most important differential diagnosis is with lymphocyte-predominant Hodgkin lymphoma. Although the distinction can be quite difficult, it is usually straightforward. In lymphocyte-predominant Hodgkin lymphoma, the area of lymphoma is usually distinct from any residual areas of reactive follicular hyperplasia, and one almost always does not see an isolated nodule of lymphocyte predominance surrounded by reactive follicles, which is typical for progressive transformation. Of course, the critical distinction is the presence of true L&H cells in lymphocyte predominance, identified by their large size and nuclear multilobulation; their localization in, around, and outside of follicles; and their CD20 positivity surrounded by a rim of T-cells that often express CD57 and bcl-6. Follicular lymphoma, particularly the floral variant, may be confused with progressive transformation. Typically, in follicular lymphoma, all the follicles are abnormal, and there are usually no interspersed benign follicles. Immunohistochemical studies for bcl-2 as well as molecular analyses (immunoglobulin and bcl-2 rearrangement studies) can be helpful in sorting this out. Finally, mantle cell lymphoma may be mimicked due to the extensive mantle cell proliferation; the absence of cytologic atypia in the mantle cells and the absence of nuclear cyclin D1 staining in the mantle cells in progressive transformation should resolve this dilemma.

Table 8. Reactive Lymphadenopathies with a Primary Paracortical Pattern

- Nonspecific reactive paracortical hyperplasia
- Viral
  - Epstein–Barr
  - CMV
  - Herpesvirus
- Postvaccinial
- Drug-induced
- Dermatopathic lymphadenitis

REACTIVE PARACORTICAL HYPERPLASIA[13]

Reactive paracortical hyperplasia is a relatively common lymph node pattern. I would like to stress once again that virtually never is the process exclusively that of reactive paracortical hyperplasia but usually includes hyperplasia of other compartments, particularly the follicles but also often the sinuses. However, this section will consider those diseases in which reactive paracortical hyperplasia represents the dominant histologic pattern. This is important to consider from a differential diagnostic viewpoint as well as possibly suggesting a specific diagnosis.

A specific etiology cannot be determined for the large majority of cases of reactive paracortical hyperplasia. Similar to reactive follicular hyperplasia, reactive paracortical hyperplasia occurs in all age groups, but is more common in young patients. Table 8 lists the most common diseases that give rise to histologic findings that may suggest the specific etiology of the paracortical hyperplasia.

In reactive paracortical hyperplasia, one sees expansion of the paracortical areas by a mixed infiltrate, often imparting a mottled appearance (Figure 6). The cortical regions usually participate to some extent in the hyperplasia. At high magnification, the paracortical areas usually show a mixture of small and large lymphoid cells, but without cytologic atypia (the latter manifested by highly irregular or hyperchromatic nuclei) (Figure 36). There are often immunoblasts, which are usually relatively evenly dispersed, and large numbers of plasma cells, eosinophils, and histiocytes are typical. Vascularity is often increased, usually with prominent high endothelial venules.

The major and most important differential diagnosis is with a peripheral T-cell lymphoma. Histologically, obliteration or marked diminution of the cortical region would favor a diagnosis of T-cell lymphoma, as the cortical region usually also undergoes hyperplasia in most cases of reactive paracortical hyperplasia. The most important criterion is the presence of a spectrum of atypical cells in T-cell lymphoma. In reactive paracortical hyperplasia, there is often an admixture of cell types, including immunoblasts, but a continuous spectrum of cytologic atypia among the lymphoid cells would certainly favor a T-cell lymphoma. A diminution of the B-cell compartments (cortical and subcapsular areas) seen by immunohistochemical studies would favor a T-cell lymphoma, while peripheral T-cell lymphoma may certainly contain B-cells, including B-immunoblasts, the greater the number of admixed B-cells of both large and small size, the more likely a diagnosis of reactive paracortical hyperplasia. The demonstration of T-cell phenotypic abnormalities such as loss of one or more pan-T-cell antigens or abnormal expression of other antigens (such as loss of bcl-2 or gain of CD10 or bcl-6) would favor a diagnosis of T-cell lymphoma. Finally, the molecular detection of clonal T-cell receptor gene rearrangements would provide strong evidence for a diagnosis of T-cell lymphoma.

Reactive follicular hyperplasia and Hodgkin lymphoma may also be difficult to distinguish from one another. In the interfollicular variant of Hodgkin

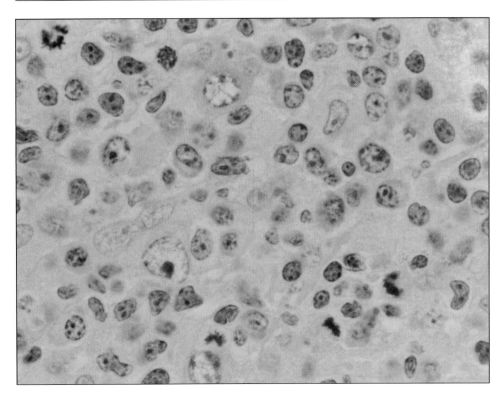

Figure 36. Reactive paracortical hyperplasia. A mixture of immunoblasts, lymphocytes, plasma cells, and plasmacytoid lymphocytes is seen.

lymphoma, the Hodgkin cells are found in between hyperplastic follicles. Sometimes, areas that are more typical of Hodgkin lymphoma are seen elsewhere in the biopsy. Hodgkin cells tend to cluster, are not usually associated with typical immunoblasts in a *reactive milieu*, but tend to be found in their characteristic background. Careful cytologic evaluation of the large atypical cells together with immunohistochemical studies seeking the typical phenotype of Hodgkin cells should resolve most cases.

Acute Infectious Mononucleosis[69–73]

Most initial infections with EBV occur asymptomatically in children under the age of 5, even in Western countries. Symptomatic acute infectious mononucleosis occurs in all age groups except childhood. Approximately one-third of EBV infections occurring in adolescents are symptomatic, with a continuum of increasing percentage and severity of symptoms as initial infection occurs at older ages. The most common symptoms include sore throat, fever, and lymphadenopathy, particularly anterior or posterior cervical lymphadenopathy. However, many other lymph node groups may be affected. Markedly enlarged tonsils are almost always present, splenomegaly is found in 50% of cases, and hepatomegaly occurs in about 10%. Hematologic examination usually reveals lymphocytosis, with at least 10% atypical lymphocytes (95% T-cells). If the diagnosis is suspected clinically, the diagnosis can be confirmed serologically, either by IgM monospot test or by more specific EBV antibody studies. However, the diagnosis is invariably not considered clinically in cases that come to

Figure 37. Acute infectious mononucleosis. Although the paracortical region is greatly expanded, reactive follicles are still present albeit somewhat obscured.

Figure 38. Acute infectious mononucleosis. A proliferation of immunoblasts is seen, closely simulating a high-grade diffuse large B-cell lymphoma.

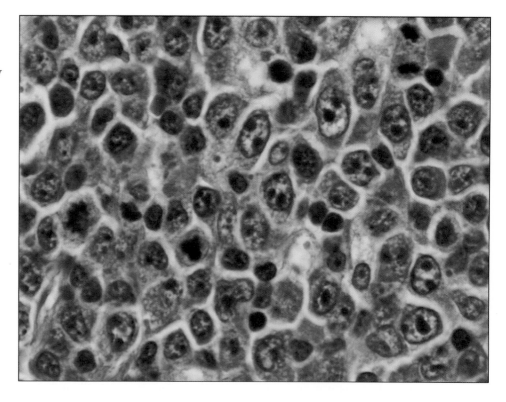

biopsy. Other diseases that may have an identical clinical and laboratory profile include cytomegalovirus (CMV) or HHV-6 infection.

The earliest manifestation of acute infectious mononucleosis may be a prominent monocytoid B-cell proliferation, along with reactive follicular hyperplasia. However, soon after, there is an immunoblastic proliferation, which may be

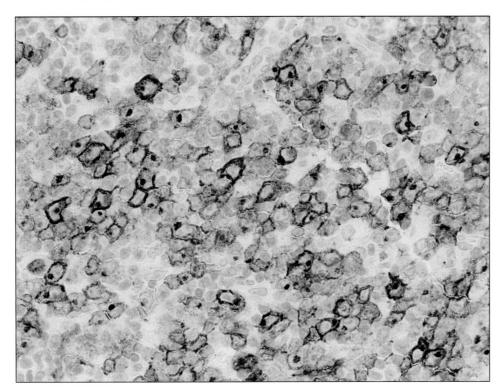

Figure 39. EBV-associated acute infectious mononucleosis. Numerous CD30-positive cells are seen, a finding that should not be confused with anaplastic large-cell lymphoma.

quite striking (Figures 37 and 38). These cells typically have prominent nucleoli and abundant cytoplasm. They have a high mitotic rate and may form sheets, may be found in sinuses, and may be multinucleated, mimicking either non-Hodgkin lymphoma or Hodgkin lymphoma. There are usually abundant plasma cells, and there may be eosinophils or epithelioid histiocytes. Necrosis may be absent, focal, or extensive. Follicles usually show striking reactive follicular hyperplasia, but may be overshadowed by the paracortical hyperplasia.

Immunohistochemical studies are nonspecific. The monocytoid cells in the sinuses mark as B-cells, the reactive germinal centers are bcl-2 negative, and the immunoblasts are a mixture of T- and B-cells. One may see coexpression of CD43 and CD20 on the immunoblasts, a finding that does not equate to a diagnosis of lymphoma in this setting. Many of the immunoblasts may be CD30 positive, including sheets of cells, a finding that does not equate to a diagnosis of anaplastic large-cell lymphoma in this setting (and ALK staining is negative) (Figure 39). The most useful studies are those for identifying EBV. Virtually all cases have varying number of EBV–latent membrane protein (LMP)–positive cells, usually immunoblasts. EBV-encoded RNA (EBER) in situ hybridizations label many more EBV-positive cells, including numerous large and small cells in the paracortical areas and scattered cells in the germinal centers and monocytoid B-cell areas (Figure 40).

The differential diagnosis includes both non-Hodgkin lymphoma and Hodgkin lymphoma. Misdiagnosis of acute infectious mononucleosis as non-Hodgkin lymphoma is the most frequent error in lymph node pathology in my experience. Simply stated, one should not diagnose a diffuse large-cell lymphoma in either the tonsil or cervical lymph nodes in a child or adolescent without first

Figure 40. Acute infectious mononucleosis, EBER stain. Note that both small and large cells show nuclear positivity and that most of the cells are still EBV negative. A much higher proportion of the cells would be expected to be positive in an EBV-associated B-cell lymphoma.

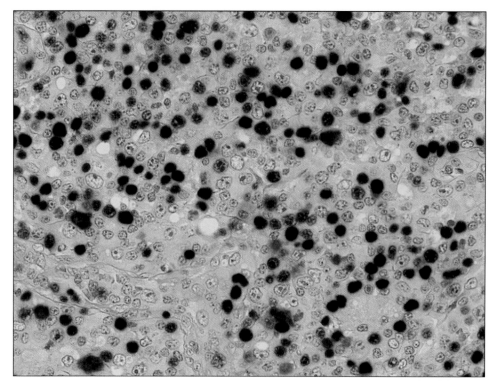

considering and ruling out a possible diagnosis of acute infectious mononucleosis! In situ hybridization using EBER probes is the most helpful ancillary study for the tissue diagnosis of acute infectious mononucleosis. In EBV-positive diffuse large B-cell lymphomas, the EBV is uniformly present in the large neoplastic cells and absent or virtually absent in the small lymphocytes, while in infectious mononucleosis, the positive cells are a subset of both large and small lymphocytes. Gene rearrangement studies may also be of use; however, both immunoglobulin and T-cell receptor studies may show oligoclonal patterns of gene rearrangement. A diagnosis of Hodgkin lymphoma may be considered if one focuses carefully on the high magnification appearance of the immunoblasts, but the overall context is not that of Hodgkin lymphoma, with a high mitotic rate and usually an accompanying florid reactive follicular hyperplasia. In situ hybridization may show EBV positivity in Hodgkin lymphoma (particularly in cases occurring in patients under the age of 21), but only the Hodgkin cells are positive – many fewer positive cells than seen in acute infectious mononucleosis. In contrast to classical Hodgkin lymphoma, immunohistochemical studies do not show CD15 reactivity in the large cells in acute infectious mononucleosis, although many may express CD30 and lack CD45 expression, similar to Hodgkin lymphoma.

CMV Lymphadenitis[74–76]

CMV lymphadenitis can be seen in both immunocompetent and immunosuppressed patients. Because of the differences in immune status in various patients, the histologic findings can be quite variable. As in EBV-associated acute infectious mononucleosis, the earliest change may be a reactive monocytoid B-cell

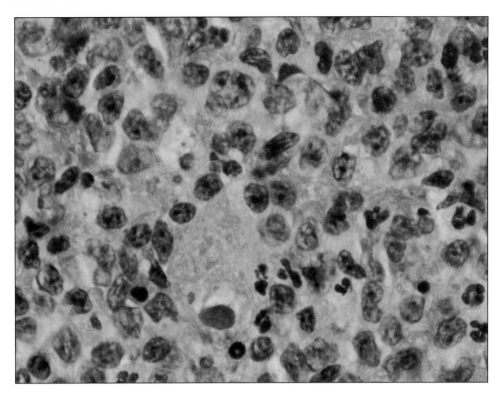

Figure 41. CMV lymphadenitis. A typical cytomegaloviral inclusion is seen within monocytoid B-cell hyperplasia.

hyperplasia, along with reactive follicular hyperplasia. However, the dominant histologic picture evolves to a prominent reactive paracortical hyperplasia, including numerous immunoblasts and prominent hypervascularity. The most intense reactions, including foci of necrosis, are seen in immunocompromised patients. Cytomegaly with viral inclusions may be seen within the monocytoid B-cell areas (more common in immunocompetent hosts) or the paracortical areas (more common in immunocompromised hosts) (Figure 41). The inclusions may be seen in endothelial cells or T-lymphocytes and may be typical (in untreated patients) or atypical (in patients who have received antiviral drugs). The differential diagnosis centers upon the specific identification of CMV-infected cells. While Hodgkin lymphoma may rarely show localization of the Hodgkin cells to monocytoid B-cell areas and CMV-infected cells may be CD15 positive, CMV-infected cells are not usually CD30 positive and immunohistochemical or in situ hybridization studies for CMV should proviclde confirmation of the diagnosis in any problematic cases.

Herpes Simplex Lymphadenitis[77–79]

Herpes simplex lymphadenitis is not uncommon, but is usually not biopsied, since patients almost invariably have clinically obvious skin lesions. Biopsied lymph nodes usually derive from the inguinal region in patients in whom a thorough anogenital examination has not been performed. Patients may be immunocompetent or immunosuppressed. Most cases show a striking reactive paracortical hyerplasia. In addition, there are usually discrete foci of necrosis. Herpetic inclusions are usually easily seen and are generally present at the

Figure 42. Herpes lymphadenitis. A herpetic inclusion is seen at the interface between the necrotic and nonnecrotic areas.

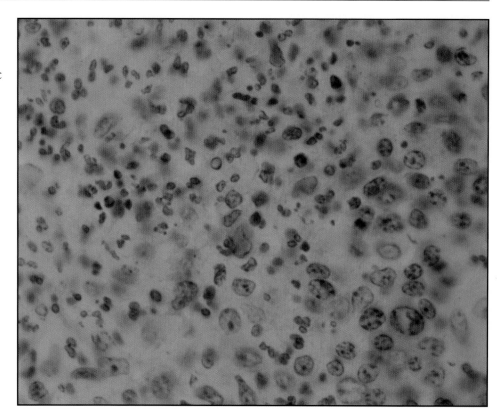

junction between the necrotic and viable areas (Figure 42). These inclusions are most frequently ground-glass nuclei, but intranuclear eosinophilic inclusions with halos, chromatin margination, and multinucleated cells may all be seen. If there is any doubt as to the specific diagnosis, immunohistochemical or in situ hybridization studies should be definitive. The diagnosis may also be established by serologic studies.

Postvaccinial Reactive Paracortical Hyperplasia[78]

Postvaccinial reactive paracortical hyperplasia is a rare complication of vaccination found at lymph nodes draining the site of vaccination. It may be seen following either intramuscular or subcutaneous inoculation. It is the clinical setting that provides the specific diagnosis, as the histologic findings are those of a nonspecific reactive paracortical hyperplasia. The one exception is that numerous Warthin-Finkeldey giant cells, representing infected follicular dendritic cells, may be seen following measles vaccination.

Drug-Induced Reactive Paracortical Hyperplasia[80–82]

Reactive paracortical hyperplasia may be induced by a wide variety of drugs, but has been most commonly documented with phenytoin. The lymphadenopathy may occur almost immediately after taking the drug, although it more commonly appears after several weeks. There may be accompanying systemic symptoms, including malaise, fever, rash, joint pain, or even hepatosplenomegaly.

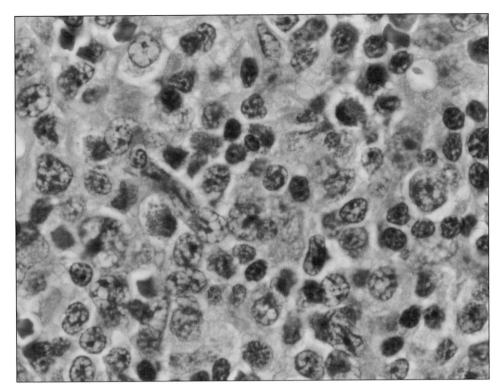

Figure 43. Reactive paracortical hyperplasia due to dilantin. There is a proliferation of reactive immunoblasts and eosinophils, along scattered plasma cells.

The peripheral blood may show eosinophilia, consistent with an allergic phenomenon. The lymphadenopathy typically resolves when the drug is removed. Histologically, one sees a reactive paracortical hyperplasia, distinctive by the presence of variable numbers of eosinophils (Figure 43). The cortical region may be hyperplastic, and atrophic obliterative vasculitis has also been reported. Some lymph nodes may show an angioimmunoblastic lymphadenopathy–like appearance. It has been reported that the immunoblasts in this condition are less likely to be CD30 positive than other types of reactive paracortical hyperplasia such as EBV-associated acute infectious mononucleosis.

Dermatopathic Lymphadenitis[70,83,84]

Dermatopathic lymphadenitis occurs in lymph nodes draining areas in which there has been disruption or irritation of the skin barrier due to any process, benign or malignant. Some patients have no more history than pruritis with scratching. In about 10% of cases, there is no history elicited, but the likelihood is that even in these cases there was a prior insult to the skin barrier that is no longer recalled. Patients present with isolated or generalized lymph node enlargement. Consistent with the pathogenesis described above, axillary and inguinal lymph nodes are most commonly affected. A subset of patients may have peripheral blood eosinophilia, consistent with an allergic phenotype.

On low magnification, the overall lymph node architecture is preserved, although the cortical area is compressed against the capsule, due to the often-massive expansion of the paracortical areas (Figure 44). The expansion in the paracortical area may be diffuse or somewhat nodular. In distinction to the other

Figure 44. Dermatopathic lymphadenitis. An exquisite paracortical distribution is seen, isolating the cortical region with scattered germinal centers against the capsule. Note the pigment.

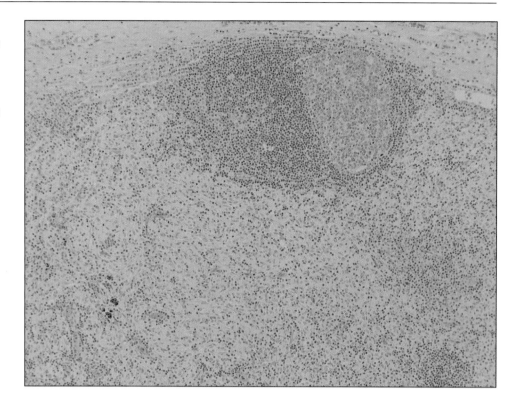

Figure 45. Dermatopathic lymphadenitis. Numerous reactive Langerhans cells and interdigitating dendritic cells are seen in the paracortex.

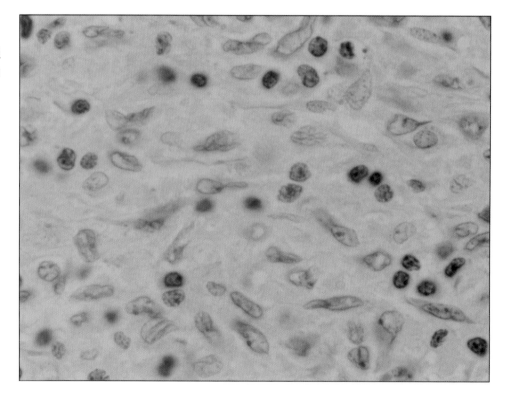

causes of paracortical hyperplasia, dermatopathic lymphadenitis shows a proliferation of dendritic cells, including both Langerhans cells and interdigitating cells (Figure 45). Langerhans cells and interdigitating cells appear similar on routine histologic sections, but can be collectively identified by their intermediate nuclear size, fine chromatin pattern, and nuclear membrane irregularities,

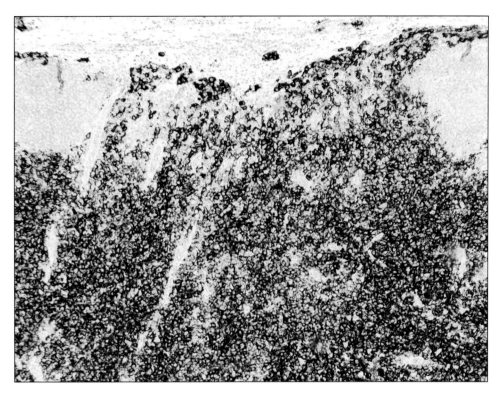

Figure 46. Dermatopathic lymphadenitis, CD1 stain. The numerous Langerhans cells are stained. Note the paracortical distribution, in contrast to the dominant sinusoidal localization in Langerhans cell histiocytosis.

including a *coffee-bean* appearance. In addition, there are numerous histiocytes, including foamy histiocytes, as well as large numbers of plasma cells and variable numbers of eosinophils. Small lymphocytes and immunoblasts are also present, and there may be significant nuclear irregularities in the small lymphoid cells. Finally, scattered melanin pigment is usually seen, usually within histiocytes. The overall appearance, with the heterogeneity of cell types, gives a mottled low-magnification appearance to the lymph node.

Immunophenotypic studies show that there are numerous Langerhans cells (CD1 and S-100 protein positive), numerous interdigitating cells (CD1 negative and S-100 positive), numerous macrophages (CD163 positive), and numerous T-cells (CD3 positive), usually of helper/inducer type (CD4 positive) (Figure 46). There may be some loss of CD7, which if that is the only phenotypic abnormality, does not indicate the presence of a T-cell lymphoma. B-cells are generally restricted to the follicles, with few B-cells seen in the paracortical areas.

The crucial entity in the differential diagnosis is lymph node involvement by mycosis fungoides, particularly given the frequent history of longstanding skin lesions. In addition, patients with mycosis fungoides may frequently have lymph nodes showing dermatopathic changes, whether or not there is involvement by lymphoma in addition. In patients with any history or clinical suspicion of mycosis fungoides, a high threshold of tolerance for atypia in the lymphoid population is recommended. However, in the setting of mycosis fungoides or a clinical suspicion of mycosis fungoides, I recommend a low threshold for ordering T-cell receptor gene rearrangements. Although there are often immunophenotypic differences between dermatopathic lymph nodes with and without involvement by mycosis fungoides (e.g., loss of CD7 or other

Table 9. Reactive Lymphadenopathies with a Primary Sinus Pattern

- Nonspecific sinus histiocytosis
- Monocytoid B-cell hyperplasia
- Whipple lymphadenopathy
- Exogenous material
- Endogenous lipid material
- Rosai-Dorfman disease
- Hemophagocytic lymphohistiocytosis

pan-T-markers), the findings may be hard to interpret and there is some overlap. Another consideration in the differential diagnosis is Langerhans cell histiocytosis. Both Langerhans cell histiocytosis and dermatopathic lymphadenitis feature proliferations of Langerhans cells, the former neoplastic and the latter reactive. In Langerhans cell histiocytosis, the proliferation occurs in the sinuses and adjacent areas, while in dermatopathic lymphadenitis the proliferation is paracortical.

SINUS HYPERPLASIA

Reactive sinus hyperplasia may occur alone or in conjunction with reactive follicular hyperplasia and/or reactive paracortical hyperplasia. It may be caused by two nonspecific histologic patterns, as well as a variety of specific diseases, summarized in Table 9.

Nonspecific Sinus Histiocytosis[85,86]

Nonspecific sinus histiocytosis is a very common phenomenon, typically seen in lymph nodes draining sites of inflammation, neoplasms, and prostheses. It is particularly common in lymph nodes in the mesenteric area draining the gut, possibly due to abundant fluids absorbed from the gastrointestinal tract. Histologically, one sees cytologically bland histiocytes with abundant cytoplasm filling and expanding the sinuses. Usually, all sinuses are involved, including subcapsular, trabecular, and medullary sinuses. Rarely (and inexplicably), the histiocytes may show cytophagocytosis, most often erythrophagocytosis, or a peculiar signet-ring cell change (Figure 47). In any cases of doubt, keratin or stains can be used to rule out the possibility of carcinoma in these latter cases. Another rare finding is a sinus eosinophilia, which may suggest a possible allergic or parasitic etiology (Figure 48).

Monocytoid B-Cell Hyperplasia[87–89]

Monocytoid B-cell hyperplasia is a relatively specific disease pattern that raises specific entities in the differential diagnosis, including toxoplasmosis (all cases), HIV lymphadenopathy, viral infection, or suppurative granulomatous lymphadenitis. When present as an isolated feature, it may be an early manifestation of EBV or CMV infection. Monocytoid cells have medium-sized nuclei about twice the diameter of small lymphocytes (Figures 9 and 49). Their chromatin is open with an inconspicuous nucleolus, and they have abundant pale cytoplasm. They are found primarily in sinuses, including subcapsular and trabecular sinuses, but may be seen adjacent to sinuses in the paracortical regions or adjacent to follicles in the cortex. They are usually admixed with neutrophils and may be associated with scattered plasma cells and large transformed cells with prominent nucleoli.

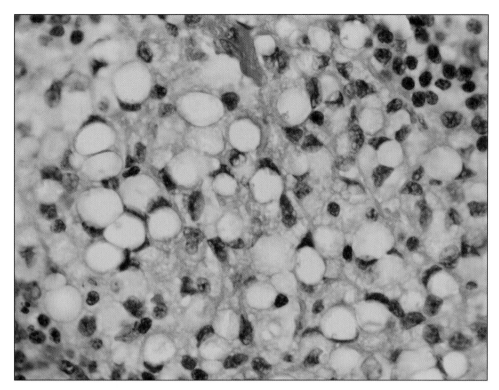

Figure 47. Signet-ring cell histiocytosis. The sinus histiocytes show a peculiar vacuolization imparting a signet-ring cell appearance. Keratin stains were performed to rule out the possibility of metastatic carcinoma.

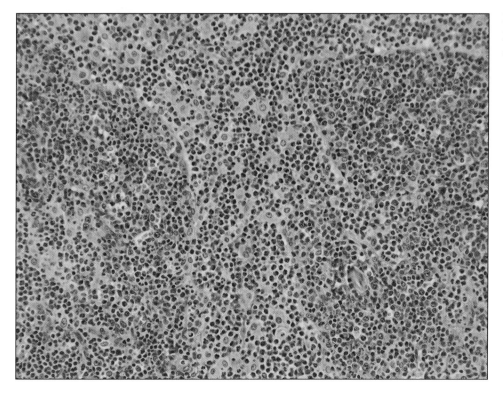

Figure 48. Sinus eosinophilia. In this case, no specific etiology was identified.

Table 10 summarizes the distinction between monocytoid B-cell hyperplasia and nodal marginal zone B-cell lymphoma. In general, the more extensive the proliferation, particularly in the absence of other reactive features, the more likely one is dealing with lymphoma. Although marginal zone B-cell lymphoma may feature bland cells, there is still a greater degree of nuclear variability than

Figure 49. Reactive monocytoid B-cell hyperplasia. A sheet of monocytoid B-cells are seen adjacent to a lymph node trabeculum.

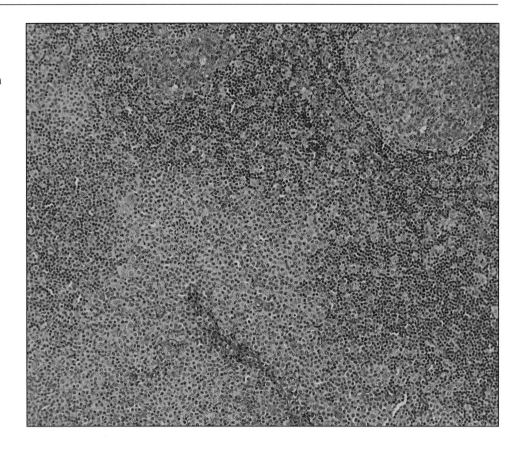

Table 10. Differential Diagnosis of Monocytoid B-Cell Hyperplasia vs. Nodal Marginal Zone B-Cell Lymphoma

Monocytoid B-Cell Hyperplasia	Nodal Marginal Zone B-Cell Lymphoma
Usually comprises <50% of node	Usually comprises >50% of node
Lacks nuclear atypia	May have nuclear atypia
Usually contains scattered neutrophils	Usually has cells with plasmacytic differentiation
Usually bcl-2 positive	Usually bcl-2 negative
Polytypic light chains	Often monotypic light chains
CD43 negative	May be CD43 positive

monocytoid B-cell hyperplasia. Nodal marginal zone B-cell lymphoma rarely has admixed neutrophils but commonly shows areas of frank plasmacytic differentiation. The bcl-2 stain is negative in monocytoid B-cell hyperplasia, but almost always expressed in marginal zone B-cell lymphoma (Figure 50). The pitfall in this stain is that one needs to be sure the bcl-2 is being assessed in monocytoid B-cells, as enlarged reactive mantle zones may abut the capsule and be mistaken for monocytoid B-cells; these cells are bcl-2 positive, and one may be misled to a mistaken diagnosis of lymphoma. Cases of marginal zone B-cell lymphoma may show monotypic light chain staining, particularly in areas showing frank plasmacytoid features (although occasionally the plasmacytoid areas may represent a reactive plasmacytic component admixed with the lymphoma).

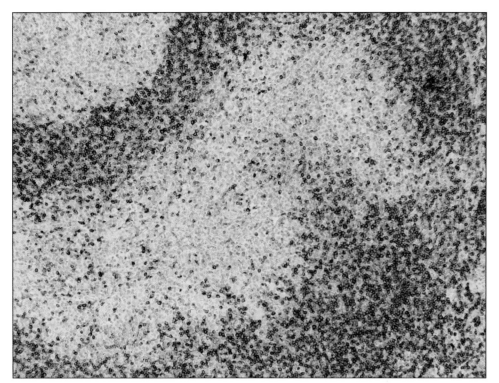

Figure 50. Reactive monocytoid B-cell hyperplasia, bcl-2 stain. In contrast to marginal zone B-cell lymphoma, reactive monocytoid proliferations are invariably bcl-2 negative.

Finally, about 50% of cases of nodal marginal zone B-cell lymphoma may have aberrant expression of CD43, a finding that is never seen in reactive monocytoid B-cells.

Whipple Lymphadenopathy[90–92]

Whipple disease (intestinal lipodystrophy) is a bacterial infection primarily involving the small intestine caused by the bacterium *Tropheryma whippelii*. It usually affects men in adulthood. Symptoms include diarrhea, weight loss, and malaise, but may also include fever, inflamed joints, pleuritis, and neurologic symptoms, as other organs may be affected. Treatment with antibiotics usually results in a rapid response, although it may still recur. Regional lymph node involvement is uniformly seen, but involvement of peripheral lymph nodes may be seen in up to 50% of cases and may be the presenting sign of the disease. Involved lymph nodes show dilation of the sinuses with histiocytes and large round empty spaces. The histiocytes contain periodic acid-Schiff (PAS) diastase-positive acid-fast–negative rods. The organisms can also be identified by electron microscopy. The differential diagnosis includes *Mycobacterium avium*, which is acid-fast positive.

Lymphadenopathy Due to Deposition of Exogenous Material[93–95]

A wide variety of exogenous materials may be present in the human body and find their way into the lymph nodes. Historically, lymphangiography

Figure 51. Lymphangiography changes. Extracellular spaces representing washed out lipid material lined by histiocytes are present.

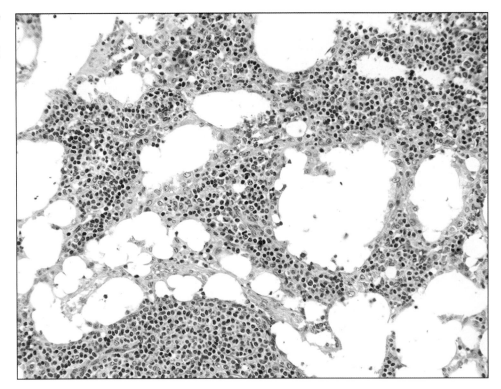

dye has been among the commonest material, although this is not often seen now since lymphangiography is no longer routinely performed as a staging tool for Hodgkin lymphoma. The dye is an oily base, which leaves holes in the tissue sections after routine processing. Left behind is a classical foreign-body giant-cell reaction, often with numerous giant cells adjacent to the spaces (Figure 51). Similar findings may be seen with silicone, which is still used in some breast implants, as well as in some orthopedic prostheses. However, the longer the silicone has been around, the more likely it is ingested by macrophages, seen as multiple fine vacuolations in histiocyte cytoplasm (Figure 52). Silicone is less likely than lymphangiography dye to be retained during tissue processing and is a nonbirefringent but refractile material. Definitive diagnosis may be made by x-ray microanalysis. Regional lymph nodes draining prostheses may show a wide variety of features, depending on the specific materials present in the prosthesis, including the cement. These changes range from holes in the tissue to extracellular and intracellular material that may or may not be refractile or birefringent to a histiocyte proliferation which may or may not show vacuoles. Particularly common is a coarsely granular PAS-positive substance in histiocytes. Tattoo pigment manifest as a jet-black pigment within macrophages in the sinuses. Clofazimine may cause a black discoloration of lymph nodes, with scattered crystals seen in histiocytes, with an accompanying paracortical plasmacytosis. The crystals are clear in paraffin sections, but red in frozen sections. Patients who have received polyvinylpyrrolidone as a plasma expander may show collections of histiocytes in the sinuses with abundant bubbly histiocytes containing a blue-gray, mucicarmine-positive, but PAS-negative, material.

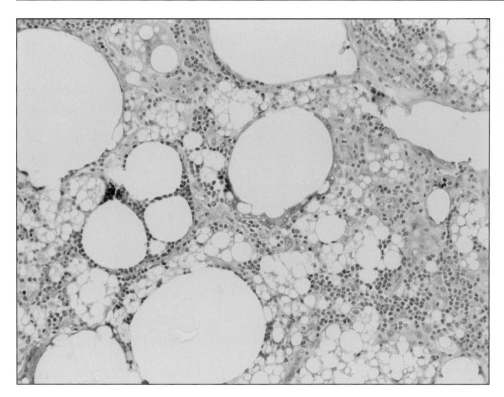

Figure 52. Silicone lymphadenopathy. Both intracellular and extracellular spaces are seen. Giant cells are present lining much of the extracellular spaces.

Lymphadenopathy Due to Deposition of Endogenous Lipid Material[96]

Lymphadenopathy due to deposition of endogenous lipid material (lipogranulo-matosis or lipophagic granuloma) is most commonly seen in lymph nodes in the porta hepatis and celiac axis. The lipid collection may be due to a wide variety of causes, including mineral oil ingestion, total parenteral nutrition, hematomas, tumors, cholesterol deposits, xanthomatous lesions, fat embolism, and fat necrosis. It manifests as vacuolization of sinus histiocytes, eventually with the formation of small lipid granulomas with multinucleated giant cells (Figure 53). The vacuoles are typically much smaller than those seen with exogenous lipid material.

Rosai-Dorfman Disease[97–106]

Rosai-Dorfman disease (sinus histiocytosis with massive lymphadenopathy) represents a peculiar proliferation of histiocyte-like cells. Of unknown etiology, a reactive proliferation is favored over a true neoplastic process, although the evidence is not conclusive. It is most commonly seen in children, although it may affect all age groups; there is no sex predilection. The disease is much more commonly seen in blacks. About 90% of patients present with multiple, massive, painless cervical lymph nodes. Other lymph nodes may also be involved, includ-ing axillary, inguinal, para-aortic, and mediastinal lymph nodes, and occasion-ally may be the presenting site. In about 40% of cases, extranodal sites are involved, including skin, upper respiratory tract, soft tissue (including orbit), bone, and rarely other sites. Patients often have constitutional symptoms and

Figure 53.
Lipogranulomatosis. When
the lipid accumulates slowly,
as in lipogranulomatosis, the
vacuoles tend to be primarily
intracellular and only later
become aggregated into larger
extracellular deposits.

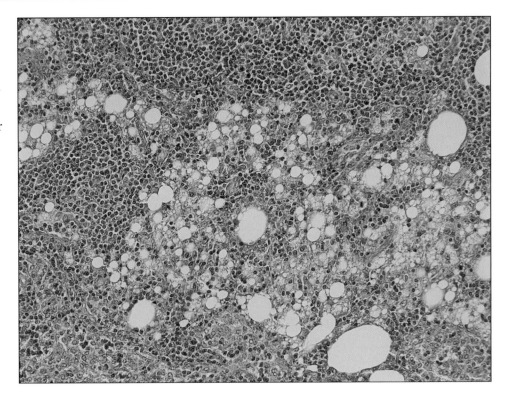

may have a wide variety of laboratory abnormalities, including leukocytosis and polyclonal hypergammaglobulinemia. Some patients may have immune dysfunction, and some patients with autoimmune lymphoproliferative disease may show focal changes of Rosai-Dorfman disease in their lymph nodes, suggesting an immune dysfunction pathogenesis. HUMARA assays performed to date are consistent with a polyclonal process, and there is no evidence of viruses, including EBV, HHV-6, and human T-cell leukemia virus (HTLV). Most patients undergo slow spontaneous remission, occurring over a period of months to years. Surgery is reserved for those cases in which a mass effect leads to compromise of the patient. Although usually benign, fatalities may occur, either due to mass effect or the accompanying immune dysfunction.

Grossly, the excised lymph node is usually very large and is often matted to overlying soft tissues or adjacent lymph nodes. At low magnification, one sees a thickened capsule as the source of the matting (Figure 54). The lymph node architecture is dominated by a striking sinus expansion, filled with the characteristic proliferating histiocyte-like cells. These cells have an intermediate- to large-sized round nucleus, a delicate nuclear membrane, and a vesicular chromatin pattern with one to a few moderately prominent nucleoli (Figure 55). Cytoplasm is abundant, amphophilic to eosinophilic, and occasionally foamy. The cytoplasm often contains phagocytosed intact small lymphocytes (lymphophagocytosis) or a variety of cells, including red blood cells, neutrophils, or plasma cells (emperipolesis). Typically, there are multiple ingested cells, forming a partial or complete ring around the nuclei. Plasma cells are abundant, both adjacent to the proliferating histiocytes within the sinuses as well as within the adjacent expanded medullary cords (Figure 56). Late lesions may show extensive fibrosis

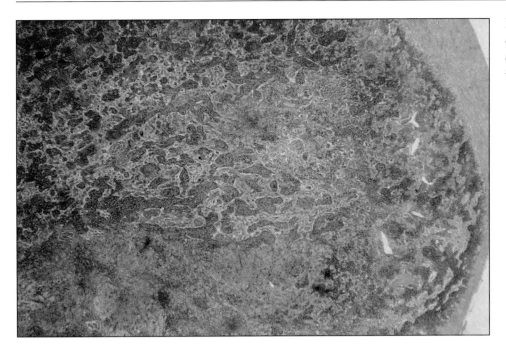

Figure 54. Rosai-Dorfman disease. A sinusoidal pattern of involvement is seen. Note the capsular fibrosis.

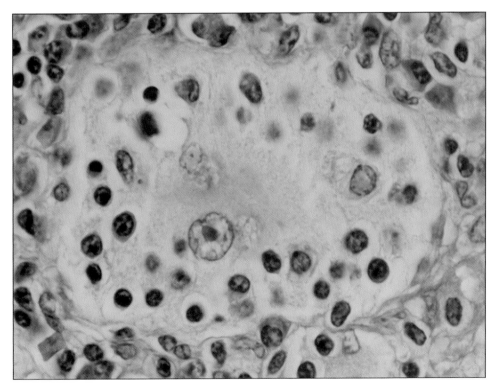

Figure 55. Rosai-Dorfman disease. The lesional cell is enormous in size, with a round nucleus, a distinct, but thin nuclear membrane, and a moderately prominent eosinophilic nucleolus. Note the abundant emperipolesis of lymphocytes and plasma cells and the infiltrate of plasma cells adjacent to the large cell.

(Figure 57). Immunohistochemical studies show that the proliferating cells express the histiocytic markers CD163 and CD68 as well as S-100 protein (Figure 58). They are negative for the Langerhans cells marker CD1a as well as the dendritic markers CD21 and CD35. They lack almost all lymphoid markers, although they may express CD30 in up to one-half of cases, and show a germline configuration of their antigen receptor genes. They lack Birbeck granules on ultrastructural examination.

Figure 56. Rosai-Dorfman disease. The atypical cells (showing characteristic nuclei and lymphophagocytosis) are present in the sinuses, while the intervening cords show a marked plasmacytosis.

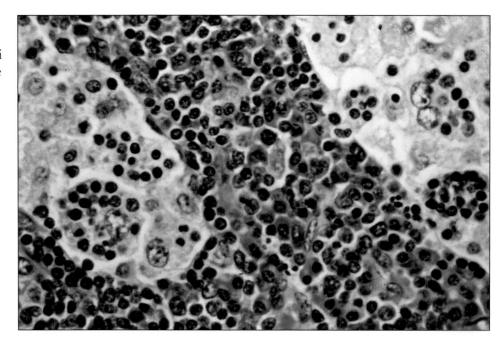

Figure 57. Rosai-Dorfman disease. This late lesion shows extensive fibrosis.

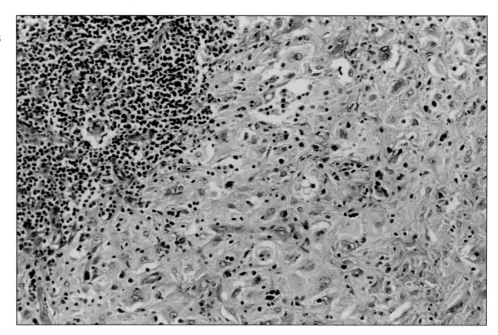

Once the possibility of lymph node involvement by Rosai-Dorfman disease is considered, there is little else in the differential diagnosis. Nonspecific reactive sinus hyperplasia lacks the distinctive large histiocytes with a vesicular chromatin pattern and relatively prominent nucleoli of Rosai-Dorfman. In cases with uncertainty, S-100 protein stains are very helpful. Although scattered reactive histiocytes may express S-100 protein, there is invariably strong and consistent staining of all the proliferating histiocytes of Rosai-Dorfman disease. Although the proliferating histiocytes of Langerhans cell histiocytosis are also localized to the sinuses and are S-100 protein positive, they have the nuclear irregularities and grooves characteristic of Langerhans cells and lack

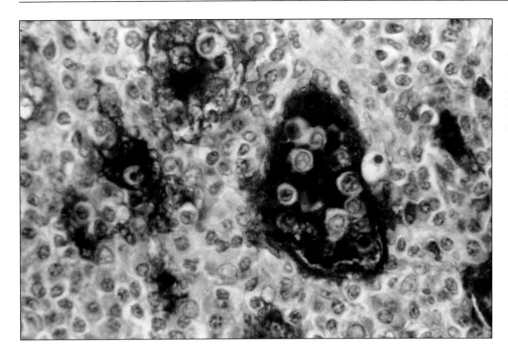

Figure 58. Rosai-Dorfman disease, S-100 protein stain. The atypical cells show nuclear and cytoplasmic positivity for S-100 protein. Note the negatively stained engulfed lymphocytes.

Table 11. Classification and Underlying Conditions of Hemophagocytic Lymphohistiocytosis (HLH)[107]

Genetic HLH

    Familial HLH (Farquhar disease)

    Immune deficiency syndromes

        Chédiak-Higashi syndrome

        Griscelli syndrome

        X-linked lymphoproliferative syndrome

Acquired HLH

    Exogenous agents (infection-associated hemophagocytic syndrome, toxins)

    Endogenous products (product of tissue destruction, metabolic products)

    Rheumatic diseases

        Macrophage activation syndrome

    Malignancies with hemophagocytosis

    Malignancies associated with hemophagocytosis

the peculiar cytologic features of the histiocytes of Rosai-Dorfman disease. Rarely, I have seen metastatic neoplasms, particularly malignant melanoma mimic Rosai-Dorfman disease. Rosai-Dorfman disease rarely has highly atypical cytologic features, which are the rule with metastatic disease. Keratin stains or specific melanocytic markers such as HMB-45 or Melan-A can also be useful in the differential diagnosis of carcinoma and melanoma, respectively. A true histiocytic sarcoma may rarely show a sinusoidal pattern. However, there should be cytologic atypia and an absence of the typical nuclei of Rosai-Dorfman disease.

Table 12. Genetic Defects in Hemophagocytic Lymphohistiocytosis[107]

Disease	Chromosome Location	Associated Gene	Gene Function
FHLH-1	9q21.3–22	Not known	Not known
FHLH-2	10q21–22	PRF1	Induction of apoptosis
FHLH-3	17q25	UNC13D	Vesicle priming
FHLH-4	6q24	STX11	Vesicle transport; t-SNARE
CHS-1	1q42.1-q42.2	LYST	Vesicle transport; not further defined
GS-2	15q21	RAB27A	Vesicle transport; small GTPase
XLP	Xq25	SH2D1A	Signal transduction and activation of lymphocytes

Abbreviations: CHS, Chédiak-Higashi syndrome; FHLH, familial hemophagocytic lymphohistiocytosis; GS, Griscelli syndrome; XLP, X-linked lymphoproliferative disorder.

Table 13. Clinical and Laboratory Criteria for Hemophagocytic Lymphohistiocytosis (five of eight criteria)[117]

1 Fever
2 Splenomegaly
3 Cytopenia ≥2 cell lines
4 Hypertriglyceridemia and/or hypofibrinogenemia
5 Ferritin ≥500 μg/L
6 sCD25 ≥2400 U/mL
7 Decreased NK-cell activity
8 Hemophagocytosis documented morphologically

Hemophagocytic Lymphohistiocytosis[107–116]

Hemophagocytic lymphohistiocytosis is a clinicopathologic syndrome characterized by uncontrolled hyperinflammation caused by a variety of inherited or acquired immune deficiencies. A classification of the syndrome is given in Table 11, while the known genetic defects are summarized in Table 12. Most of the genetic defects involve defects in granule-mediated cytotoxicity and NK-cell function. Familial hemophagocytic lymphohistiocytosis usually presents within the first year of life, with a symptom-free interval after birth typically seen. EBV is the triggering agent in about 75% of cases of infection-associated hemophagocytic lymphohistiocytosis. The terminal stages of any malignancy, including malignant lymphoma, may be associated with hemophagocytic lymphohistiocytosis. However, EBV-associated T/NK-neoplasms are particularly common, and the accompanying hemophagocytic syndrome may occur at an early stage and may even be the presenting feature of the lymphoma. Patients with hemophagocytic lymphohistiocytosis usually present with fever, hepatosplenomegaly, and cytopenias, and central nervous system symptoms are also common. Laboratory abnormalities include cytopenias of two or more cell lines, hypertriglyceridemia and/or hypofibrinogenemia, and an increase in serum ferritin and serum CD25. The specific clinical diagnostic criteria are given in Table 13.[117] The prognosis is poor, with the immediate aim of therapy being to suppress the increased inflammatory response by immunosuppressive/immunomodulatory agents and cytotoxic drugs. Identification of a specific infectious agent is helpful and should prompt specific treatment, but does not obviate the need for treatment of the syndrome. The prognosis is poor, with overall survival of about 50%. Stem cell transplantation may be curative in patients with a genetic etiology.

Early in the disease course, biopsied lymph nodes may show a marked immunoblastic proliferation in the paracortex, with only minor hyperplasia of histiocytes noted in the sinuses. Later on, however, there is a massive infiltration of the sinusoids by benign-appearing histiocytes (Figure 59). They may show prominent hemophagocytosis and platelet phagocytosis. There are also usually scattered to

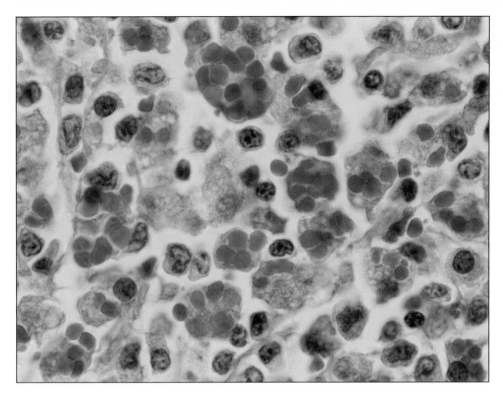

Figure 59. Hemophagocytic lymphohistiocytosis. Prominent erythrophagocytosis is seen in this dilated lymph node sinus.

abundant plasma cells. The cortical and paracortical regions become comparatively diminished in size and stimulation. Finally, the lymph node may show lymphocyte depletion, with marked histiocytic hyperplasia with abundant phagocytosis in sinusoids. The hemophagocytic lymphohistiocytosis syndrome is usually established on clinical criteria, with lymph node biopsy performed to rule out coexisting malignant lymphoma. Therefore, one should examine the lymph node biopsy carefully for an occult NK/T-cell lymphoma. In situ hybridization studies may be useful; EBV will be present in virtually all tumor cells in EBV-associated NK/T-cell lymphoma, while it may also be present in scattered cells, of both B- and T-lineages, in EBV-associated hemophagocytic lymphohistiocytosis.

BENIGN LYMPHADENOPATHY WITH EXTENSIVE NECROSIS

Any benign lymphadenopathy may at times show necrosis, either focal or extensive. This section will cover those benign lymphadenopathies in which extensive (or complete) necrosis is the characteristic feature of the disease.

Complete Necrosis[118–120]

Occasionally, a lymph node may show complete necrosis. Although often impossible to distinguish from one another, I find it helpful to try to distinguish whether the necrosis is liquefactive or infarctive. In liquefactive necrosis, the necrosis is due to the breakdown of tissue caused by enzymes and other factors secreted by inflammatory cells, usually neutrophils. There is usually a massive

Figure 60. Liquefactive necrosis. Note the numerous inflammatory cells. This pattern of necrosis is typical of infection.

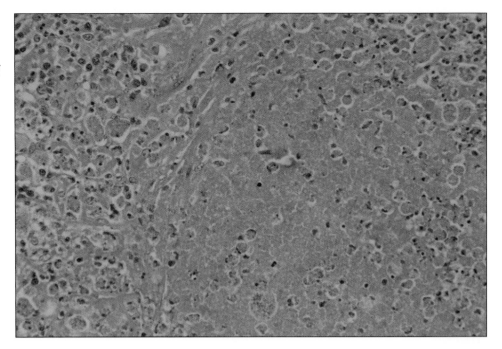

Figure 61. Infarcted lymph node. In this case, there were histiocytes at the rim, but few inflammatory cells in the infarcted area. The ghost outlines of dead cells can be seen.

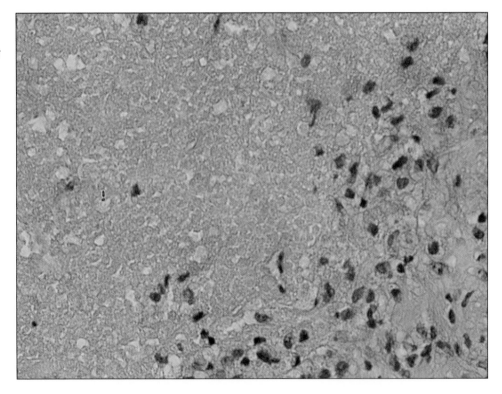

infection, such as that may be seen in AIDS, and may be due to a bacterial, or less frequently an invasive fungal, infection. One usually sees abundant karyorrhectic debris and fragments of cells, particularly neutrophils, often organized into an abscess (Figure 60). Because the process is usually fulminant, one does not typically see a rim of fibrosis and granulation tissue.

In infarctive necrosis, one sees the ghost outlines of cells, often without an inflammatory background (Figure 61). The rim of the lymph node may be

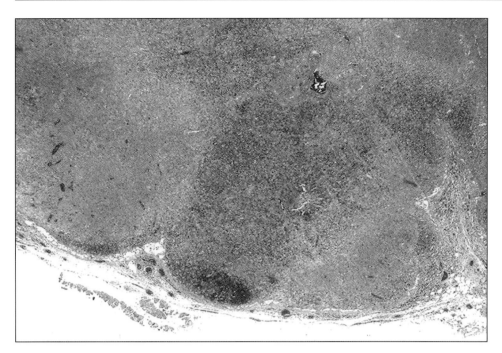

Figure 62. Kikuchi histiocytic necrotizing lymphadenitis. A patchy area of necrosis is seen adjacent to several reactive germinal centers.

viable, and because the process is often subacute, a surrounding zone of fibrosis and granulation tissue may be seen. The most important cause of infarctive necrosis is a non-Hodgkin lymphoma, which is usually high grade, but may be low grade. Viable lymphoma cells may be present at the periphery. Alternatively, occasionally the membranes of the infarcted cells may be left intact, and immunohistochemical studies (interpreted carefully) may show sheets of B-cells consistent with a B-cell lymphoma. Rebiopsy, either immediately or after an interval, may show more definitive evidence of lymphoma at another site.

Kikuchi Histiocytic Necrotizing Lymphadenitis[110,121–126]

Kikuchi histiocytic necrotizing lymphadenitis is an inflammatory disorder of unknown etiology. It most commonly affects young Asian women and may occur in both sexes and in all age groups and ethnicities. Patients most often present with isolated cervical lymphadenopathy, which may be tender, of several months duration. They sometimes have a history of a fever with upper respiratory symptoms; less commonly, they may have systemic symptoms, such as malaise and weight loss. The prognosis is excellent, with resolution usually occurring within 1–4 months, although some patients may relapse. No association with viruses has been found, and an autoimmune pathogenesis has been proposed, given the similar histologic appearance seen in lymph nodes involved by systemic lupus erythematosus (see the section Systemic Lupus Erythematosus).

Grossly, involved lymph nodes are usually only mildly enlarged. Histologically, three phases have been described. In the first phase, the proliferative phase, there are patchy areas of involvement, with adjacent areas showing a nonstimulated appearance or a nonspecific reactive follicular and/or paracortical hyperplasia (Figure 62). In the areas of involvement, there is a proliferation of

Figure 63. Kikuchi histiocytic necrotizing lymphadenitis. An exuberant immunoblastic process is seen at the periphery of the necrotic areas, which can closely mimic a diffuse large-cell lymphoma.

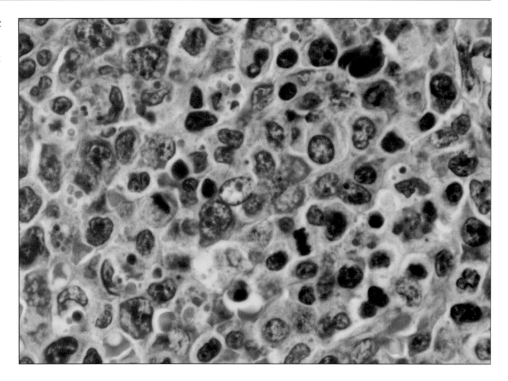

Figure 64. Kikuchi histiocytic necrotizing lymphadenitis. Numerous histiocytes are seen along with apoptotic debris, including histiocytes with crescentic-shaped nuclei.

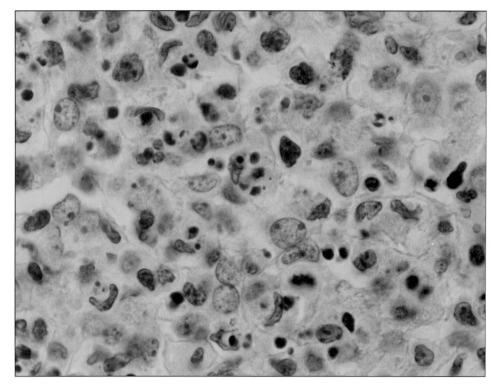

medium-to-large lymphoid cells, histiocytes, and plasmacytoid monocytic/dendritic cells (Figure 63). Scattered small lymphocytes may be present, but do not dominate the histologic picture. The histiocytes have a bland chromatin pattern, but may have highly irregular nuclear outlines (e.g., crescentic, twisted, or even signet-ring–shaped nuclei) (Figure 64). They often contain phagocytosed cellular fragments. The plasmacytoid monocytic/dendritic cells are hard to identify

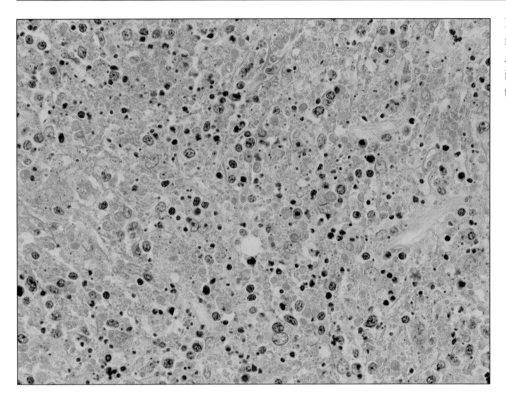

Figure 65. Kikuchi histiocytic necrotizing lymphadenitis. Apoptotic debris without intact neutrophils are seen in the areas of necrosis.

when present singly, but tend to cluster, particularly at the edges of the lesion. Mature neutrophils, eosinophils, and plasma cells are rare. There is usually no widespread necrosis at this stage, although single-cell necrosis and karyorrhectic debris may be present and even prominent. In the second phase – the necrotic phase – focal to extensive areas of geographic necrosis are present. These areas show an eosinophilic appearance, often with admixed karyorrhectic debris (Figure 65). Once again, mature neutrophils are rare, and medium- to large-sized lymphoid cells and histiocytes are usually present at the margins of the necrosis. In the final phase, the resolution stage, large numbers of foamy macrophages may be seen. Immunohistochemical studies show a predominance of T-cells and macrophages. Helper/inducer (CD3-positive/CD4-positive) cells predominate in the early phase, while cytotoxic/suppressor (CD3-positive/CD8-positive) cells predominate in the more commonly biopsied necrotic stage (Figure 66). Only scattered CD20-positive B-immunoblasts are present.

The typical clinical setting of Kikuchi necrotizing histiocytic lymphadenitis should be kept in mind in the differential diagnosis with non-Hodgkin lymphoma. The proliferative stage of the disease, in particular, may be easily mistaken for a diffuse large-cell lymphoma, with its predominance of medium-to-large lymphoid cells, histiocytes, and plasmacytoid monocytic/dendritic cells. The presence of abundant karyorrhectic debris should raise suspicion of histiocytic necrotizing lymphadenitis. Immunohistochemical studies showing few B-cells will rule out the possibility of a B-cell lymphoma, and a predominance of CD8-positive cells, if found, would be unusual for a peripheral T-cell lymphoma. The presence of focal necrosis raises the differential diagnosis with Hodgkin lymphoma, but the absence of morphologic and immunohistologic evidence

Figure 66. Kikuchi histiocytic necrotizing lymphadenitis, CD8 stain. There is often a predominance of CD8-positive T-suppressor cells, an unusual finding in peripheral T-cell lymphoma.

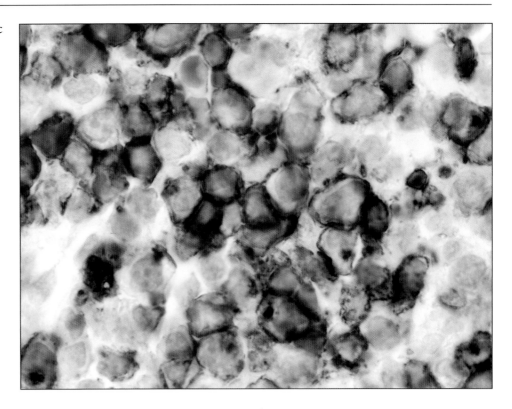

Table 14. American College of Rheumatology Classification Criteria for Systemic Lupus Erythematosus (at least four criteria needed for diagnosis)[128]

1	Malar rash
2	Discoid rash
3	Photosensitivity
4	Oral ulcers
5	Arthritis
6	Serositis
7	Renal disorder
8	Neurologic disorder
9	Hematologic disorder
10	Immunologic disorder
11	Antinuclear antibodies

of Hodgkin cells at the border of the necrosis would make this diagnosis unlikely. Granulomatous necrotizing lymphadenitis has greater numbers of neutrophils and epithelioid histiocytes, forming stellate microabscesses as opposed to patchy areas of necrosis. Systemic lupus erythematosus may have additional features that distinguish it from Kikuchi histiocytic necrotizing lymphadenitis, but at times may have an identical histologic appearance (see the section Systemic Lupus Erythematosus). For this reason, appropriate serologic and other studies should always be performed in all potential cases of Kikuchi histiocytic necrotizing lymphadenitis to rule out this possibility. Finally, Kawasaki disease can be distinguished by its clinical setting and greater extent of vascular changes (see section Kawaski Disease).

Systemic Lupus Erythematosus[127]

Systemic lupus erythematosus is a multisystem disease of as yet unknown etiology, but thought to have an autoimmune pathogenesis. There are wide varieties of abnormal clinical and laboratory findings, and the current recommended diagnostic criteria are summarized in Table 14.[128] The histologic features in lymph nodes may be identical to those seen in Kikuchi histiocytic necrotizing lymphadenitis (see above). Therefore, laboratory testing to rule out lupus should be performed in all cases diagnosed as Kikuchi histiocytic necrotizing lymphadenitis. However, there are additional histologic features in lupus that may distinguish it from Kikuchi disease. First, the presence of hematoxylin (basophilic) bodies or the deposition of a hematoxiphilic substance on necrotic foci is characteristic of lupus, but not seen in Kikuchi histiocytic necrotizing lymphadenitis (Figure 67).

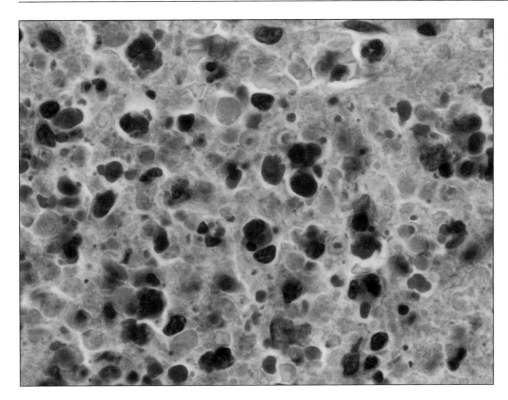

Figure 67. Acute lupus lymphadenitis. Several hematoxylophilic bodies are seen.

Hematoxylin bodies are homogeneous purple bodies on H&E-stained sections of about 10 μm in size; they are also PAS and Feulgen positive. They are usually present within or adjacent to necrotic foci and may also be present in the sinuses. In addition, the presence of abundant plasma cells, a prominent reactive follicular hyperplasia, an arteritis, or significant capsular or pericapsular inflammation should raise particular concern for systemic lupus erythematosus.

Kawasaki Disease[129,130]

Kawasaki disease (mucocutaneous lymph node syndrome) is a rare inflammatory disorder that mainly affects Asian children under the age of 5. It usually presents in two phases of disease. The first phase involves a high fever for at least 5 days, conjunctivitis, a rash, distal extremity lesions, inflammation of the oral mucosal membranes, and lymphadenopathy; the presence of at least five of these six criteria usually establishes the diagnosis. The second phase begins within a couple of weeks and includes peeling of skin, especially on the hands and feet, along with joint pain, diarrhea and vomiting, or abdominal pain. Left untreated, major and potentially life-threatening complications may develop, including a vasculitis, which often involves coronary arteries, endocarditis, myocarditis, or pericarditis. Treatment usually consists of prompt administration of intravenous doses of gamma globulin and/or high-dose aspirin.

Histologically, Kawasaki disease usually shows widespread geographic necrosis in involved lymph nodes. The areas of necrosis generally have abundant fibrin deposition, karyorrhectic debris, and neutrophils (Figure 68). Fibrin thrombi are seen in small vessels, within, adjacent to, and outside of the areas of

Figure 68. Kawasaki disease. Small vessels with fibrin thrombi are seen adjacent to areas of necrosis.

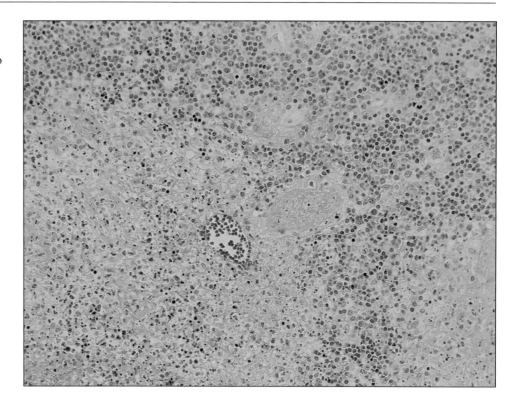

necrosis. In addition, an arteritis with fibrinoid necrosis may be present, along with inflammation of the lymph node capsule. The prominent infiltration with neutrophils, the presence of numerous fibrin thrombi (particularly outside the areas of necrosis), and arteritis are all histologic features unusual for Kikuchi histiocytic necrotizing lymphadenitis, and should raise specific concern for Kawasaki disease. The clinical history, particularly the age of the patient, can also be quite helpful in raising concern for Kawasaki disease. The presence of fibrin thrombi in small vessels is not specific to Kawasaki disease, however, as thrombotic thrombocytopenic purpura and rickettsial infection may also show these features.

REACTIVE LYMPHADENOPATHIES WITH A PRIMARY GRANULOMATOUS PATTERN: NONINFECTIOUS

The granuloma is the body's reaction to a foreign substance that is neither destroyed by the acute inflammatory response nor easily neutralized by individual phagocytes. It consists of a cluster of macrophages that have undergone transformation to epithelioid histiocytes, cells with a larger cytoplasm than macrophages with increased secretory and killing capability but decreased phagocytic capability. The epithelioid histiocytes are usually associated with helper/inducer T-cells, present through the granuloma, as well as cytotoxic/suppressor T-cells, usually concentrated at the periphery of the granuloma. Occasional giant cells are also often present in granulomas, which have evolved from fusion of epithelioid histiocytes. Giant cells early in the formation have nuclei randomly distributed in the cytoplasm (foreign-body type) and, over time, develop nuclei that align toward the periphery (Langhan type). Giant cells may have peculiar inclusions, which, although not associated with specific etiologies, are usually found in high-stimulated processes. These include calcium oxalate or calcium carbonate crystals (birefringent), Schumann or conchoidal bodies (calcium crystals in a mucopolysaccharide matrix), asteroid bodies (functionally obsolescent cell organelles; primarily microfilaments, microtubules, and centrioles), and Hamazaki-Wesenberg bodies (yellow-brown pseudofungal forms representing degenerating giant lysosomes).

Reactive lymphadenopathies with a primary granulomatous pattern can be divided into noninfectious and infectious types. Noninfectious causes of reactive lymphadenopathy with a primary granulomatous pattern include neoplasms, sarcoidosis, berylliosis, and Crohn disease.

Granulomatous Inflammation in Malignant Neoplasms[131–133]

Both malignant lymphoma and carcinoma have been associated with the occurrence of noncaseating granulomas in lymph nodes. The granulomas are not distinctive and are usually present in the paracortical areas. It is not necessary to perform special stains for organisms in the absence of necrosis, as these studies are invariably negative. The occurrence of noncaseating granulomas has been particularly well studied in Hodgkin lymphoma, in which the granulomas may occur at both involved as well as noninvolved sites. Early studies found this phenomenon to be associated with a better prognosis, although this is no longer seen since the prognosis of Hodgkin lymphoma is so uniformly good. Noncaseating granulomas may also be seen in association with a wide variety of non-Hodgkin lymphomas.

Sarcoidosis

In sarcoidosis, the granulomas may be seen in any lymph node, but mediastinal and hilar lymph nodes are by far most commonly involved. The lymph node may be partially or wholly replaced by noncaseating granulomas (Figure 69). Occasional granulomas may show central foci of fibrinoid necrosis (Figure 70); even though these granulomas are perfectly consistent with sarcoidosis, it is probably prudent to perform acid-fast and fungal stains to rule out the possibility of an infectious etiology. They are most often seen in highly active cases, of recent onset. A positive skin (Kveim) test and elevated serum angiotensin–converting enzyme levels will support the diagnosis of sarcoidosis, which is essentially established by clinicopathologic correlation.

REACTIVE LYMPHADENOPATHIES WITH A PRIMARY GRANULOMATOUS PATTERN: INFECTIOUS[123]

Infectious causes can be divided into those that are typically associated with nonsuppurative inflammation and those that are typically associated with

Figure 69. Sarcoidosis. In most lymph node excisions showing sarcoidosis, there are usually confluent granulomas.

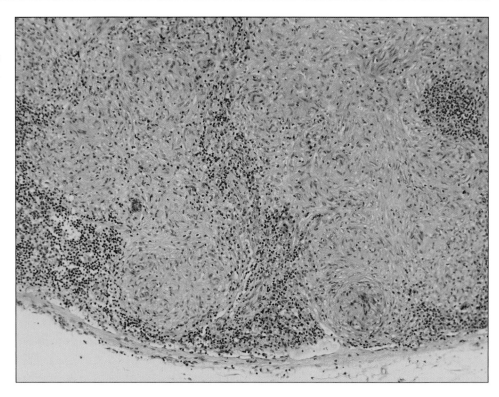

Figure 70. Sarcoidosis. Some granulomas in sarcoidosis may show a central area of necrosis mimicking an infective granuloma.

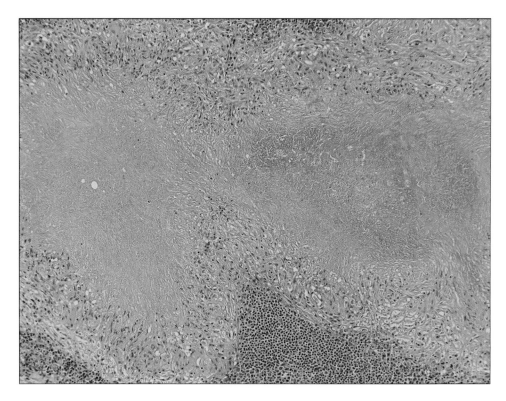

suppurative inflammation. Examples of the former include tuberculosis, atypical mycobacterial infection, leprosy, most fungal infections, and pneumocystis infection. Examples of the latter include cat scratch disease, lymphogranuloma venereum, and Yersinia lymphadenitis. With nonsuppurative granulomatous inflammation, there is a predominance of histiocytes with lesser numbers of T-cells and dendritic cells. Mantle B-cells are found at the periphery of, but not inside, the granulomas. With suppurative granulomatous inflammation, there is also a predominance of histiocytes. However, the centers of the granulomas have neutrophils and monocytoid B-cells. In addition, there are variable numbers of B-cells, either at the periphery or in the center of the suppurative granulomas, in addition to T-cells and dendritic cells.

Tuberculosis

Tuberculosis is the archetypical example of nonsuppurative infectious granulomatous lymphadenopathy. Lymph node involvement by tuberculosis is most often seen in cases with concurrent pulmonary involvement and is most often seen in hilar, mediastinal, and cervical lymph nodes. When occurring as an isolated phenomenon, the cervical region is the most common site. The histologic findings may be indistinguishable from sarcoidosis, but usually, the granulomas are caseating, that is, show a central area of necrosis in which cell outlines are not discernible. There may also be broad areas of caseation, with a granulomatous rim. The organisms may usually be identified by acid-fast stains (but only in cases with large numbers of organisms) or culture. PCR studies for tuberculosis performed in formalin-fixed paraffin-embedded tissues may be positive in up to 80% of cases.

Atypical Mycobacterial Infection[134,135]

Isolated lymphadenopathy is more commonly seen in atypical mycobacterial infection than classical tuberculosis; again the cervical region is the most common site. It may be histologically indistinguishable from tuberculosis; however, there are usually less granulomatous changes and more acute inflammation, sometimes with abscess formation. Patients with immunocompromise such as HIV infection may show a histiocytic proliferation, which may be foamy cell or even spindled. The latter proliferation, when marked, may closely simulate an inflammatory pseudotumor (Figure 71). Acid-fast stains usually readily demonstrate organisms, and cultures may be confirmatory.

Lepromatous Lymphadenitis[136]

Lymph node involvement is not common in leprosy, which usually involves the cooler acral regions. The histologic findings vary with the immune status of the patient. In patients with a relatively intact cellular immunity, the lymph nodes are usually uninvolved. With borderline immunity, numerous noncaseating granulomas are seen; acid-fast organisms may or may not be identified by Fite stain. In patients with defective cellular immunity (lepromatous leprosy), generalized lymphadenopathy is often seen, and there are numerous foamy macrophages replacing the paracortical regions (Figure 72). Organisms are usually easily seen on Fite stain.

Figure 71. Atypical mycobacterial infection. A benign spindle-cell proliferation is seen, which could be mistaken for an inflammatory pseudotumor. Fite stains revealed numerous organisms.

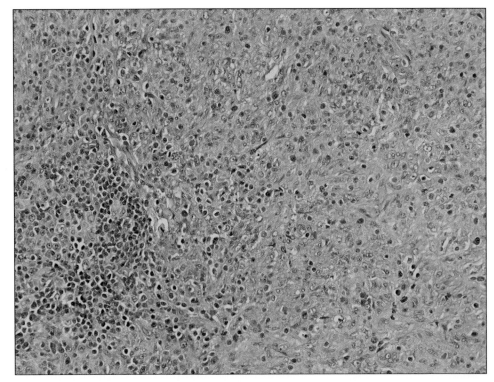

Figure 72. Lepromatous leprosy. When immunity is low, many foamy cells are seen, each containing abundant intracellular organisms.

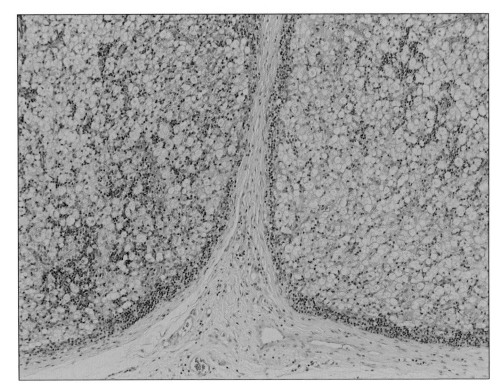

Fungal Lymphadenitis

Fungi do not usually give rise to isolated lymphadenitis, but lymphadenitis may be seen as part of a systemic infection. Histologically, one sees granulomatous inflammation often with the formation of central stellate microabscesses. The diagnosis is established by fungal stains along with appropriate cultures.

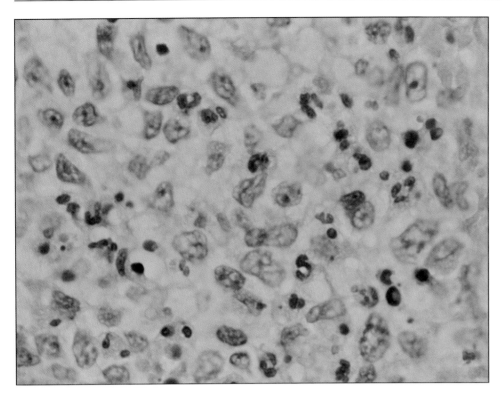

Figure 73. Cat scratch disease. The focus of monocytoid B-cell hyperplasia shows a cluster of neutrophils, suggesting early microabscess formation.

Cat Scratch Lymphadenitis[137–141]

Cat scratch lymphadenitis is the most common specific cause of suppurative granuloma in Western populations. It is an infectious disease due to infection by the gram-negative bacterium *Bartonella henselae*, usually introduced through the skin following a cat (kittens more likely to be infected) bite or contact with saliva on broken skin or conjunctiva (the latter may result in oculoglandular syndrome). Patients, usually children or young adults, present several weeks later with lymphadenopathy, usually in the axillary, cervical, or submandibular regions. Culture is difficult, but a skin test is positive in about 90% of cases. It is usually a self-limited disease, even without treatment, although some cases may have severe complications, including encephalitis and neuroretinitis. Antibiotics are curative in severe cases or in cases with complications.

Early on in the course, involved lymph nodes may show a nonspecific florid reactive follicular hyperplasia with monocytoid B-cell hyperplasia. Small foci of necrosis first develop in the midst of the monocytoid B-cell hyperplasia, particularly near the capsule, usually associated with small clusters of neutrophils and histiocytes, forming microabscesses (Figure 73). Microabscesses may also form within the germinal centers. Organisms are most numerous at this stage, detectable by Warthin-Starry stain or by specific immunohistochemical stains. Organisms are most frequently found within the wall of capillaries, histiocytes, and in the areas of necrosis as clumps of pleomorphic coccibacilli with occasional chains or L-forms. Later, granulomas develop in and adjacent to the monocytoid B-cell areas, consisting a central area of abscess surrounded by palisading histiocytes (Figures 74 and 75). Eventually, there are geographic areas of abscess

Figure 74. Cat scratch disease. A necrotizing abscess is seen in the center.

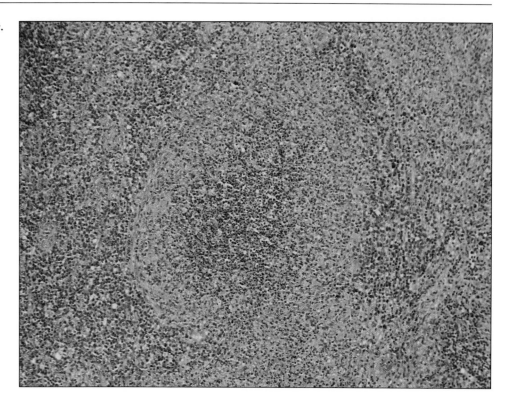

Figure 75. Cat scratch disease. The edge of a necrotizing abscess is shown, containing histiocytes and lacking atypical cells, in distinction to the syncytial variant of nodular sclerosing Hodgkin lymphoma.

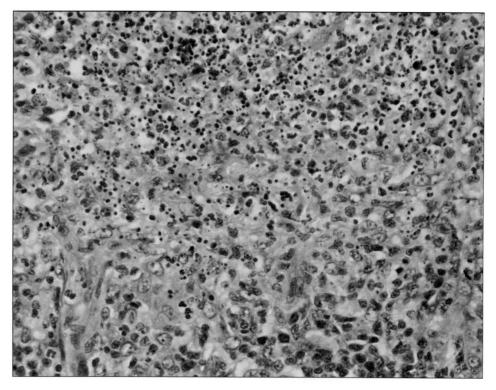

consisting of neutrophils and necrotic or fibrinoid material, which in 10 to 40% of cases may extend through the lymph node capsule, causing pericapsular inflammation and fibrosis, and may even form a fistula with the overlying skin. Multinucleated histiocytes are unusual at all stages of the process, but plasma cells and immunoblasts are common.

The distinction of cat scratch disease from Kikuchi histiocytic necrotizing lymphadenitis is usually quite easy, as cat scratch disease features microabscesses and larger abscesses with a center of neutrophils; large collections of neutrophils are never seen in Kikuchi disease. A more difficult differential diagnosis is with non-suppurative forms of granulomatous inflammation, including tuberculous and fungal infections. These diseases usually have a greater degree of necrosis and a lesser degree of neutrophilic infiltration. In addition, immunohistochemical stains show a greater infiltrate of B-cells (including monocytoid B-cells) in cat scratch disease than in tuberculosis or fungal infections. Finally, the specific identification of *Bartonella henselae* can distinguish cat scratch disease from other diseases with a very similar suppurative granulomatous inflammation such as lymphogranuloma venereum, *Yersinia* infection, tularemia, and brucellosis (see below).

Lymphogranuloma Venereum[142]

Lymphogranuloma venereum is a sexually transmitted disease caused by *Chlamydia trachomatis*. It almost always presents in inguinal lymph nodes. The diagnosis is best established by serologic testing. The histologic findings are those of suppurative granulomatous inflammation similar to that seen in cat scratch disease, although patients usually present at a later stage of disease and with a higher incidence of pericapsular inflammation and fistula formation to skin. One characteristic finding in lymphogranuloma venereum is the presence of vacuolated macrophages, which contain the organisms, present in and around the monocytoid B-cell hyperplasia and areas of necrosis and abscess formation (Figure 76). The organisms may be identified by Giemsa or Warthin-Starry stain as fine, sandlike organisms; alternatively, the disease may be confirmed by direct culture or molecular studies.

Yersinial Lymphadenitis[143]

Yersinial lymphadenitis is usually caused by *Yersinia enterocolitica* or, less frequently, *Yersinia pseudotuberculosis*. It most frequently occurs in children or young adults who present with symptoms indistinguishable from acute appendicitis. At the time of laparotomy, markedly enlarged mesenteric lymph nodes draining the ileocecal region, with a normal-appearing appendix. Histologically, one sees suppurative granulomatous inflammation along with small granulomas. One characteristic feature is the frequent localization of microabscesses within germinal centers (Figure 77). There is also usually a prominent capsulitis with capsular thickening. The diagnosis may be established by the identification of gram-negative acid-fasts diplobacilli, or by cultures and serology.

LYMPHADENOPATHY DUE TO ALTERATION OF THE CONNECTIVE TISSUE FRAMEWORK

Lymphadenopathy due to alteration of the connective tissue framework is uncommon. The most common cause is a reactive proliferation of sinusoidal

Figure 76. Lymphogranuloma venereum. Several vacuolated macrophages are seen in this focus of monocytoid B-cell hyperplasia undergoing necrosis.

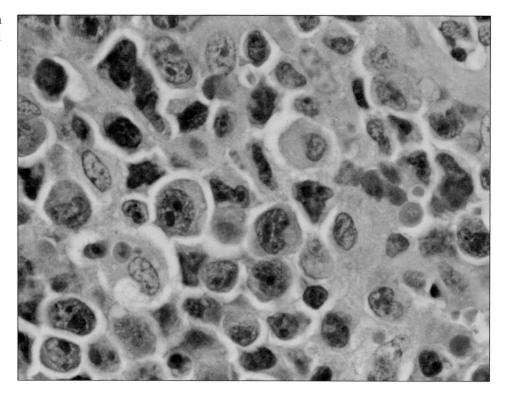

Figure 77. Yersinia lymphadenitis. This reactive germinal center shows a focus of acute necrosis.

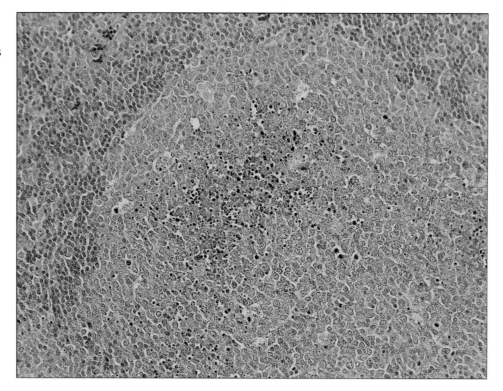

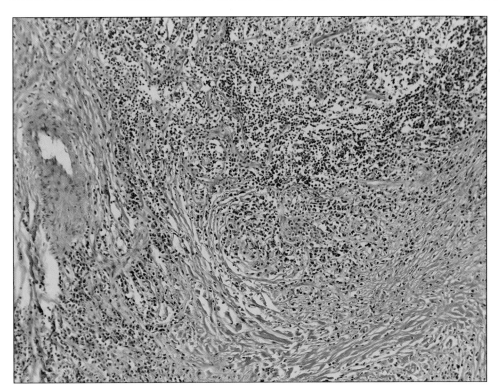

Figure 78. Inflammatory pseudotumor. A reactive germinal center is seen at top, while the paracortical region shows fibrosis and inflammatory cells.

vessels, a process termed vascular transformation of the sinuses. More rare is an inflammatory disorder primarily affecting the lymph node framework: inflammatory pseudotumor of lymph nodes.

Inflammatory Pseudotumor of Lymph Nodes[144–146]

Inflammatory pseudotumor of lymph nodes is a rare idiopathic inflammatory disorder that primarily affects the lymph node framework. It affects predominantly young adults of both sexes. Patients usually present with prominent lymphadenopathy, involving either a single lymph node or multiple sites. This is often associated with constitutional symptoms, such as malaise, fever, and night sweats. Abnormal laboratory findings may include anemia and hyperglobulinemia. In contrast to inflammatory pseudotumors occurring at other sites, there is no association with either EBV or ALK translocation. In fact, it is likely that inflammatory pseudotumor of lymph nodes is a disease process that is distinct from other diseases termed inflammatory pseudotumor at other sites. Inflammatory pseudotumor is a true inflammatory process, while inflammatory pseudotumor at most other sites probably represents a clonal proliferation. The course of inflammatory pseudotumor of lymph nodes is usually benign, although the disease may persist or relapse in a subset of patients.

Histologically, one sees an inflammatory process centered upon the lymph node capsule, trabeculae and hilum, with spillover into the perinodal soft tissues (Figure 78). These structures are edematous to fibrotic and contain a spindle-cell proliferation, an infiltrate of inflammatory cells, and a proliferation of small blood vessels. The spindle cells include myofibroblasts and spindled histiocytes.

Figure 79. Inflammatory pseudotumor. An intense plasmacytic infiltrate surrounds blood vessels in the paracortical region.

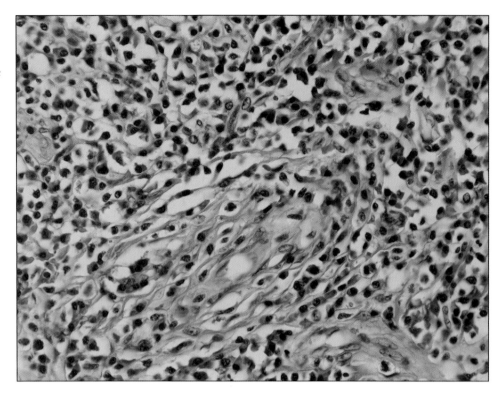

The inflammatory cells include small lymphocytes, plasma cells, immunoblasts, histiocytes, eosinophils, and neutrophils (Figure 79). The vessels are generally small and may show fibro-obliteration. The subjacent sinuses are still patent, and the underlying lymphoid parenchyma is still intact and may show mildly reactive features. Immunohistochemical studies reveal no phenotypic abnormalities.

The most important disease in the differential diagnosis is Kaposi sarcoma. Kaposi sarcoma is HHV-8 positive and lacks the mixed inflammatory infiltrate. Dendritic cell tumors do not preferentially involve the lymph node capsule. Mycobacterial infections can show spindle-cell proliferations that may simulate inflammatory pseudotumor; however, it also does not preferentially involve the lymph node capsule, and acid-fast stains will reveal numerous organisms. The lack of cytologic atypia and the preferential capsular localization should rule out the possibility of a malignant lymphoma.

Vascular Transformation of Lymph Node Sinuses[147,148]

Vascular transformation of lymph node sinuses is a reactive proliferation of vessels in the lymph node sinuses due to obstruction of efferent lymphatics. It may be due to obstruction caused by local tumors, vascular thrombosis, previous surgery, or even severe heart failure. The inguinal lymph nodes are most frequently affected, but it may involve any lymph node group. Patients may present with lymphadenopathy or the lesion may be discovered as an incidental finding in an excision performed for another reason.

Histologically, one sees a proliferation of small blood vessels involving the hilar sinuses, the hilar and medullary sinuses, or all sinuses (Figure 80). The capsule is

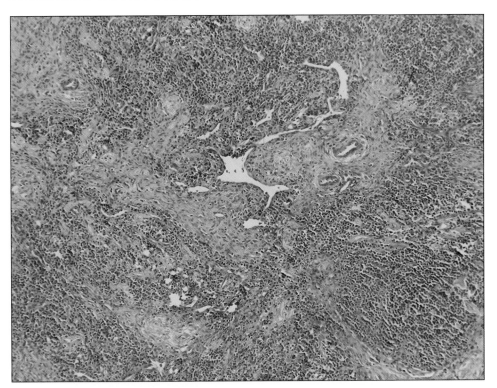

Figure 80. Vascular transformation of lymph node sinuses. The medullary area is replaced by cellular fibrous tissue containing proliferating blood vessels.

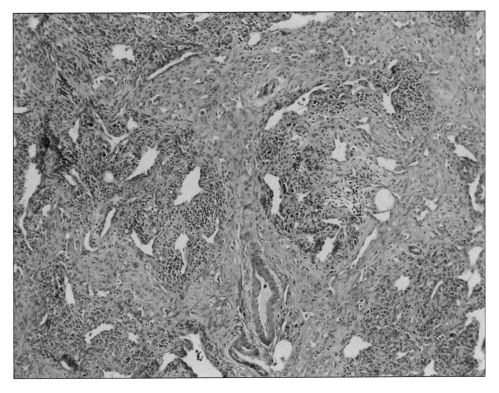

Figure 81. Vascular transformation of lymph node sinuses. The vessels have a vaguely lobular configuration, separated by fibrous tissue.

uninvolved. The expanded sinuses are sclerotic and the intervening lymphoid tissues may be atrophic. The vessels are greatly increased in number and may have slitlike spaces or be open (Figure 81). Solid areas may be present, representing nodules of compressed blood vessels. The appearance may mimic a vascular malformation. There is a variant, termed the nodular spindle-cell variant, in which

Figure 82. Nodular variant of vascular transformation of the sinuses. The dilated sinuses are lined by a pericytic proliferation of epithelioid cells. This proliferation may be confused with metastatic urothelial carcinoma.

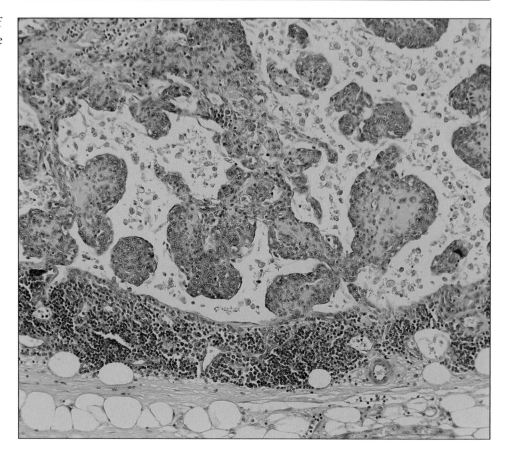

spindle and epithelioid cells (probably representing pericytes) form cuffs surrounding vascular channels (Figure 82). This pattern is most often seen in retroperitoneal lymph nodes, often draining, and not to be mistaken for metastatic carcinoma.

Kaposi sarcoma is the most important entity to distinguish from vascular transformation of lymph node sinuses. In Kaposi sarcoma, there is a primary spindle-cell proliferation with poorly formed vessels and with frequent extension to the capsule, all features lacking in vascular transformation. In cases of doubt, Kaposi sarcoma expresses HHV-8–associated antigens. Inflammatory pseudotumor has a prominent inflammatory component, which is lacking in vascular transformation. Bacillary angiomatosis forms nodules within the lymph node parenchyma and does not preferentially involve the sinuses.

Bacillary Angiomatosis[149,150]

Bacillary angiomatosis is a form of *Bartonella hensalae* infection (the causative agent of cat scratch disease) that occurs in the setting of immunosuppression, especially in the context of AIDS. It usually presents as multiple skin nodules, but any organ may be involved, and lymph nodes may rarely be the presenting site or even the sole manifestation of the disease. Once recognized, there is an excellent response to antibiotics.

Histologically, one sees multiple coalescent nodules of proliferating vessels throughout the lymph node parenchyma. These nodules are composed of

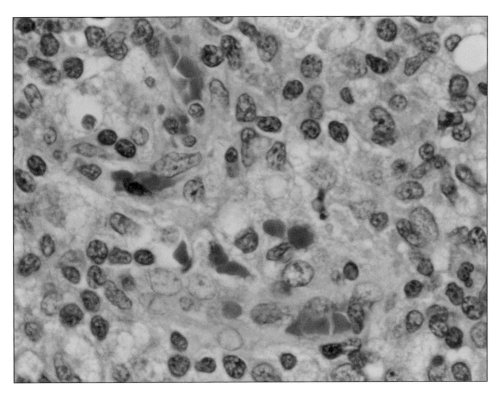

Figure 83. Bacillary angiomatosis. Blood vessels lined by prominent endothelial cells are seen. The interstitium is granular – this is the area where the organisms are best identified.

proliferating blood vessels, from capillaries to small veins. The vessels are lined by very plump endothelial cells with pale or freely vacuolated cytoplasm. The interstitium between the blood vessels contains numerous acute inflammatory cells and an abundant amorphous to granular interstitial material (Figure 83). Warthin-Starry, Giemsa, and immunohistochemical stains employing specific antibodies against the organism reveal numerous coccibacilli, usually forming aggregates.

The differential diagnosis includes Kaposi sarcoma and nodal angiomatosis. Kaposi sarcoma lacks the amorphous interstitial material, lacks abundant acute inflammation, and expresses HHV-8–associated antigens by immunohistochemistry. Nodal angiomatosis similarly lacks the amorphous interstitial material and inflammatory features and usually forms one mass, as opposed to several discrete nodules.

DEPOSITION OF INTERSTITIAL SUBSTANCE

These benign lymphadenopathies are rare and essentially consist of proteinaceous lymphadenopathy, amyloidosis, and pneumocystis infection.

Proteinaceous Lymphadenopathy[145,151]

Proteinaceous lymphadenopathy (angiocentric sclerosing lymphadenopathy) is a rare disease of unknown etiology. Originally, it was thought to represent a variant of a light chain deposition disease, but it probably is a unique idiopathic

Figure 84. Proteinaceous lymphadenopathy. There are concentric rings of fibrous tissue centered around blood vessels. The overall appearance is extremely cell poor, with only scattered lymphocytes.

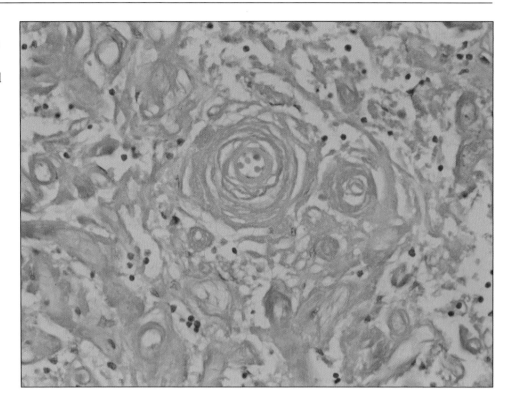

disease with no evidence of a clonal proliferation. Patients typically present with generalized lymphadenopathy. They often also have systemic symptoms, including malaise, fever, and myalgia. A polyclonal hypergammaglobulinemia is often found.

Involved lymph nodes show an extensive deposition of a nonamyloid material obliterating the architecture (similar changes can be seen in other involved organs). The material is formed by dense concentric bundles of fine reticulin fibers along involved vessel walls (Figure 84). The deposits are very hypocellular, with few lymphocytes and plasma cells. The differential diagnosis includes immunoglobulin deposits (see below), which are usually associated with a monoclonal proliferation of plasma cells, do not show concentric bundles of fibers, and are often congophilic.

Immunoglobulin Deposition Lymphadenopathy[152–154]

Patients with immunoglobulin deposition lymphadenopathy have an underlying plasma cell dyscrasia or, much less commonly, a lymphoplasmacytic lymphoma, with or without systemic amyloidosis. There is often accompanying renal disease. The clinical presentation is determined by the underlying disease, and the lymph node is only rarely the presenting site. Involved lymph nodes may show either of two histologic patterns. In the amyloid type, the deposits have the typical appearance of amyloid, with deposition of a homogeneous pink material with irregular borders, occasionally ringed by multinucleated giant cells (Figure 85). The deposits are congophilic, with characteristic apple green birefringence, and stain for monotypic immunoglobulin (light chains only or complete

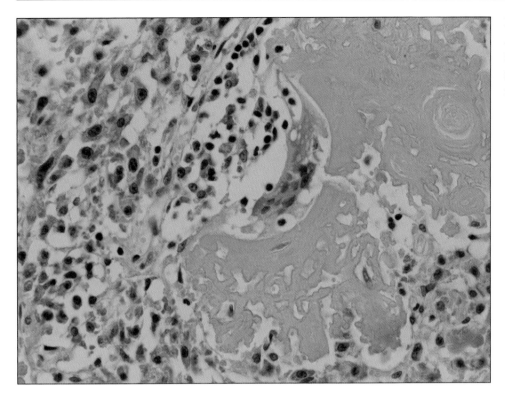

Figure 85. Amyloidosis. Amyloid deposits are seen rimmed by a multinucleate giant cell and surrounded by numerous plasma cells.

immunoglobulin). The material is usually accompanied by a plasma cell infiltrate. In the nonamyloid type, the material is noncongophilic, but still stains for monotypic immunoglobulin, and an accompanying plasma cell infiltrate is still seen. The differential diagnosis of this latter pattern includes the nonamyloid deposits that are occasionally seen in angioimmunoblastic lymphadenopathy or Hodgkin lymphoma. In these diseases, the deposits are usually not extensive. The sclerosis commonly found in pelvic lymph nodes usually is not as solid as that seen in immunoglobulin deposition lymphadenopathy, is not associated with a plasma cell infiltrate, and does not stain for immunoglobulin.

Pneumocytis Lymphadenitis[155]

Lymph node involvement by *Pneumocytis carinii* is one of the most common extrapulmonary forms of the infection. Rarely, patients who have received aerosolized prophylaxis against pulmonary disease may present with lymphadenopathy, usually in the mediastinum. Histologically, one sees PAS-positive pink, bubbly exudates, in which one can identify light basophilic dots, which represent the organisms. The exudate usually lacks an accompanying inflammatory infiltrate. Once the diagnosis is considered, a silver stain reveals numerous typical organisms.

4 EPITHELIAL AND NEVOMELANOCYTIC LESIONS OF LYMPH NODES

Epithelial Lesions   82
   Benign Epithelial Inclusions   82
   Carcinoma   84
Nevomelanocytic Lesions   87

EPITHELIAL LESIONS

Epithelial lesions range from benign inclusions to metastatic carcinoma.

Benign Epithelial Inclusions[156–158]

There are a variety of benign epithelial inclusions. They are uncommon lesions, but commonly raise differential diagnostic problems with metastatic carcinoma. Glandular inclusions include Mullerian inclusions, salivary gland inclusions, breast inclusions, and thyroid inclusions. Mullerian inclusions usually occur in the pelvic and para-aortic lymph nodes of postmenarchial women, occurring in up to 40% of patients in carefully performed studies. They probably represent a metaplastic phenomenon. They are usually clinically silent, until a staging or other lymph node biopsy is performed, and have little clinical significance other than their distinction from carcinoma. They usually occur in the capsule, trabeculae, or cortical region, but they may occur anywhere in the lymph node parenchyma, including the subcapsular sinuses (Figure 86). They consist of single or multiple glands that are usually lined by a single layer of bland cells, most often of ciliated and/or columnar type. Occasionally, papillary or cerebriform patterns may be seen, and there may be associated psammoma bodies. There is usually a basement membrane surrounding the inclusions, with a variable amount of underlying connective tissue. Occasionally, endometrial stroma, sometimes with accompanying hemosiderin deposition, is found associated with inclusions, warranting the diagnosis of endometriosis. The endometrial stroma may decidualize during pregnancy; in addition, isolated areas of deciduosis unassociated with glands may also be encountered. The bland cytologic features of all these proliferations help to distinguish them from carcinoma. The presence of a basement membrane and the absence of a fibrous or desmoplastic response are also helpful

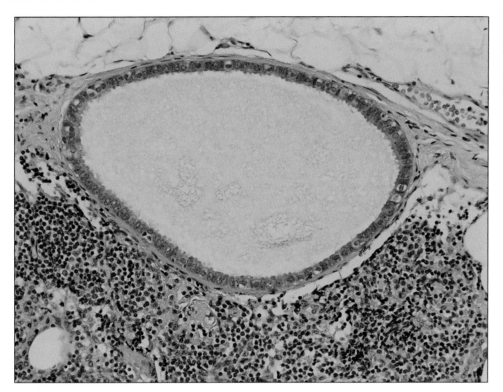

Figure 86. Endosalpingiosis in a pelvic lymph node. The localization may be capsular, as in this case, or intraparenchymal.

features. Nonetheless, at times the distinction between Mullerian inclusions, involvement by borderline tumors, and carcinoma may be extremely difficult. It has been recommended that no additional treatment be given in cases in which the distinction cannot be made with confidence. Deciduosis can be easily distinguished from squamous carcinoma by keratin immunostaining.

Ectopic salivary gland tissue is very commonly seen in lymph nodes adjacent to and within the major salivary glands and can be considered to be a normal occurrence. Both ducts and acini may be seen. These inclusions are probably the source of the lymphoepithelial lesions of Sjogren disease as well as the lymphoepithelial cysts that occur in HIV-infected patients. They also seem to give rise to an inordinate number and variety of neoplasms, most commonly Warthin tumors. Benign thyroid inclusions may rarely occur in cervical lymph nodes. They are small, up to thirty follicles, without papillae, psammoma bodies, or any nuclear atypia. Nonetheless, the most common cause of thyroid tissue in neck lymph nodes is metastatic thyroid carcinoma, no matter how bland the thyroid tissue appears to be. Some recommend subtotal thyroidectomy to rule out the possibility of metastatic thyroid carcinoma when potential thyroid inclusions are encountered in neck lymph nodes.

Benign mammary epithelial inclusions are rarely encountered in axillary lymph nodes, but are well documented, particularly in the current era of sentinel lymph node biopsy. They may show normal epithelium, fibrocystic changes, or even carcinoma in situ. The key to their identification is the localization to the lymph node capsule. Any epithelial cells localized to the sinuses are more likely to represent a true metastasis or benign mechanical transport of breast epithelial cells.

Rarely, ectopic pancreatic cells have been found in abdominal lymph nodes, colonic cells have been found in lymph nodes draining the colon (after surgery),

Figure 87. Merkel cell carcinoma. The morphologic appearance is that of an undifferentiated malignant neoplasm. Although the cytologic features do not look very lymphoid, stains should still be performed to rule out the latter possibility.

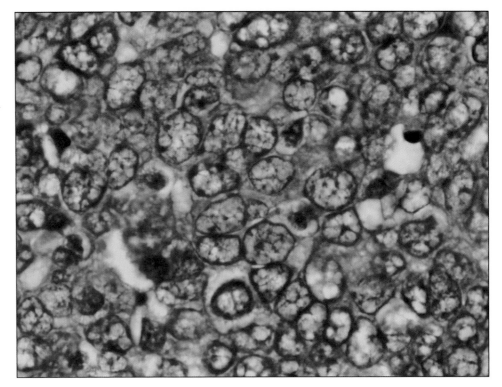

and complexes of renal epithelial cells and Tamm-Horsfall protein (apparently derived from nephrons damaged by obstruction) have been found in lymph nodes draining the kidney.

Hyperplastic mesothelial cells have been reported in mediastinal and abdominal lymph nodes. The cells are present in the lymph node sinuses, as single cells or small clusters, and are often only detected after keratin immunostaining. In many patients, there is a history of pleural or pericardial effusion or inflammation. In some cases, the distinction from metastatic mesothelioma can only be made by careful clinical follow-up.

Carcinoma[159,160]

Carcinoma is by far the most common neoplasm affecting lymph nodes. There have been occasional series of primary neuroendocrine carcinomas with features of Merkel cell occurring as a primary lesion in inguinal, or less commonly, axillary lymph nodes, although it is difficult to completely rule out the possibility of an occult primary tumor in the skin or another site (Figures 87 and 88). Nonetheless, the presence of carcinoma in lymph nodes is almost synonymous with metastatic carcinoma. All major carcinomas commonly metastasize to lymph nodes and may mimic either diffuse large B-cell lymphoma or Hodgkin lymphoma (Figure 89). For lymph node dissections, ADASP recommends that the number of positive lymph nodes and total number of lymph nodes should be reported. For positive cases, the size of the largest positive node should be given, if clinically indicated. The presence of extranodal extension should be given, if clinically indicated, and if the only tumor is seen in extranodal vessels, this

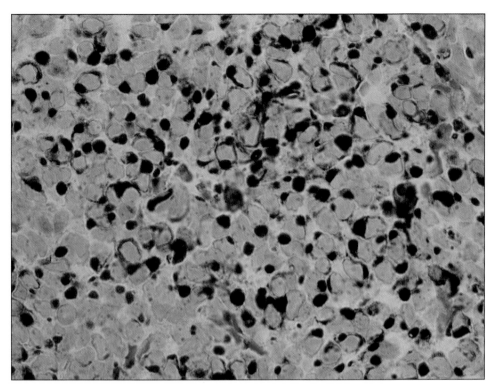

Figure 88. Merkel cell carcinoma, cytokeratin 20 (same case as previous figure). This case shows strong ball-like cytoplasmic staining for cytokeratin 20, consistent with a neuroendocrine carcinoma.

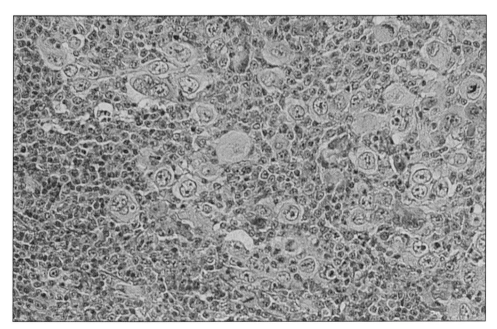

Figure 89. Nasopharyngeal carcinoma, metastatic to a cervical lymph node. This case was originally misdiagnosed as nodular sclerosing Hodgkin lymphoma, which is understandable given the morphologic features of the neoplastic cells and their distribution. Immunostains were only performed after there was a poor response to therapy for Hodgkin lymphoma.

should be specifically stated. For sentinel lymph node biopsies, others have recommended that the lymph node be sliced into 1.5-mm- to 2.0-mm-thick sections. When frozen sections are performed, some have recommended that each 2.0-mm slice be cut at three levels. It has also been recommended that each paraffin block be cut at three levels. The use of immunohistochemistry is deemed to be optional at the current time. At my institution, we routinely bivalve sentinel lymph nodes. One-half is subjected to frozen section, cutting at least

Figure 90. Isolated tumor cells. There is a focus of carcinoma, less than 0.2 mm in size in the subcapsular sinus. Keratin stains were helpful in confirming the diagnosis. Note the keratin-positive stromal cells at the bottom of the field.

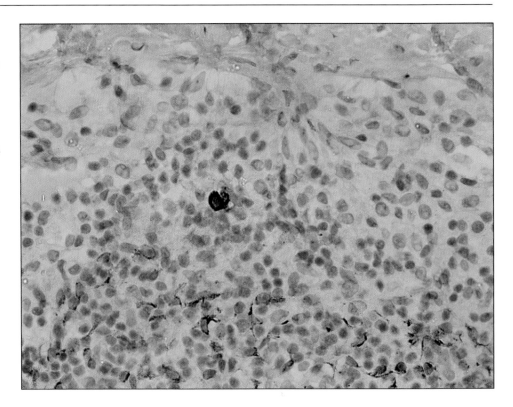

two levels. The frozen section remnant and the remainder of the lymph node are embedded in paraffin, with three levels prepared. In addition, each block is subjected to keratin (or S-100 protein) immunohistochemistry at one level cut between the levels prepared for H&E examination.

It is important to distinguish metastasis from micrometastasis (usually defined as greater than 0.2 mm and no greater than 2.0 mm, respectively) and from isolated tumor cells (usually defined as no cell cluster greater than 0.2 mm), whether identified by H&E section or by immunohistochemistry (Figure 90). The clinical significance of the finding of isolated tumor cells is not yet clear. The presence of metastases greater than 2.0 mm, the size of the greatest metastasis, and the presence of extranodal extension usually portend a poorer prognosis, although this may depend on the site of the primary tumor. There is not yet convincing evidence that shows a survival difference for breast cancer patients with micrometastases vs. node-negative patients. The significance of isolated tumor cells is even more unclear at present. Many investigators have hypothesized that many isolated tumor cells represent benign mechanical transport of cells due to surgical compression during biopsy, breast massage, or use of a substance to facilitate the localization of sentinel lymph nodes and may not have the metastatic potential of *true* metastases.

NEVOMELANOCYTIC LESIONS[161-165]

Nevus cell aggregates are uncommon, but not rare, findings in lymph node dissections, not only occurring most often in the axillary region, but also seen

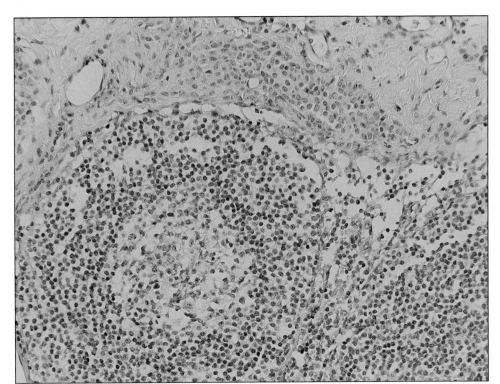

Figure 91. Benign neval cell aggregates in a lymph node. Note the capsular rather than subcapsular localization. Ki-67 stains may be useful, rarely showing any positive cells in nevus.

in inguinal and cervical lymph nodes. They are usually located in the capsule, with possible extension to the trabeculae or perinodal soft tissues (Figure 91). They may occasionally be found in the lymph node parenchyma or even subcapsular lymphatics, but this is usually found in conjunction with capsular infiltration. The nevus cells are bland and form typical nevus nests. Their pattern of localization suggests a developmental pathogenesis. Spitz nevus aggregates may also be seen in lymph nodes in patients with Spitz nevus. This is being seen in increasing frequency now that some surgeons are performing sentinel lymph node biopsies for atypical Spitz nevi of the skin. About one-third of these patients have foci of atypical Spitz nevi in the sentinel lymph nodes, usually in subcapsular and parenchymal areas. Despite this, patients with lymph node spread generally do not have the dire prognosis of typical melanoma patients with lymph node metastases, raising the consideration that these deposits may not represent true metastases. Blue nevi may also be found in lymph nodes, either as an incidental finding, usually in axillary lymph nodes, or in nodes draining sites of skin involvement. Lymph node deposits may also be seen in lymph nodes draining sites of cellular blue nevi; similar to patients with atypical Spitz nevi and lymph node deposits, these patients do not have a poor prognosis.

The regional lymph nodes are the most frequent site of metastasis in malignant melanoma and may be the presenting site of disease. Malignant melanoma can have virtually any appearance, including a close resemblance to malignant melanoma (Figure 92). Lymph node involvement by malignant melanoma has a very adverse affect on prognosis. Patients with palpable lymph node metastases have a worse prognosis than those patients with only nonpalpable metastases,

Figure 92. Metastatic malignant melanoma to a lymph node. These cells have lymphoid cytologic features. The correct diagnosis was established by appropriate immunostains, after all lymphoid markers were negative. The history of prior malignant melanoma was not available at the time the biopsy was originally evaluated.

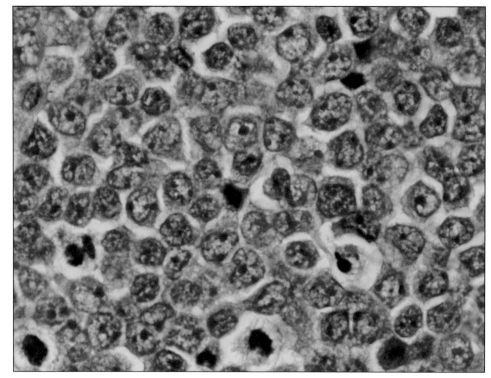

and a poorer survival is seen with an increasing number of positive lymph nodes. Sentinel lymph node biopsies are being performed in patients with malignant lymphoma in the appropriate clinical setting. However, the clinical utility is perhaps not as clear as in the case of breast carcinoma. Some laboratories use S-100 protein staining to help identify microscopic deposits, and a few laboratories supplement S-100 protein staining with another antibody such as Melan-A or HMB-45, due to the potential staining of dendritic cells by S-100 protein. However, S-100–positive dendritic cells are usually seen as single cells in the paracortex with a dendritic morphology and are usually easily distinguishable from melanoma cells, which usually have a more epithelioid morphology and are usually first seen in the subcapsular sinuses.

5 STROMAL TUMORS AND TUMORLIKE LESIONS OF LYMPH NODES

Lipomatosis	**89**
Palisaded Myofibroblastoma	**90**
Smooth Muscle Neoplasms	**90**
Vascular Tumors and Tumorlike Lesions	**93**
Angiomyomatous Hamartoma	93
Epithelioid Hemangioma	95
Vascular Lesion Arising in Castleman Disease	96
Hemangioendothelioma	97
Kaposi Sarcoma	98
High-Grade Angiosarcoma	100

A classification of primary stromal tumors and tumorlike lesions of lymph nodes is given in Table 15. They include myofibroblastic, smooth muscle, fibrohistiocytic, neural, and vascular lesions. Of course, sarcomas may also metastasize to lymph nodes, although this is not a common phenomenon. Approximately 3–5% of patients with sarcoma show metastasis in lymph nodes at some course in their disease, usually at a late stage. Thus, the presentation of a sarcoma of unknown origin would be extremely unusual, and most malignant spindle-cell neoplasms with this presentation turn out to be spindled metastatic carcinoma or malignant melanoma. Lymph node metastases are most frequently seen in patients with epithelioid sarcoma, rhabdomyosarcoma, leiomyosarcoma, clear cell sarcoma, synovial sarcoma, and angiosarcoma.

LIPOMATOSIS

Lipomatosis represents one of the commonest histologic findings seen in lymph nodes. In fact, it may represent a normal phenomenon, more marked in obese individuals, and it may occasionally give rise to lymphadenopathy. It is commonly seen in axillary and pelvic lymph nodes. Histologically, much of the lymph node parenchyma is replaced by mature adipose tissue, starting from the hilum and extending toward the capsule.

Table 15. Nonlymphoid Lesions of Lymph Nodes

Epithelial lesions
    Benign epithelial inclusions
    Carcinoma
Nevomelanocytic lesions
Stromal tumors and tumor-like lesions
    Lipomatosis
    Palisaded myofibroblastoma
    Smooth muscle neoplasms
Vascular tumors and tumor-like lesions
    Angiomyomatous hamartoma
    Epithelioid hemangioma
    Vascular lesion arising in Castleman disease
    Hemangioendothelioma
    Kaposi sarcoma
    High-grade angiosarcoma

Figure 93. Palisaded myofibroblastoma. There is a rim of uninvolved lymph node, separated from the spindle-cell proliferation by fibrous tissue containing numerous hemosiderin-laden macrophages.

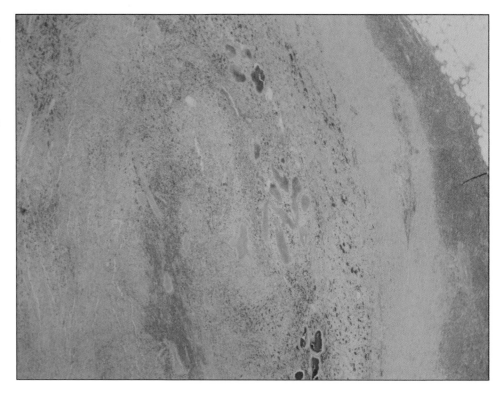

PALISADED MYOFIBROBLASTOMA[166–168]

Palisaded myofibroblastoma (intranodal hemorrhagic spindle-cell tumor with amianthoid fibers) is a rare primary tumor that is unique to lymph nodes. The tumor occurs over a wide age range, with a slight male predominance. Patients usually present with a solitary mass involving inguinal or, less commonly, submandibular lymph nodes. The clinical course is benign, with no recurrences or metastases reported to date. At low magnification, a spindle-cell proliferation is seen, typically with a rim of uninvolved lymph node and a hemorrhagic zone present at the interface (Figure 93). The tumor is composed of fascicles of spindle cells that intersect at right angles, often with thick collagenized areas (Figure 94). These areas have a central zone of dense collagen, which may be calcified surrounded by a paler zone. The spindle cells are bland and show vaguely palisaded nuclei, and mitotic figures are rare. The spindle cells express actin and vimentin, but not desmin, consistent with myofibroblasts. The differential diagnosis includes benign schwannoma, which is invariably S-100 protein positive, and Kaposi sarcoma, which expresses vascular markers in addition to HHV-associated antigens.

SMOOTH MUSCLE NEOPLASMS[169]

A variety of smooth muscle neoplasms may involve the lymph node. Isolated intranodal leiomyoma is extraordinarily rare and is usually confused with a reactive smooth muscle proliferation of the nodal hilum. This latter proliferation

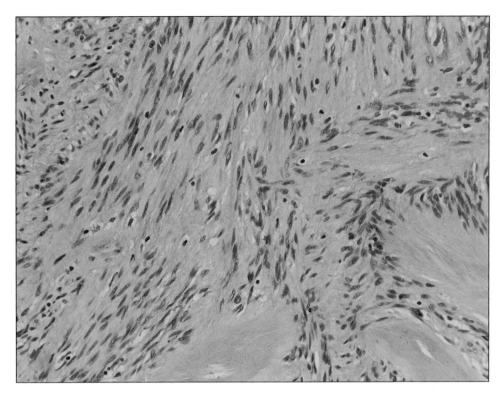

Figure 94. Palisaded myofibroblastoma. The spindle-cell proliferation is bland and resembles that seen in benign schwannoma, although the S-100 protein stain is negative. Note the focal areas of hyalinized collagen.

is commonly seen in inguinal and axillary lymph nodes and consists of disorganized bundles of smooth muscle in a fibrous stroma. Histologically, bland smooth muscle proliferations can be seen in the pelvic and para-aortic lymph nodes of women. They may represent metastases from uterine leiomyosarcoma, metastatic uterine *leiomyoma*, part of leiomyomatosis peritonealis disseminata, or as a metaplastic phenomenon associated with or evolving from endometriosis.

Angiomyolipomas, identical to the more common hamartomatous lesions of the kidney, may occur in retroperitoneal lymph nodes. They are usually associated with tumor in the kidney or retroperitoneum, interpreted as multicentric rather than metastatic disease. A subset of patients have tuberous sclerosis. Histologically, they involve the subcapsular sinus, with variable extension into the lymph node parenchyma. They feature combinations of vacuolated smooth muscle, abnormal vessels, and mature adipose tissue (Figure 95). The smooth muscle stains for typical markers of smooth muscle as well as for HMB-45.

Lymphangiomyomatosis (lymphangioleiomyomatosis, lymphangiomyoma, and leiomyomatosis) is a hamartomatous proliferation of lymphatic vessels and smooth muscle. It occurs exclusively in women, usually during their reproductive years. Patients usually present with dyspnea due to a similar involvement of the lungs, and a significant subset of patients have tuberous sclerosis. There is frequent involvement of multiple pulmonary hilar, posterior mediastinal, and retroperitoneal lymph nodes, although other, primarily centrally located, lymph node groups may also be affected. Rarely, there may be solitary lymph node involvement. Patients usually die of respiratory failure within a decade; treatment with progesterone or oophorectomy may be of some benefit. At low

Figure 95. Angiomyolipoma. In this case, the smooth muscle cells show prominent epithelioid features. The patient had a simultaneous angiomyolipoma in the kidney. The epithelioid cells were positive for HMB-45.

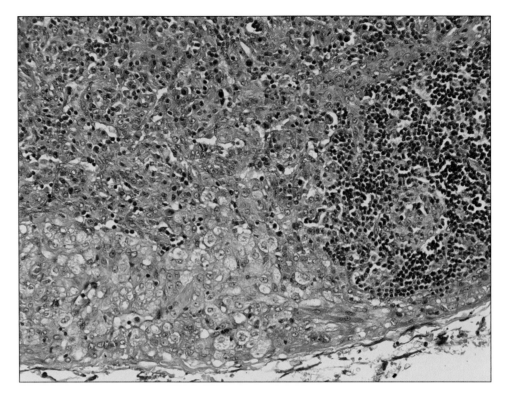

Figure 96. Lymphangiomyomatosis. Collapsed lymphatics are surrounded by fascicles of benign smooth muscle cells.

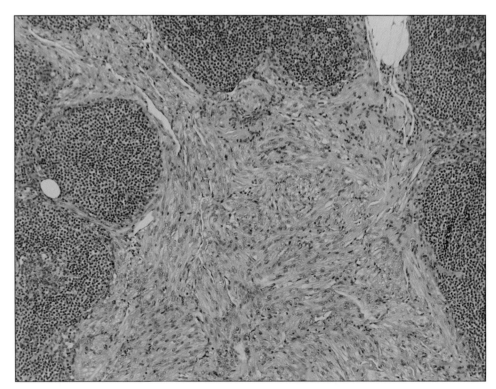

magnification, the proliferation starts in the subcapsular region and progresses toward the hilum (Figure 96). It is composed predominantly of vacuolated smooth muscle cells with clear cytoplasm along with a variable number of anastomosing lymphatics. The smooth muscle stains for typical markers of smooth muscle as well as for HMB-45. The clinical setting and the

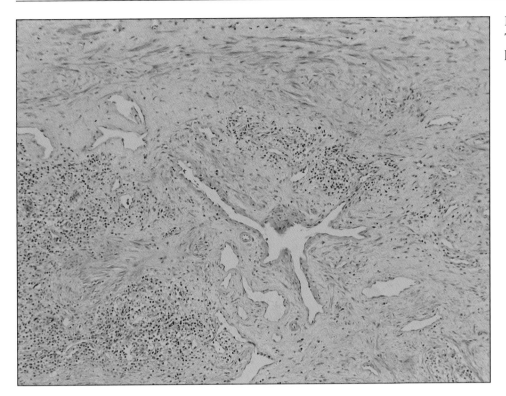

Figure 97. Lymphangioma. This patient had systemic lymphangiomatosis.

staining for HMB-45 should provide distinction from metastatic smooth muscle tumors.

VASCULAR TUMORS AND TUMORLIKE LESIONS[170]

A variety of vascular lesions may occur in lymph nodes. Lymphangioma of lymph node is almost always part of a systemic lymphangiomatosis, a syndrome involving multiple organs, including the spleen, and is usually associated with lymphangioma of the adjacent soft tissue. The histologic appearance is similar to other lymphangiomas, with dilated spaces filled with proteinaceous fluid and lymphocytes lined by bland endothelial cells (Figure 97). Hemangioma of lymph node is usually an incidental finding, but may present as isolated lymphadenopathy. It is occasionally associated with vascular lesions at other sites. Histologically, one sees a space-occupying lesion that is usually well circumscribed (Figure 98). It may be capillary, cavernous, or a combination of the two patterns. Rarely (particularly in children), one may see the histologic features of cellular capillary hemangioma.

Angiomyomatous Hamartoma[170]

Angiomyomatous hamartoma is a peculiar, benign vascular lesion exclusively affecting inguinal lymph nodes. There is a wide age range with a male predominance. Patients present with lymphadenopathy, often of long duration. Edema of the ipsilateral leg may also be present. It probably represents a reactive condition

Figure 98. Capillary hemangioma. This lesion forms a mass that focally obliterates the lymph node architecture.

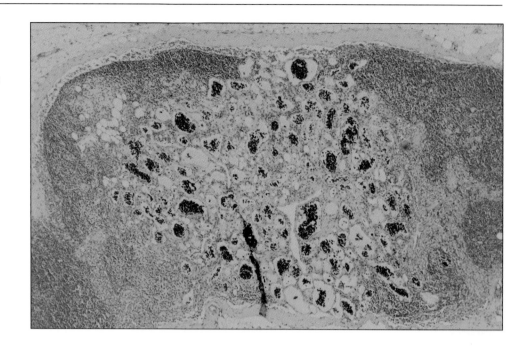

Figure 99. Angiomyoma. This lesion extends from the hilum to the capsule, isolating areas of residual cortex.

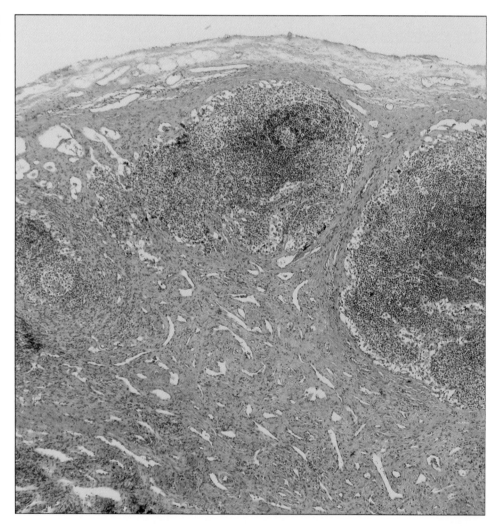

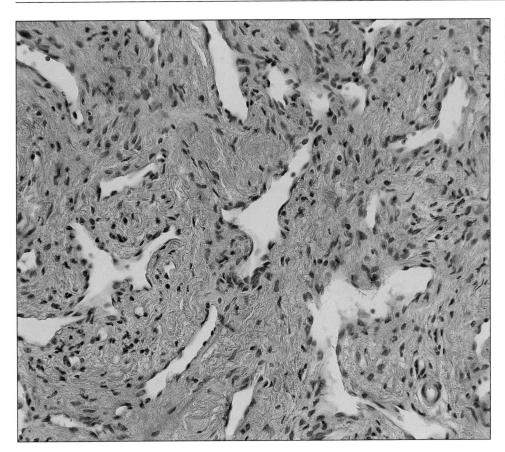

Figure 100. Angiomyoma. The vascular channels are lined by endothelial cells, with intervening fibrous tissue containing bland spindle cells.

rather than a true neoplasm and may be a more advanced stage of reactive smooth muscle proliferation of the lymph node hilum. The histologic appearance is very distinctive. At low magnification, the lesion involves the hilum and medullary areas, extending through the lymph node parenchyma to the capsule (Figure 99). At higher magnification, there are multiple thick and ecstatic thin-walled vessels, whose muscle coats merge imperceptibly with a surrounding sclerotic stroma (Figure 100). The sclerotic stroma contains scattered smooth muscle cells and rarely may include interspersed adiposities.

Epithelioid Hemangioma[170]

Epithelioid hemangioma (angiolymphoid hyperplasia with eosinophils, NOT Kimura disease) is usually an isolated finding, presenting as lymphadenopathy at one site. Clinically, it is benign. The histologic appearance is identical to that seen at other sites. One sees epithelioid endothelium-lined, well-formed blood vessels, often arising from or closely associated with a hilar blood vessel (Figure 101). Characteristically, the stroma includes inflammatory cells, particularly eosinophils (Figure 102). Kimura disease can be distinguished from epithelioid hemangioma by its characteristic clinical features, its primary inflammatory nature, and the absence of proliferation of epithelioid endothelial cells in blood vessels. Hemangiothelioma has a greater degree of cytologic atypia and usually lacks an accompanying eosinophilic infiltrate.

Figure 101. Epithelioid hemangioma with eosinophils. This lesion is centered upon the lymph node hilum.

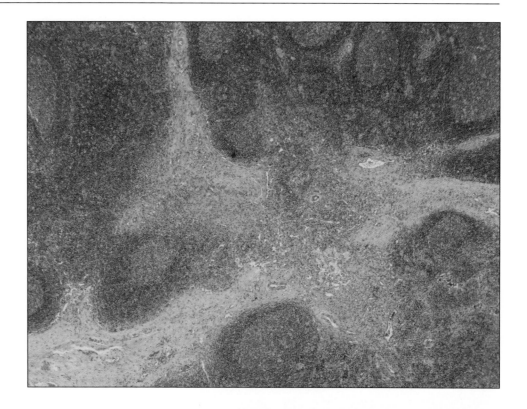

Figure 102. Epithelioid hemangioma with eosinophils. The irregular vascular channels are lined by plump endothelial cells. Note the numerous eosinophils in the stroma.

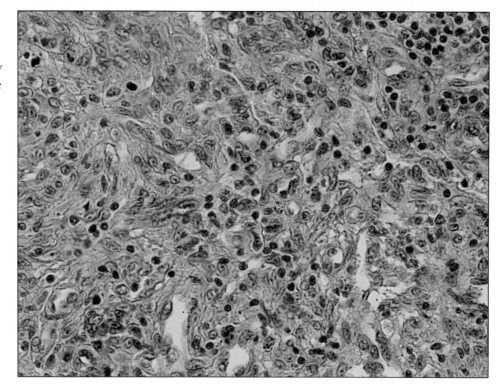

Vascular Lesion Arising in Castleman Disease[39,171]

The vascular lesion arising in Castleman disease is one of several neoplasms that may complicate this disease. It is rare and only occurs in univocal hyaline-vascular Castleman disease. Thus, it is clearly distinct from Kaposi sarcoma,

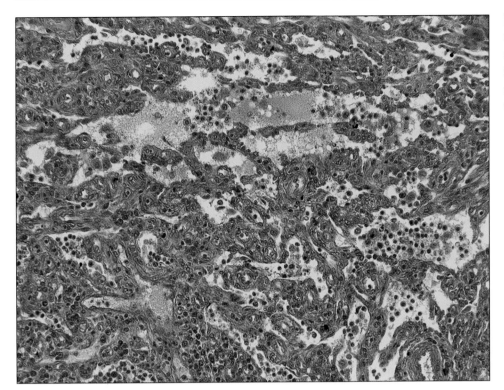

Figure 103. Vascular lesion occurring in Castleman disease. Angiomatoid spaces that are lined by bland endothelial cells are seen in this example.

which is associated with multicentric cell Castleman disease, two diseases that share an HHV-8 pathogenesis. It usually occurs in relation to larger lesions of hyaline-vascular Castleman disease; therefore, it occurs most frequently in the retroperitoneum and mediastinum. The clinical course is variable, with at least some behaving in a malignant fashion. It may be identified grossly as a focal hemorrhagic area. Histologically, it may form discrete nodules or it may blend into the paracortical vascular proliferation characteristic of the hyaline-vascular variant of Castleman disease. The vascular proliferation varies from vessels closely resembling high endothelial venules to retiform channels with slitlike spaces to fascicles of spindle cells that only occasionally form vascular lumina (Figure 103). The nuclei of the proliferating cells also vary, from bland to highly pleomorphic, with a corresponding variation in the mitotic rate. Immunohistochemical studies are often not helpful, with the proliferative cells showing a vascular phenotype in only focal areas. The most important distinction is with Kaposi sarcoma, which occurs in a different clinical setting and expresses HHV-8–associated antigens, and follicular dendritic cells tumor (another neoplasm that may be associated with Castleman disease), which lacks a vascular proliferation and expresses the follicular dendritic cell markers CD21 and/or CD35.

Hemangioendothelioma[172]

Hemangioendothelioma (low-grade angiosarcoma) may rarely occur as a primary lesion in lymph nodes. It is usually an isolated finding, presenting as lymphadenopathy at one site. It is usually clinically benign, but it may recur, or rarely, metastasize. The most common histologic appearance is that of

Figure 104. Epithelioid hemangioendothelioma, polymorphous type. This variant has a predilection for occurrence in lymph nodes. Note the atypical cells lining the subcapsular sinuses.

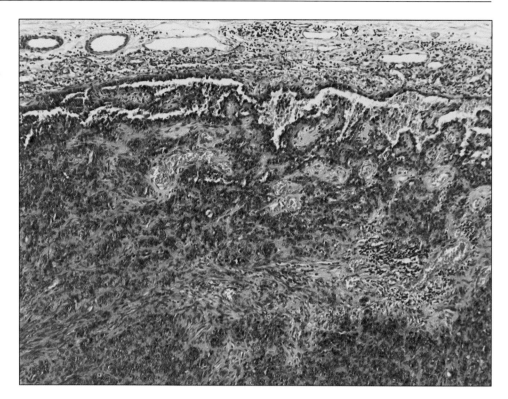

classical epithelioid hemangioendothelioma, as seen at other sites. A mixed spindle and epithelioid hemangioendothelioma has also been described. The most difficult to diagnose variant is the polymorphous hemangioendothelioma, which features a variety of histologic patterns, ranging from solid to papillary to angiomatous (Figure 104). In fact, the vascular nature may be only discernible in a small portion of the tumor. The expression of vascular markers will confirm the diagnosis of hemangioendothelioma, remembering that some cases may also express keratin. Given its rarity as a primary lesion of lymph node, one should rule out the possibility of a metastatic lesion.

Kaposi Sarcoma[173]

Kaposi sarcoma is a vascular neoplasm invariably associated with HHV-8 infection in the neoplastic cells. Lymph node involvement is seen in several clinicopathologic settings. In classical Kaposi sarcoma occurring predominantly in elderly Jewish or Mediterranean males with skin lesions, usually confined to the lower extremities, lymph node involvement is uncommon but may occur in draining lymph nodes. The clinical course is generally indolent. In African (epidemic) Kaposi sarcoma, there is a lymphadenopathic form occurring mainly in male children and young adults; the prognosis is poor in this group. In Kaposi sarcoma associated with HIV infection, lymph node involvement usually occurs in association with disseminated disease, and prognosis is dependent on the overall immune status of the patient. It is particularly common in those patients with multicentric Castleman disease, another HHV-8–associated neoplasm, and is often seen concurrently in the involved lymph node. Kaposi sarcoma also

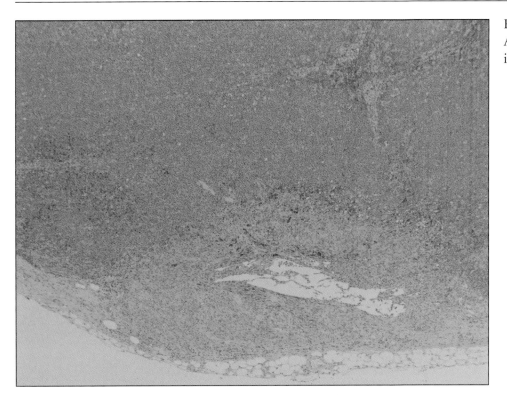

Figure 105. Kaposi sarcoma. A capsular localization is seen in this case.

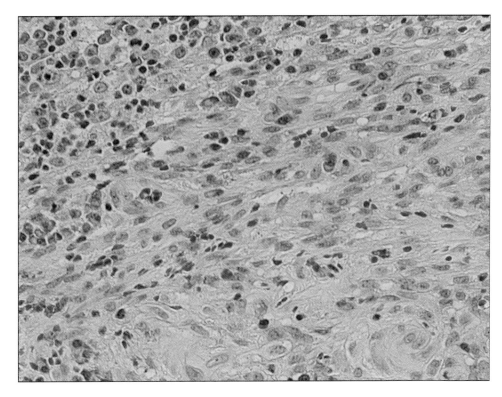

Figure 106. Kaposi sarcoma. At high magnification, a classical appearance is seen (same case as Figure 105). Note the scattered plasma cells.

occurs in other settings of immunosuppression, such as posttransplant, occurring in about 0.5% of renal transplant patients; however, it is uncommonly seen in lymph nodes in the absence of disseminated disease.

The histologic features are similar regardless of the clinical setting. Kaposi may show focal or diffuse effacement, by single or multiple nodules.

Figure 107. Angiosarcoma, involving lymph node. A pleomorphic neoplasm is seen. Irregular vascular channels are seen at the interface between the neoplasm and the lymphoid tissue. The tumor expressed CD31 and CD34 and lacked other specific differentiation markers.

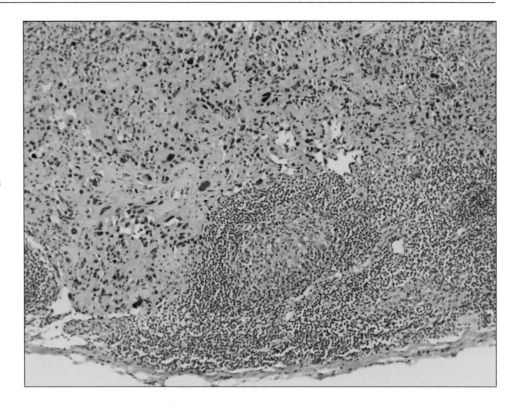

It often appears to start in the subcapsular sinuses or the capsule, with progression to the rest of the lymph node parenchyma (Figure 105). The high-magnification appearance is identical to that seen in skin and other sites (Figure 106). A number of fibrous and vascular proliferations may be confused with Kaposi sarcoma. The most effective means of diagnosis is immunohistochemistry for the detection of HHV-8–associated antigens; no other proliferation in the differential diagnosis will have staining in the proliferating elements.

High-Grade Angiosarcoma

Angiosarcoma is extremely rare as a primary neoplasm of lymph nodes; secondary involvement via metastasis from another primary site is much more common. It may show a spindled or epithelioid histology, similar to that seen in other organs (Figure 107). There is usually total replacement of the lymphoid parenchyma, with atypia and mitoses the rule. The expression of vascular markers, along with ruling out the possibility of metastasis from another site, establishes the diagnosis. The prognosis is poor, even in patients with seemingly limited disease at presentation.

6 HODGKIN LYMPHOMA

Classical Hodgkin Lymphoma	101
Nodular Lymphocyte–Predominant Hodgkin Lymphoma	115

Hodgkin lymphoma consists of two distinct neoplasms with the common feature that the neoplastic element comprises less than 1% of the overall cellular elements at involved sites of disease. In the World Health Organization (WHO) Classification, Hodgkin lymphoma is separated into classical Hodgkin lymphoma and nodular lymphocyte–predominant Hodgkin lymphoma (Table 16). Classical Hodgkin lymphoma is discussed in the first section, while nodular lymphocyte predominance is discussed in the section Nodular Lymphocyte–Predominant Hodgkin Lymphoma.

CLASSICAL HODGKIN LYMPHOMA[174–196]

Classical Hodgkin lymphoma comprises greater than 25% of all malignant lymphomas in Western countries. There is a well-known bimodal peak of incidence, with peaks in young adulthood and older age. Some have speculated that this is actually due to three patho-etiologies of classical Hodgkin lymphoma, with one occurring in childhood, with a male predominance, associated with EBV, large family size, and a lower socioeconomic status; a second occurring in young adulthood, with a slight female predominance, with a high incidence of mediastinal masses, not associated with EBV, and occurring in individuals from small families and of a higher socioeconomic status; and a third occurring in older individuals, with a male predominance, and associated with EBV. There is an increased concordance rate for Hodgkin lymphoma among identical twins as opposed to dizygotic twins, suggesting a genetic component. There is also an increased risk of classical Hodgkin lymphoma in patients with immunodeficiencies, whether congenital or acquired.

Classical Hodgkin lymphoma represents a clonal neoplasm of germinal center cell–derived B-cells. Hodgkin precursor cells undergo immunoglobulin rearrangement, enter the germinal center, and participate in the germinal center process of somatic hypermutation. However, instead of undergoing the normal mechanism of apoptosis as a result of developing nonfunctional mutations,

Table 16. WHO Classification of Hodgkin Lymphoma[213]

Classical Hodgkin lymphoma
    Nodular sclerosis
    Mixed cellularity
    Lymphocyte-rich
    Lymphocyte-depleted
Nodular lymphocyte–predominant Hodgkin lymphoma

Table 17. Cotswolds Modification to Ann Arbor Staging System for Hodgkin Lymphoma[197]

Stage	Definition
I	Involvement of a single lymph node region or lymphoid organ
II	Involvement of two or more lymph node regions on the same side of the diaphragm
III	Involvement of lymph node regions or organs on both sides of the diaphragm
III_1	Without para-aortic, iliac, or mesenteric nodes
III_2	With para-aortic, iliac, or mesenteric nodes
IV	Involvement of extranodal site(s) beyond that designated E

X, bulky disease, >1/3 widening of mediastinum or >10 cm nodal mass; E, involvement of a single extranodal site, contiguous or proximal to known nodal site.

Hodgkin cells somehow escape cell death and continue to proliferate, possibly mediated via the nuclear factor-kappa B (NF-κB) pathway.

Patients usually present with either enlarged, nontender, peripheral lymphadenopathy (70% of cases) or a mediastinal mass. The most commonly involved lymph node sites include the cervical and axillary groups, the left side slightly more than right side. B symptoms, comprising documented fever greater than 38° during the previous month, drenching night sweats, or unexplained weight loss greater than 10% in the preceding 6 months, are seen in about 30% of patients. The fever tends to be worse in the evening and may be intermittent (Pel-Ebstein fever). Patients may also have pruritis or pain in affected lymph nodes following alcohol ingestion. Abnormal laboratory studies may include a normochromic, normocytic anemia or a Coombs positive hemolytic anemia. The current staging system for Hodgkin lymphoma is given in Table 17. Hodgkin lymphoma spreads through the lymph nodes in a contiguous fashion, before disseminating to distant nonadjacent sites through the blood. The majority of patients present in stage I or II. Five-year survival rates now exceed 80%, attributable to the improved treatments. One of the major goals of treatment is to minimize late effects, particularly the incidence of second cancers, including leukemia, non-Hodgkin lymphoma, and solid tumors such as breast or lung cancer. Adverse clinical prognostic factors include bulky disease; involvement of multiple sites, and B symptoms for those with low-stage disease; and low albumin, low hemoglobin, male sex, older age, stage IV disease, leukocytosis, and lymphocytopenia for those with advanced disease. These latter factors have been combined into a prognostic score for patients with advanced disease. The success of modern treatment regimens has negated the prognostic significance of histologic subtyping or other histologic factors, with the exception of grading in nodular sclerosis when large numbers of patients are studied.

Biopsies taken for a possible diagnosis of classical Hodgkin lymphoma may be processed according to the principles outlined at the beginning of the book. Frozen section diagnosis is possible, but should be rendered only if an immediate

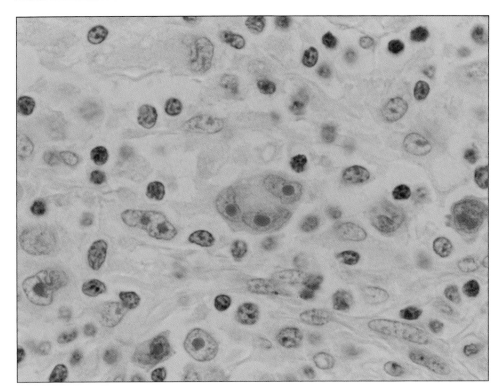

Figure 108. Classical Hodgkin lymphoma. A classical or diagnostic Reed-Sternberg cell is seen, with several nuclei or lobes, each of which containing a prominent eosinophilic nucleolus approaching the size of a normal lymphocyte nucleus. Several other Hodgkin cells are also seen in this field.

clinical decision (such as insertion of a catheter) depends upon rapid diagnosis. Frozen sections provide good assessment of architecture, such as the presence of fibrous bands, while touch or scrape (preferred by me) preparations are often adequate for cytologic detail. Grossly, lymph nodes involved by Hodgkin lymphoma are enlarged and may show a vague (mixed cellularity) or distinct (nodular sclerosis) nodular pattern, and the nodules are typically larger than the pattern seen in follicular lymphoma. Immunohistochemical studies are an important adjunct to the diagnosis of Hodgkin lymphoma. Flow cytometry studies are not as useful, but can be helpful in showing the absence of a monotypic B-cell population.

The histologic diagnosis of Hodgkin lymphoma depends on the definitive recognition of the neoplastic element (Hodgkin cells) in the appropriate cellular milieu. Hodgkin cells are uninucleated or multinucleated cells with large nuclei. The nuclei are often multilobated and have large, prominent eosinophilic nucleoli approaching the size of small lymphocytes. The nuclear membranes are prominent and have rounded outlines. So-called diagnostic Reed-Sternberg cells are multinucleated cells or cells with multilobated nuclei, which each nucleus or nuclear lobe containing prominent eosinophilic nucleoli (Figure 108). The cytoplasm of Hodgkin cells is abundant and amphophilic to slightly basophilic and lacks a paranuclear hof. Mitoses, including atypical mitoses, are not common, although apoptotic *mummified* cells are typically easy to identify. Hodgkin cells are always few in number, overall usually comprising less than 1% of the total cellular population. However, they typically cluster together and may form small sheets adjacent to areas of necrosis. They are usually identified in diffuse areas of effacement of lymph node architecture, although they rarely may be identified

Figure 109. Classical Hodgkin lymphoma. Occasionally, an interfollicular pattern is seen, with the Hodgkin cells found outside or directly adjacent to reactive follicles. This is seen most often in mixed cellularity.

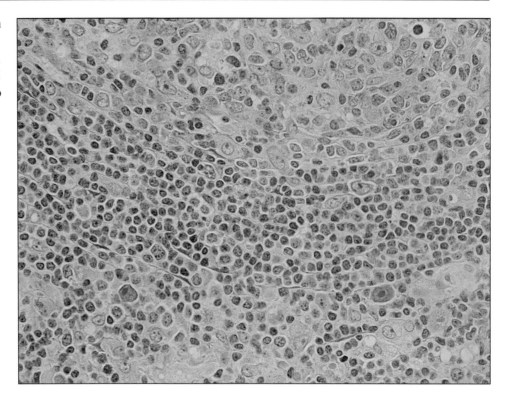

Figure 110. Successfully treated Hodgkin lymphoma. There is dense acellular fibrous tissue with scattered small lymphocytes.

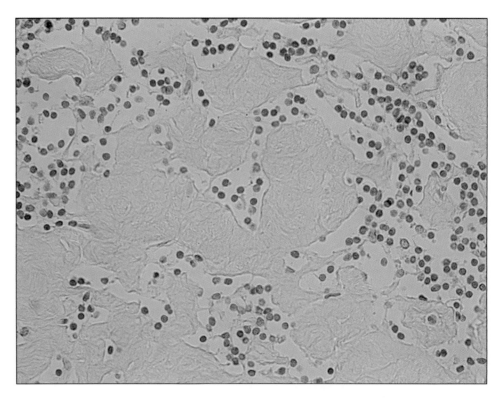

at the edges of follicles or between reactive follicles (interfollicular Hodgkin lymphoma) more rarely in association with monocytoid B-cell hyperplasia, or even more rarely in sinuses (Figure 109). They are typically found in greater numbers in recurrences as opposed to initial biopsies. There is also tendency for an increase in pleomorphism in recurrences, particularly in sites that have been

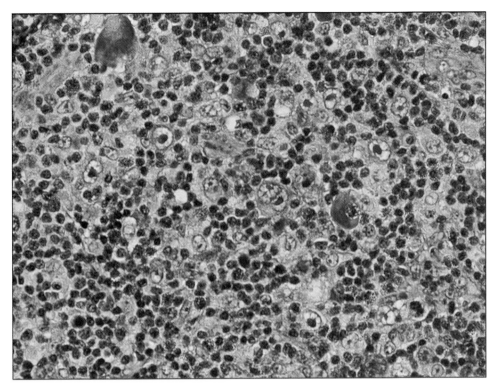

Figure 111. Classical Hodgkin lymphoma, mixed cellularity type. There are scattered Hodgkin cells, including *mummified* apoptotic forms, in a background of small lymphocytes, eosinophils, and histiocytes.

previously radiated. Successfully treated sites show dense acellular fibrous tissue (Figure 110).

The cellular milieu in which the Hodgkin cells are found varies with the histologic subtype as well as within a given case and typically consists of a mixture of small mature lymphocytes, generally of T-helper/inducer type, histiocytes, eosinophils, neutrophils, and plasma cells (Figure 111). The small lymphocytes tend to immediately surround the Hodgkin cells. Immunoblasts are generally not seen, and small lymphocytes of B-lineage are not found in large numbers, except in the lymphocyte-rich subtype (see below). The histiocytes are usually nonactivated, but clusters of epithelioid histiocytes, or even well-formed granulomas, may be seen in some cases (Figure 112). Eosinophils can vary markedly in numbers from case to case. Plasma cells are usually not overly abundant in number, with the exception of rare cases.

The overall histologic appearance of classical Hodgkin lymphoma varies with the histologic subtype. The subtypes currently recognized by the WHO are given in Table 16. In general, they correspond to the subtypes originally described by Lukes. Nodular sclerosis is the most frequent subtype, occurring in approximately 70% of cases in Western populations. It is by far the most common subtype seen in the young adult epidemiologic grouping of classical Hodgkin lymphoma and does not have a strong association with EBV infection. Patients typically present with a mediastinal mass, with or without concurrent cervical and/or axillary adenopathy. Thus, most patients present in stage II. Histologically, nodular sclerosis is defined by the presence of one or more broad fibrous bands, typically radiating from a thickened lymph node capsule (Figure 113). The bands are densely collagenized and relatively acellular. Possibly

Figure 112. Classical Hodgkin lymphoma. Occasionally, Hodgkin cells are seen in or adjacent to granulomas.

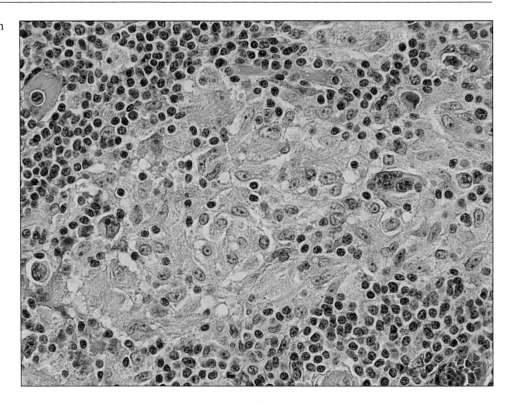

Figure 113. Classical Hodgkin lymphoma, nodular sclerosing type. Nodules separated by broad fibrous bands are seen, in a classic appearance of nodular sclerosis.

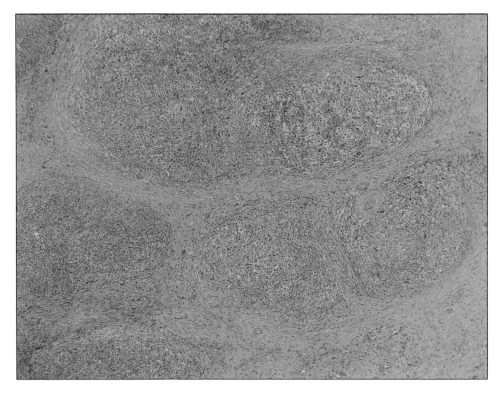

because these bands impart a relative rigidity to the lymph node, the Hodgkin cells may show artifactual cytoplasmic retraction (lacunar cells) (Figure 114). Eosinophils tend to be numerous in this subtype. In addition, large areas of necrosis are particularly common, with the Hodgkin cells frequently forming large clusters or sheets at the edges of the necrosis, an appearance that has been

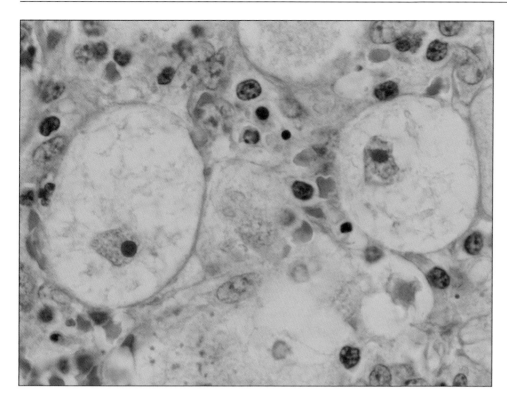

Figure 114. Classical Hodgkin lymphoma, nodular sclerosing type. The lacunar cells have voluminous clear cytoplasm.

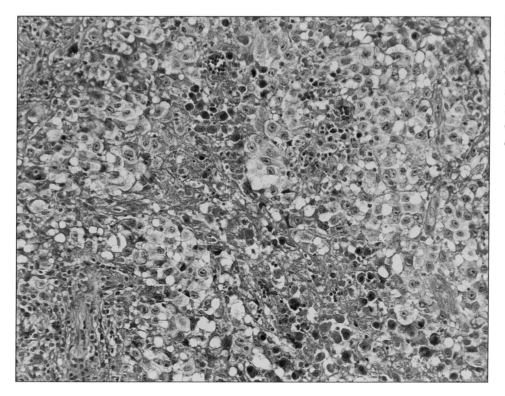

Figure 115. Classical Hodgkin lymphoma, nodular sclerosing type, syncytial variant (type 2 nodular sclerosing). Central foci of necrosis are rimmed by sheets of lacunar cells, mimicking a carcinoma.

termed the syncytial variant (Figure 115). Since nodular sclerosis is so common, an attempt has been made to subclassify it. The British National Lymphoma Investigation has established two grades (Table 18). Although study of large numbers of cases has shown survival differences between these two groups of cases, there is no great clinical utility in the evaluation of individual patients

Table 18. Grading of Nodular Sclerosis Hodgkin Lymphoma[183,185]

Grade II if

>25% nodules show reticular or pleomorphic lymphocyte depletion

>80% of the nodules show fibrohistiocytic lymphocyte depletion

>25% nodules contain bizarre and highly anaplastic Hodgkin cells with lymphocyte depletion

Grade I: All other cases

outside the setting of a clinical study; therefore, most hematopathologists do not routinely provide a subclassification of individual cases on this basis.

Mixed cellularity is the next most frequent subtype of classical Hodgkin lymphoma, seen in about 25% of cases. It represents the most common subtype seen in Hodgkin lymphoma occurring in children and older adults and is associated with EBV in over 50% of cases. Patients may present in any stage, and this is the most common subtype seen in patients who present in stages III and IV. By definition, mixed cellularity lacks any thick fibrous bands, although a vaguely nodular appearance may still be evident. Architectural effacement is almost always present, although rarely an interfollicular pattern of involvement may be present, either focally or throughout the lymph node. The histologic appearance is highly variable, with widely varying numbers of Hodgkin cells and types and numbers of background cells.

The lymphocyte-rich subtype is uncommon, seen in less than 5% of cases. There is a male predominance, and it may affect an older age group than other subtypes of Hodgkin lymphoma. At low magnification, either of two patterns may be seen. In the more frequent pattern, there is an overall nodular architecture, imparted by the presence of numerous expanded follicles with prominent mantle zones and absent, inconspicuous, or regressed germinal centers (Figure 116). The paracortical region is correspondingly diminished in size. The Hodgkin cells are usually located in or around the prominent mantle zones. The mantle zones are composed primarily of typically mantle zone B-cells, while the paracortical regions usually lack the admixture of eosinophils and neutrophils often seen in other subtypes of Hodgkin lymphoma. In the diffuse pattern, follicles with prominent mantle zones are not seen. Nonetheless, the areas of diffuse effacement lack large numbers of Hodgkin cells and again lack a significant admixture of eosinophils and neutrophils (Figure 117). In contrast, the number of histiocytes, including epithelioid histiocytes, is typically greater than seen in other subtypes.

The lymphocyte depletion subtype is the rarest subtype of classical Hodgkin lymphoma in Western populations, seen in less than 1% of cases, although it is more commonly seen in developing countries. There is a marked male predominance and a high incidence of association with EBV. A significant number of cases are also associated with HIV infection. It generally is associated with high stage and the presence of B symptoms. Histologically, there is invariably diffuse

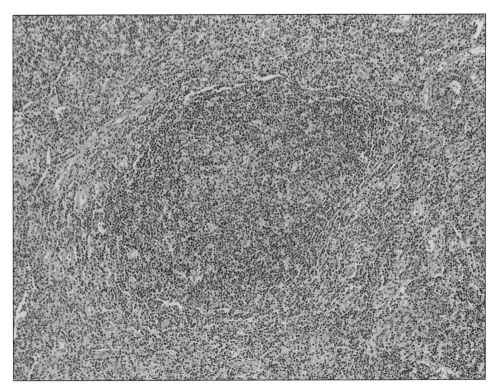

Figure 116. Classical Hodgkin lymphoma, lymphocyte-rich type. A vague nodule is seen in the center of the field, mimicking nodular lymphocyte–predominant Hodgkin lymphoma.

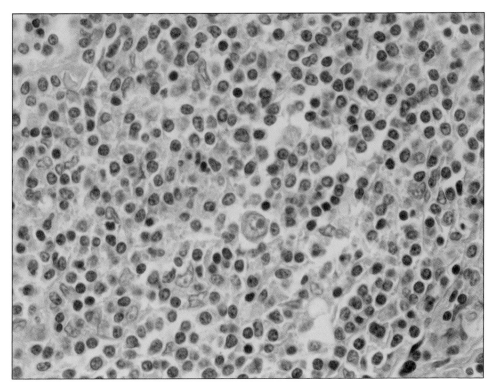

Figure 117. Classical Hodgkin lymphoma, lymphocyte-rich type. A single Hodgkin cell is seen in this field, in a background of small lymphocytes and occasional histocytes, and rare plasma cells and eosinophils.

effacement of architecture, without the presence of any thick fibrous bands. There is often a cell-poor appearance, imparted by the presence of a fine fibrosis that envelops individual cells. At high magnification, there are usually a relatively large number of Hodgkin cells, although some cases with fine fibrosis may lack this feature (Figure 118). The Hodgkin cells may not only show typical

Figure 118. Classical Hodgkin lymphoma, lymphocyte depletion type. A Reed-Sternberg cell is seen in the center of the field, in a cell-poor background dominated by histiocytes and a fine fibrosis.

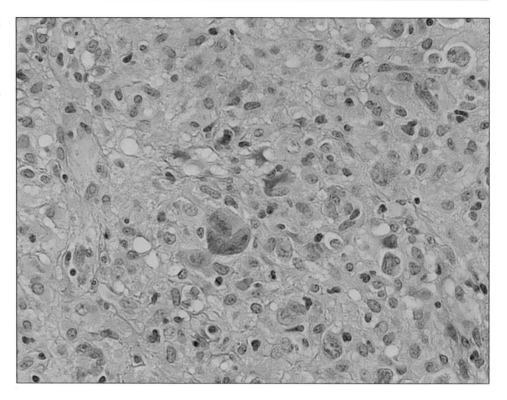

Figure 119. Classical Hodgkin lymphoma, lymphocyte depletion type. Numerous pleomorphic Hodgkin cells are seen. The phenotype was typical of Hodgkin cells.

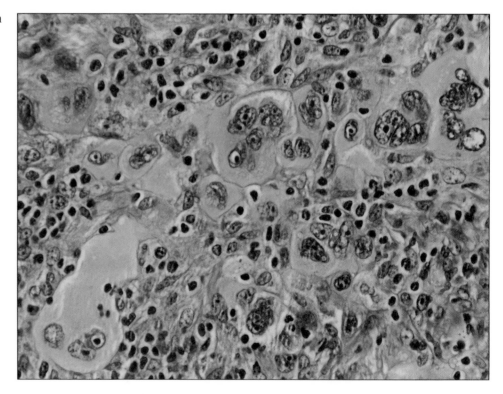

cytologic findings but also show pleomorphic forms, occasionally in large numbers (Figure 119). There is usually a relative paucity of small mature lymphocytes and a large number of histiocytes and other inflammatory cells.

The role of immunohistochemical studies is to provide a specific immunophenotypic identification of Hodgkin cells, as well as to rule out the diagnosis of non-Hodgkin lymphoma. Hodgkin cells have a characteristic phenotype, which is not shared by any other normal or neoplastic population. Unfortunately, this phenotype is not expressed by every Hodgkin cell or even case; nonetheless, the phenotypic assessment of cases of possible Hodgkin lymphoma is highly recommended in all but the most classic of cases of nodular sclerosis. The characteristic phenotype is given in Table 19. CD30 antigen is the most consistent marker of classical Hodgkin cells, in which a membrane and/or paranuclear staining is seen (Figure 120). A similar pattern of staining is seen with CD15 antibodies, although a variable number of staining cells are typically seen in positive cases (Figure 121). CD15-negative cases tend to be found in older male patients of higher stage; these cases have a poorer prognosis than CD15-positive cases. Hodgkin cells also show consistent expression of the late centrocyte post–germinal center marker MUM-1, and about 90% of cases express the B-lineage marker PAX-5 (Figure 122). Staining for CD20 is more variable, with only 20–50% of cases positive for CD20 in the literature, with only a subset of the Hodgkin cells staining. In some studies, CD20-positive cases have a more favorable prognosis than CD20-negative cases. The plasma cell marker CD138 is positive in about 30–40% of cases. In contrast, Hodgkin cells typically lack positivity for the B-cell transcription factors BOB.1 and OCT-2, and do not express cytoplasmic or membrane immunoglobulin. Hodgkin cells are usually negative for T-cell markers, although expression of CD3 may be seen in a subset of cases. They are almost always negative for CD45 and CD43, although these stains may be extremely difficult to interpret, given the frequent ringing of Hodgkin cells by reactive T-cells (Figure 123). EBV-associated cases are consistently positive for EBV-LMP (Figure 124). In view of the variable staining with most antibodies, we recommend that a panel of antibodies be used in the evaluation of any cases in which Hodgkin lymphoma is in the differential diagnosis, including CD30, CD15, CD45, CD3, and CD20. Second-line antibodies that may be helpful include EBV-LMP, PAX-5, MUM-1, and other B- and T-cell markers.

Molecular studies are typically not helpful in the differential diagnosis of Hodgkin lymphoma, other than for the purpose of ruling out a B-cell or T-cell lymphoma. PCR performed on microdissected Hodgkin cells will show clonal rearrangements of the immunoglobulin genes, but these are not detectable in similar studies performed on whole-tissue sections. Hodgkin lymphoma is not associated with any specific translocations including the t(14;18), t(2;5), or t(3;14). Classical cytogenetic studies are usually negative, but may show hypertetraploidy with aneuploidy.

Because of the protean histologic appearance of classical Hodgkin lymphoma, the differential diagnosis is enormous and encompasses much of the surgical pathology of lymph nodes. The syncytial variant of nodular sclerosis Hodgkin lymphoma may closely simulate carcinoma and malignant melanoma, and undifferentiated nasopharyngeal carcinoma or lymphoepithelioma-like carcinomas of a variety of other sites may resemble nodular sclerosis or mixed cellularity Hodgkin lymphoma. A panel of stains including keratin and S-100

Table 19. Phenotype of Classical Hodgkin Cells

Phenotype	%
CD30	98
CD15	85
MUM-1	98
PAX-5	90
CD138	30
CD20	20–50
CD79a	10
BOB.1	10
OCT-2	10
BCL-6	40
EBV-LMP	40
T-cell markers	<5
CD43	<5
EMA	<5
Fascin	90

Figure 120. Classical Hodgkin lymphoma, CD30 stain. Note the paranuclear and membrane accentuation of staining present in several cells, important to note to rule out the possibility of artifactual cytoplasmic staining.

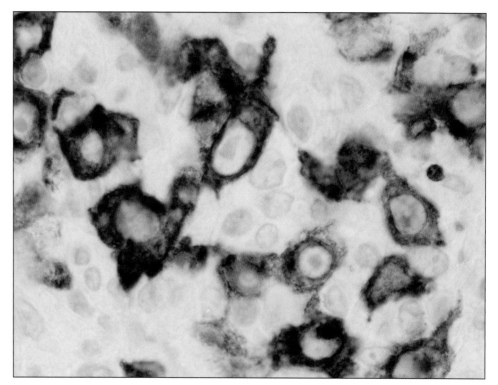

Figure 121. Classical Hodgkin lymphoma, CD15 stain. Numerous positive Hodgkin cells are seen. At least some paranuclear and/or membrane staining should be present to call a case CD15 positive.

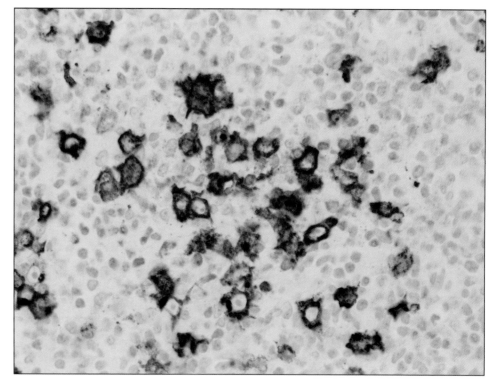

will identify cases of carcinoma and malignant melanoma, respectively, as Hodgkin cells never express these markers. Germ cell tumors of the mediastinum, particularly seminoma, may simulate nodular sclerosis Hodgkin lymphoma. OCT-4 is a consistent marker of seminoma, but it must be kept in mind that embryonal

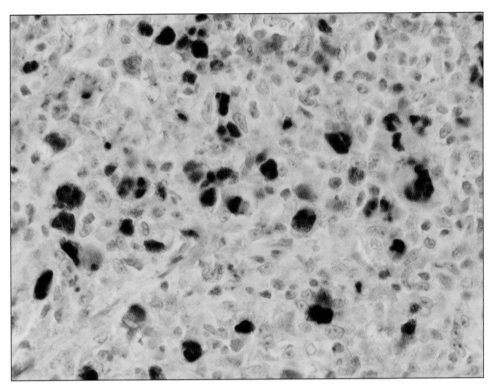

Figure 122. Classical Hodgkin lymphoma, PAX-5 stain. About 95% of cases of classical Hodgkin lymphoma have PAX-5–positive Hodgkin cells, very helpful in distinguishing cases from T-cell lymphoma, including anaplastic large-cell lymphoma.

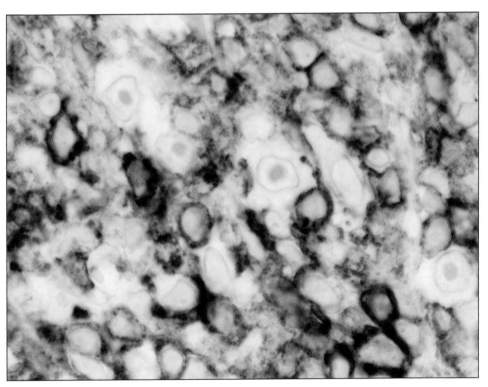

Figure 123. Classical Hodgkin lymphoma, CD45 stain. Although the surrounding lymphocytes and histiocytes show membrane reactivity for CD45, the Hodgkin cells are negative. This is best seen in the upper left, where two Hodgkin cells are abutting upon one another.

carcinomas consistently express CD30; keratin or OCT-4 stains would be definitive if the latter diagnosis is being considered.

Several types of B-cell lymphomas may be easily confused with Hodgkin lymphoma. Diffuse large B-cell lymphoma may be extremely difficult to distinguish from Hodgkin lymphoma, particularly mediastinal B-cell lymphoma vs.

Figure 124. Classical Hodgkin lymphoma, EBV-LMP stain. Despite the name *membrane protein*, LMP usually shows a paranuclear and granular cytoplasmic pattern of staining. All or virtually all of the Hodgkin cells are stained in an EBV-positive case.

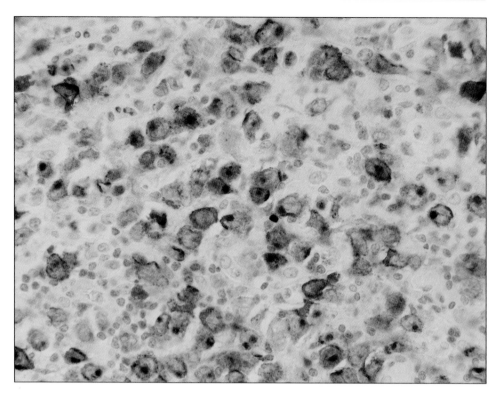

Table 20. Mixed Cellularity Hodgkin Lymphoma vs. T-cell/Histiocyte-Rich B-Cell Lymphoma

	MCHD (%)	T/HRBCL (%)
CD30	100	5
CD15	85	1
CD45	5	98
CD20	20–50	99
EBV-LMP	40	1

syncytial nodular sclerosis. The sclerosis in mediastinal B-cell lymphoma is finer than that of nodular sclerosis and compartmentalizes smaller groups of cells. Some cases of mediastinal B-cell lymphoma may express CD30, but the expression of CD45 along with the uniform expression of CD20 should distinguish the two entities in most cases. The T-cell/histiocyte-rich B-cell lymphoma may also be extremely difficult to distinguish from mixed cellularity Hodgkin lymphoma. Similar to Hodgkin lymphoma, the neoplastic cells in T-cell–rich B-cell lymphoma comprise only a small percentage of the cellular population, and these cells may show Hodgkin-like features in a significant subset of cases. The expression of CD45 along with uniform expression of CD20 would favor T-cell/histiocyte-rich B-cell lymphoma, while expression of CD30 and CD15 would favor Hodgkin lymphoma (Table 20). In addition, the neoplastic cells of T-cell/histiocyte-rich B-cell lymphoma consistently express CD45RA and the B-cell transcription factors BOB.1 and OCT-2, while Hodgkin cells typically lack expression of these markers. Finally, cases of T-cell/histiocyte-rich B-cell lymphoma often express epithelial membrane antigen, a marker positive in less than 10% of cases of classical Hodgkin lymphoma.

Peripheral T-cell lymphoma, particularly when polymorphic, can be easily confused with classical Hodgkin lymphoma. Peripheral T-cell lymphoma often contains an admixture of reactive cells, including eosinophils, histiocytes, and plasma cells. In addition, there may be expression of CD30, particularly in the large cells, giving a close resemblance to mixed cellularity Hodgkin lymphoma. A range of cytologic atypia, from small- to medium-sized to large atypical lymphoid cells, as well as a high mitotic rate would favor peripheral T-cell lymphoma. The neoplastic cells of peripheral T-cell lymphoma typically express

T-lineage antigens, including CD43, as well as CD45, while the large majority of cases of Hodgkin lymphoma express the B-lineage marker PAX-5 and may express EBV-LMP. Anaplastic large-cell lymphoma, although it consistently expresses CD30 and lacks CD45 expression in about one-third of cases, lacks expression of PAX-5 and EBV-LMP and is ALK positive in a significant subset of cases.

Reactive proliferations that may simulate Hodgkin lymphoma include cases of necrotizing granulomatous lymphadenitis, such as cat scratch disease, and reactive paracortical hyperplasia. The low-magnification appearance of necrotizing granulomatous lymphadenitis may closely resemble cases of syncytial nodular sclerosis with central necrosis. The key to the diagnosis is the close examination of the cells lining the areas of necrosis. In Hodgkin lymphoma, those cells are Hodgkin cells, while in necrotizing lymphadenitis, those cells are histiocytes, with or without epithelioid features. In cases in which the histologic differential diagnosis is not clear, immunohistochemical stains can be of great help. Although histiocytes may show a granular cytoplasmic staining for CD15, they are always CD30 negative and usually CD45 positive. In contrast, Hodgkin cells should show consistent staining for CD30 and lack CD45 staining. At times, Hodgkin lymphoma, particularly the mixed cellularity subtype, may show an interfollicular pattern, closely mimicking reactive paracortical hyperplasia. In reactive paracortical hyperplasia, the immunoblasts are usually very evenly dispersed, while in the Hodgkin lymphoma, the atypical cells tend to show irregular clustering. Immunoblasts tend to have a single nucleus with a single prominent nucleolus, but bilobated and multinucleated forms resembling Hodgkin cells may be seen in florid immunoblastic proliferations such as acute infectious mononucleosis. Immunoblasts tend to have strongly basophilic cytoplasm, often with a paranuclear hof, in contrast to Hodgkin cells, which have amphophilic to mildly basophilic cytoplasm without paranuclear hofs. Immunoblasts may show CD30 positivity, but it is often weaker and variable from cell to cell, and they may also show variable staining for CD45. In addition, immunoblasts may show immunoglobulin expression and are consistently CD15 negative.

NODULAR LYMPHOCYTE–PREDOMINANT HODGKIN LYMPHOMA[59,68,174,180,190,191,193,198–212]

Nodular lymphocyte–predominant Hodgkin lymphoma comprises less than 5% of all Hodgkin lymphomas. It affects predominantly males with a 3:1 male-to-female (M:F) ratio. The median age of incidence is about 35 years, with a wide range, and it is not uncommon in children. The majority of patients present with isolated lymphadenopathy, most often in the cervical, axillary, or inguinal regions. About one-half of patients present in stage I, and over three-quarters of patients present in either stage I or II, with only rare B symptoms. Involvement of the spleen occurs in about 10% of cases, and involvement of bone marrow or visceral organs occurs in less than 5% of cases. Patients tend to have an indolent course, with an overall good survival, despite the frequent occurrence of relapses

Figure 125. Nodular lymphocyte–predominant Hodgkin lymphoma. A vague nodular pattern is seen at low magnification. Note that the nodules are larger and more widely spaced than typically seen in follicular lymphoma.

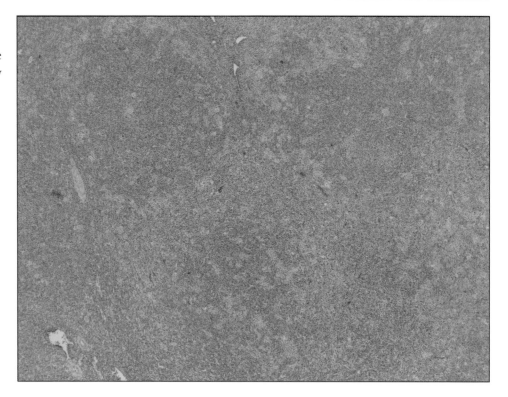

after adequate therapy. In fact, there are some data to suggest that these patients may do well without any therapy beyond excision. Nonetheless, patients treated with protocols for classical Hodgkin lymphoma have outcomes no different than patients with classical Hodgkin lymphoma. In some cases, progressive transformation of germinal centers may occur in patients who have been previously treated for nodular lymphocyte predominance. In addition, transformation to non-Hodgkin lymphoma may occur in up to 5–10% of patients; it is usually, but not always, a B-cell lymphoma, most often of diffuse large-cell type.

Molecular biologic studies have shown that nodular lymphocyte–predominant Hodgkin lymphoma is a monoclonal B-cell neoplasm of germinal center origin. The presence of ongoing mutations of the immunoglobulin genes in about 50% of cases implies a close relationship to follicular lymphoma. There is no significant association with EBV. Some cases have a preceding history of progressive transformation of germinal centers; however, there is no convincing evidence that progressive transformation of germinal centers imparts an increased risk of developing nodular lymphocyte–predominant Hodgkin lymphoma.

Grossly, involved lymph nodes tend to be larger than most other lymphomas. The cut section often reveals a vague or distinct nodular architecture, with a rim of uninvolved lymphoid tissue sometimes discernable. At low magnification, the lymph node shows partial or complete architectural effacement, and the capsule is usually intact. Uninvolved areas may show normal follicles or reactive follicular hyperplasia, with or without progressive transformation of germinal centers. Involved areas usually show replacement by vague or well-formed nodules, which may be highlighted by a wreath of epithelioid histiocytes (Figure 125). Occasionally, a nodular pattern is not easily discernible at low magnification.

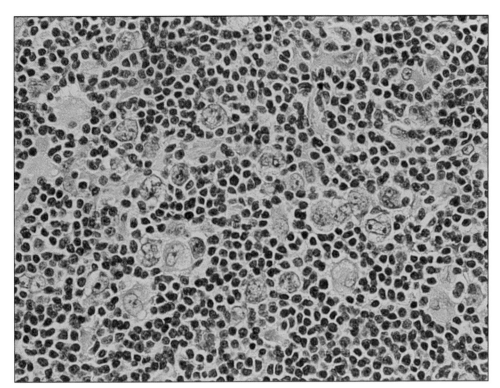

Figure 126. Nodular lymphocyte–predominant Hodgkin lymphoma. Numerous L&H cells are seen in this field, along with scattered epithelioid histiocytes.

The hallmark of nodular lymphocyte–predominant Hodgkin lymphoma is the identification of L&H cells (Figure 126). L&H cells are large cells with a distinctive appearance, although there is some resemblance to centroblasts. The most characteristic feature is the presence of multiple lobulations and other irregularities, giving rise to the alternate names of popcorn or elephant-foot cells (Figure 127). Although the chromatin pattern resembles centroblasts, there are often one or more nucleoli, which are small to medium in size and are usually present adjacent to the nuclear membrane. L&H cells are usually located in and around the nodules, in contrast to centroblasts, which are exclusively present in germinal centers. L&H cells may resemble classic Hodgkin cells, but the presence of more than a few true classical Hodgkin cells should raise suspicion of lymphocyte-rich classical Hodgkin lymphoma. Along with the L&H cells, the nodules consist of small mature lymphocytes, nonstimulated and epithelioid histiocytes, and scattered germinal center cells. They usually lack mantle zones. The internodular areas also show a predominance of small lymphocytes, along with an admixture of nonstimulated and epithelioid histiocytes, plasma cells, and varying numbers of L&H cells.

Immunohistochemical studies show that the majority of the small lymphocytes in the nodules are B-cells encased in a meshwork of CD21-positive/CD23-positive/CD35-positive follicular dendritic cells (Figure 128). In fact, these stains may be helpful in demonstrating patterns that may not be obvious on H&E staining. These patterns have been characterized as classic nodular, serpiginous/interconnected nodular, nodular with prominent extranodular L&H cells, T-cell–rich nodular, diffuse with a T-cell–rich background, and a B-cell–rich pattern. The majority of the small lymphocytes in the internodular areas are

Figure 127. Nodular lymphocyte–predominant Hodgkin lymphoma. Several L&H cells are seen; although they may have prominent nucleoli, they are still not as prominent as typically seen in classical Hodgkin lymphoma. Note highly irregular nuclear outlines.

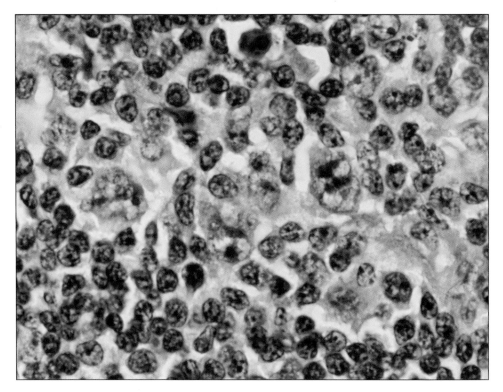

Figure 128. Nodular lymphocyte–predominant Hodgkin lymphoma, CD20 stain. The nodularity is often better seen in immunostains than in H&E-stained sections.

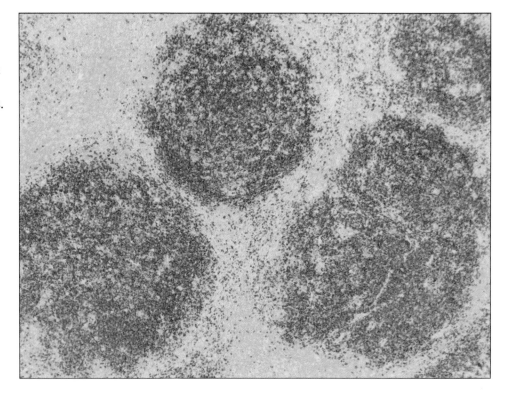

T-cells. The nodules and, to a lesser extent, the interfollicular areas also contain significant numbers of CD4-positive/CD57-positive/bcl-6–positive T-helper/inducer cells, which may form rings around the L&H cells (Figure 129). Over time, there is a tendency for progression to a more diffuse pattern. The number of T-cells tends to increase, in both the nodules and the internodular areas, while

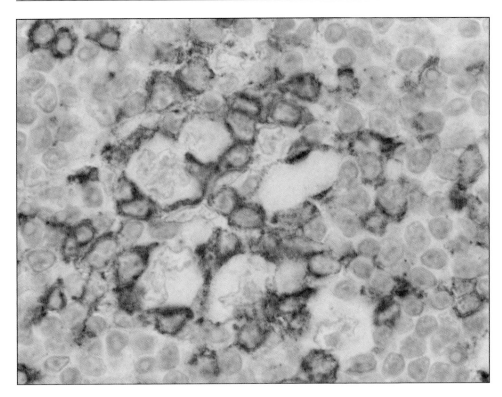

Figure 129. Nodular lymphocyte–predominant Hodgkin lymphoma, CD57 stain. There is a ringing of L&H cells by CD57-positive T-helper cells. These cells are also positive for bcl-6.

the number of CD57-positive cells decreases. Flow cytometry studies have shown large populations of dual CD4-positive and CD8-positive cells in a majority of cases. The immunophenotype of L&H cells is summarized in Table 21. They express CD45 and numerous markers of B-lineage, including CD20, PAX-5, BOB.1, and OCT-2 (Figure 130). They express the germinal center marker bcl-6; however, they are negative for the germinal center marker CD10 and are also usually negative for bcl-2, MUM-1, and CD138. They consistently express the immunoglobulin-associated protein J-chain and often express cytoplasmic immunoglobulin mRNA and protein, which is frequently monotypic for lambda light chain. L&H cells are negative for CD15 and negative to weakly positive for CD30. L&H cell may be positive for epithelial membrane antigen in a majority of cases. They are negative for T-cell and NK-cell markers. Single-cell microdissection studies have demonstrated that L&H have clonal rearrangements of their immunoglobulin genes, but this is not detectable in whole-tissue extracts. Recent FISH studies have demonstrated a t(3;14) in a subset of cases.

The differential diagnosis of nodular lymphocyte–predominant Hodgkin lymphoma includes progressive transformation of germinal center, classical Hodgkin lymphoma, and B-cell lymphoma. Progressive transformation of germinal centers may precede, coexist with, or follow nodular lymphocyte–predominant Hodgkin lymphoma. Progressive transformation always occurs in the context of reactive follicular hyperplasia, with maintenance of the overall lymph node architecture. In contrast, nodular lymphocyte predominance generally occurs in areas of loss of normal architecture and is not typically a focal phenomenon occurring amidst reactive follicles. The nodules in nodular

Table 21. Phenotype of L&H Cells

CD45	+
CD20	+
CD79a	+
PAX-5	+
BOB.1	+
OCT-2	+
Bcl-6	+
Ig J-chains	+
Bcl-2	−
CD10	−
MUM-1	−
CD138	−
CD30	−/+ (weak)
EMA	+ (75%)
T/NK markers	−

Figure 130. Nodular lymphocyte–predominant Hodgkin lymphoma, CD20 stain. The L&H cells are positive, as well as numerous small lymphoid cells in the background. This picture was taken at the edge of one of the B-cell nodules.

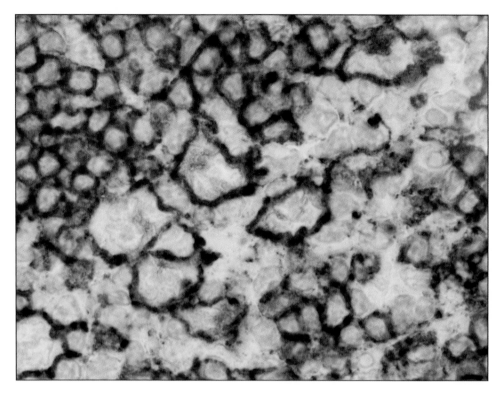

Table 22. Classical Hodgkin Lymphoma vs. Nodular Lymphocyte–Predominant Hodgkin Lymphoma

	CHD	NLPHD
CD45	−	+
CD20	−/+	+
CD30	+	−/+ (weak)
CD15	+	−
MUM-1	+	−
BOB.1	−	+
OCT-2	−	+
Bcl-6	−/+	+
EBV-LMP	+/−	−

lymphocyte predominance tend to show an irregular, *broken-up* pattern with B-lineage markers. The most important criterion, however, is the specific identification of L&H cells in nodular lymphocyte predominance. Although this distinction can usually be made on morphologic features alone, L&H cells usually show T-cell or CD57-positive rosettes highlighting the atypical cells, which are CD10 negative and may be epithelial membrane antigen positive, while centroblasts only rarely show T-cell or CD57-positive rosettes and are usually CD10 positive and consistently epithelial membrane antigen negative.

Classical Hodgkin lymphoma, specifically the lymphocyte-rich subtype, may be extremely difficult to distinguish from nodular lymphocyte predominance; in fact, they may be virtually identical histologically and only clearly separable by immunohistochemical studies. The major diagnostically useful markers are summarized in Table 22. CD45 expression may be very difficult to interpret when numerous small lymphocytes abut Hodgkin cells. CD30 expression may be a little difficult to interpret, as L&H cells may show weak CD30 expression, and scattered CD30-positive immunoblasts may be present, which must be distinguished from staining of L&H cells. Almost all cases of classical Hodgkin lymphoma express MUM-1 and lack expression of both BOB.1 and OCT-2 and most cases lack bcl-6; in contrast, L&H cells almost always lack MUM-1, while BOB.1, OCT-2, and bcl-6 are consistent markers of L&H cells.

The distinction of nodular lymphocyte–predominant Hodgkin lymphoma and B-cell lymphoma, particularly T-cell/histiocyte-rich B-cell lymphoma, can be quite confusing. The neoplastic cells of both tumors essentially have identical immunophenotypes. I make the distinction based on three criteria: First, if there is a nodular pattern, either seen histologically or with the benefit of immuno-histochemical studies, I prefer a diagnosis of nodular lymphocyte–predominant Hodgkin lymphoma. Second, if there are large numbers of CD57-positive cells, particularly if ringing is seen, I also prefer a diagnosis of nodular lymphocyte–predominant Hodgkin lymphoma. Finally, if there is a previous documented diagnosis of nodular lymphocyte predominance, I will diagnose recurrence even in the absence of the first two criteria. Not all hematopathologists agree with my approach, especially in regard to the last criterion. Some hematopathologists prefer a diagnosis of T-cell/histiocyte-rich B-cell lymphoma if there is splenic involvement, because splenic involvement imparts a worse prognosis.

Nodular lymphocyte–predominant Hodgkin lymphoma may be complicated by the occurrence of a non-Hodgkin lymphoma, usually of diffuse large B-cell type, which may occur in 1–10% of cases. The distinction between nodular lymphocyte predominance and a coexistent diffuse large-cell lymphoma may be difficult. One may see large numbers of L&H cells in nodular lymphocyte predominance, particularly within the follicles. I prefer a diagnosis of diffuse large B-cell lymphoma when sheets of large B-cells are seen outside of the follicles. Immunostains for CD20 may be helpful in evaluating the number and distribution of large B-cells.

7 NON-HODGKIN LYMPHOMA

Chronic Lymphocytic Leukemia/Small Lymphocytic
    Lymphoma — 125
Lymphoplasmacytic Lymphoma — 130
Plasmacytoma — 133
Hairy Cell Leukemia — 135
Nodal Marginal Zone B-Cell Lymphoma — 138
Extranodal Marginal Zone B-Cell Lymphoma of
    Mucosa-Associated Lymphoid Tissue (MALT)
    Involving Lymph Nodes — 142
Splenic Marginal Zone Lymphoma Involving Lymph
    Nodes and Primary Nodal Marginal Zone
    Lymphoma of Splenic Type — 143
Follicular Lymphoma — 145
Mantle Cell Lymphoma — 156
Diffuse Large B-Cell Lymphoma — 161
Burkitt Lymphoma — 175
Precursor B-Lymphoblastic Lymphoma/Leukemia — 181
Precursor T-Lymphoblastic Lymphoma/Leukemia — 183
Mature T-Cell and NK-Cell Neoplasms — 187
Angioimmunoblastic T-Cell Lymphoma — 187
Peripheral T-Cell Lymphoma, Unspecified — 190
Anaplastic Large-Cell Lymphoma, ALK-Negative Type — 197
Anaplastic Large-Cell Lymphoma, ALK-Positive Type — 200
Mycosis Fungoides/Sezary Syndrome — 205
Adult T-Cell Leukemia/Lymphoma — 208
T-Cell Prolymphocytic Leukemia — 209
Other Mature T- and NK-Cell Neoplasms — 210
    T-Cell Large Granular Lymphocytic Leukemia — 211
    Aggressive NK-Cell Leukemia — 211
    Extranodal NK/T-Cell Lymphoma, Nasal Type — 212
    Enteropathy-Associated T-Cell Lymphoma — 213
    Hepatosplenic T-Cell Lymphoma — 213
    Subcutaneous Panniculitis-Like T-Cell Lymphoma — 215

Table 23. Ann Arbor Staging System for Non-Hodgkin Lymphoma

Stage	Definition
I	Involvement of a single lymph node region or lymphoid organ or of a single extranodal organ or site (IE)
II	Involvement of two or more lymph node regions on the same side of the diaphragm, or localized involvement of an extranodal site or organ (IIE) and one or more lymph node regions on the same side of the diaphragm
III	Involvement of lymph node regions on both sides of the diaphragm, which may also be accompanied by localized involvement of an extranodal organ or site (IIIE) or spleen (IIIS) or both (IIISE)
IV	Diffuse or disseminated involvement of one or more distant extranodal organs

The spleen is considered nodal.

Non-Hodgkin lymphoma[213–219] can be defined as all neoplasms of lymphoid origin other than Hodgkin lymphoma. It represents one of the major malignancies, with about 50,000 new cases a year, roughly five times the incidence of Hodgkin lymphoma. On a biological level, it represents a heterogenous group of neoplasms of B-cell, T-cell, or NK-cell lineage. Therefore, it occurs in adults and children (with a predominance in adults) and males and females (with a 1.3:1 M:F ratio). Some cases are due to HTLV-1 infection and other cases due to HHV-8 infection, and some are associated with EBV and some are associated with hepatitis C. Some are due to immunosuppression from a wide variety of causes, and environmental factors, such as hair dyes, herbicides, and organic chemicals, may be causative in a small proportion of cases.

Patients typically present with a painless mass or multiple masses, with or without systemic symptomas and/or hepatosplenomegaly. Although presentation in lymph nodes is most common, extranodal masses are not uncommon and are particularly frequent in certain subtypes. Although progression of disease does not occur in as orderly a fashion as in Hodgkin lymphoma, the Ann Arbor staging system is still used for non-Hodgkin lymphoma (Table 23). An International Prognostic Index has been developed, based on age, stage, number of extranodal sites of disease, performance status, and serum lactate dehydrogenase levels, originally used for diffuse aggressive lymphomas but probably showing some significance in a variety of other types (see Table 24).

Pathologic classification is important in the evaluation of non-Hodgkin lymphoma. As everyone in medicine is aware, there have been numerous proposed classifications of non-Hodgkin lymphomas, based on a wide variety of criteria. Rather than this text serving as a historical record of futility, I will only present the current widely used classification, that of the WHO. This classification, originally described in 2001 and modified in 2008, represented an international effort of both pathologists and clinicians and is based on a combination of clinical, histologic, and biologic characteristics (see Table 25). It first separates the neoplasms into precursor lymphoid neoplasms, mature B-cell neoplasms, mature T-cell and NK-cell neoplasms, Hodgkin lymphoma, and histiocytic and

Table 24. International Prognostic Index For Aggressive Non-Hodgkin Lymphoma[214]

1. Age >60 years
2. Serum lactate dehydrogenase
3. Performance status >2
4. Stage: III or IV
5. Extranodal sites >1

Low risk	0–1 factors
Low-intermediate	2 factors
High-intermediate	3 factors
High risk	4–5 factors

Table 25. WHO Classification of B- and T-cell Neoplasms (as applied to lymph nodes)[213]

Mature B-cell neoplasms

Chronic lymphocytic leukemia/small lymphocytic lymphoma

Lymphoplasmacytic lymphoma

Plasmacytoma

Hairy cell leukemia

Nodal marginal zone B-cell lymphoma

Extranodal marginal zone B-cell lymphoma of mucosa-associated lymphoid tissue

Splenic marginal zone lymphoma

Follicular lymphoma

Mantle cell lymphoma

Diffuse large B-cell lymphoma, unspecified

Diffuse large B-cell lymphoma variants

    Primary mediastinal (thymic) large B-cell lymphoma

    T-cell/histiocyte-rich large B-cell lymphoma

    Intravascular large B-cell lymphoma

    ALK-positive diffuse large B-cell lymphoma

    Plasmablastic lymphoma

    Diffuse large B-cell lymphoma associated with chronic inflammation

    Primary effusion lymphoma

    Lymphoma associated with HHV-8–associated multicentric Castleman disease

Burkitt lymphoma

B-cell lymphoma with features intermediate between diffuse large B-cell lymphoma and Burkitt lymphoma

B-cell lymphoma with features intermediate between diffuse large B-cell lymphoma and classical Hodgkin lymphoma

Precursor lymphoid neoplasms

Precursor B-lymphoblastic lymphoma/leukemia

Precursor T-lymphoblastic lymphoma/leukemia

Precursor NK-lymphoblastic lymphoma/leukemia

Mature T-cell and NK-cell neoplasms

Angioimmunoblastic T-cell lymphoma

Peripheral T-cell lymphoma, unspecified

Anaplastic large-cell lymphoma, ALK-negative

Anaplastic large-cell lymphoma, ALK-positive

Mycosis fungoides/Sezary syndrome

Adult T-cell leukemia/lymphoma

T-cell prolymphocytic leukemia

Extranodal NK/T-cell lymphoma, nasal type

Enteropathy-associated T-cell lymphoma

Hepatosplenic T-cell lymphoma

Subcutaneous panniculitis-like T-cell lymphoma

Figure 131. Chronic lymphocytic leukemia/small lymphocytic lymphoma. Note the presence of scattered paler areas – the pseudoproliferation centers. This feature is distinctive for this neoplasm.

dendritic cell neoplasms. Then, within each category, it delineates specific clinicopathobiologic entities.

CHRONIC LYMPHOCYTIC LEUKEMIA/SMALL LYMPHOCYTIC LYMPHOMA[220-233]

The WHO Classification recognizes that chronic lymphocytic leukemia and small lymphocytic lymphoma essentially represent the same biologic process. It represents approximately 5–10% of malignant lymphomas in lymph node–based series and is by far the commonest chronic leukemia in hematology series. There is an M:F ratio of about 2:1. It primarily affects older adults, with a median age of incidence of about 65, and is extraordinarily rare in children. Most patients present with an asymptomatic lymphocytosis. A minority present with painless lymphadenopathy without peripheral blood involvement, which usually occurs later in the course of the disease. The cervical, supraclavicular, or axillary regions are most often involved. Patients may also have accompanying autoimmune hemolytic anemia or hepatosplenomegaly. The neoplasm is relatively indolent, but, as yet, incurable. The overall median survival is between 5 and 10 years, partially reflecting the older age group affected. Standard treatment typically includes purine nucleoside analogues such as fludarabine.

Lymph node biopsies almost always show effacement of normal architecture by a diffuse or vaguely nodular process (Figure 131). In a small minority of cases, focal or striking paracortical involvement is seen, with preservation of follicles; this appearance is not uncommon when the lymphoma is found in the course of

Figure 132. Chronic lymphocytic leukemia/small lymphocytic lymphoma. The pseudoproliferation centers contain a higher concentration of prolymphocytes than seen in the adjacent lymph node parenchyma.

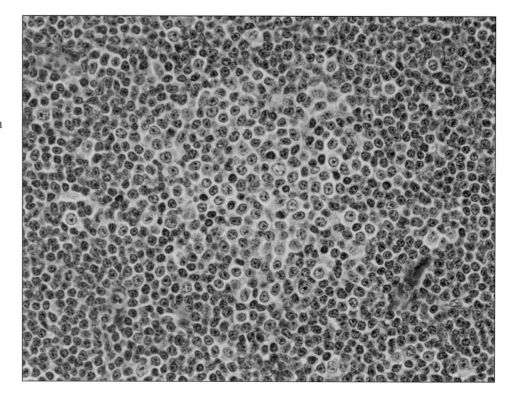

biopsies taken for other purposes (such as staging for carcinoma). The vaguely nodular appearance is imparted by the presence of pale areas called proliferation centers (pseudofollicles), which are present in nearly all cases; occasionally they are so prominent as to resemble true follicles (Figure 132). At high magnification, the most numerous cell type is a small lymphoid cell, at or slightly larger than the size of a normal resting lymphocyte (Figure 133). The chromatin pattern is either condensed or clumped, and there may be a small discernible nucleolus. The nuclear outline is usually smooth and round, although some irregularities may be seen in a subset of cases. The cytoplasm is usually scanty, but a subset of cases may show some plasmacytoid features. The small lymphoid cells are invariably accompanied by scattered larger cells, with larger nuclei with a more vesicular chromatin pattern. These cells cluster within the proliferation centers, and have been separated into medium-sized cells with small nucleoli, termed prolymphocytes, and larger cells with medium to large nucleoli and more abundant cytoplasm, termed paraimmunoblasts or immunoblasts. Mitotic figures, when seen, usually occur within the proliferation centers.

Chronic lymphocytic leukemia/small lymphocytic lymphoma shows a characteristic immunophenotype (Table 26). They consistently express pan-B-cell markers, although weak expression of CD20 may be present by flow cytometry. They also consistently aberrantly coexpress CD43 and CD5 in greater than 95% of cases (Figure 134). They are also positive for CD23, although this marker is occasionally false negative in paraffin section immunohistochemical studies (Figure 135). The neoplastic cells are usually negative for CD10 and cyclin D1, although a small subset of cases may show weak cyclin D1 positivity. Those cases with a mutator phenotype are positive for ZAP-70, although this marker may be

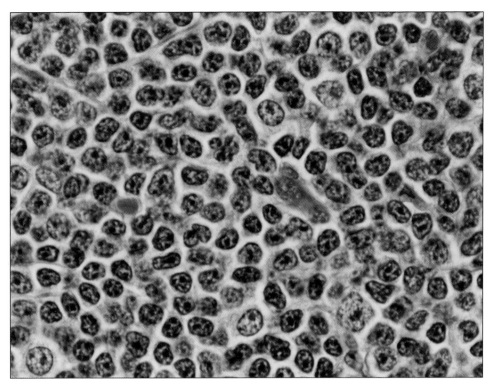

Figure 133. Chronic lymphocytic leukemia/small lymphocytic lymphoma. Most of the cells are small, with a relatively mature chromatin pattern. In addition, there are scattered slightly larger cells, with a more vesicular chromatin pattern and with more prominent single nucleoli, the prolymphocytes.

Table 26. Differential Diagnosis of Small Lymphocytic Lymphoproliferations

	SLL/CLL	Lymphoplasmacytic	Marginal	Follicular	Mantle
Ig	98%	98%	98%	90%	98%
Heavy	IgM ± IgD	IgM	IgM, D, A	IgM, G	IgM + IgD
K:L	2:1	2:1	2:1	2:1	1:1
CD20	99%	98%	98%	100%	99%
CD43	98%	60%	50%	2%	80%
CD5	98%	25%	10%	1%	90%
CD10	1%	1%	1%	95%	1%
CD23	90%	10%	5%	15%	5%
Cyclin D1	5%	5%	0%	0%	95%

problematic in paraffin section immunohistochemical studies. Ki-67 studies usually demonstrate a low proliferation rate in diffuse areas, but can be quite high (over 50%) in the proliferation centers (consistent with their name).

Molecular studies show consistent clonal rearrangement of the immunoglobulin heavy and/or light chain genes. Approximately one-half of cases show no evidence of somatic mutations in the variable region genes, consistent with a naive phenotype, while the other one-half of cases do show somatic mutations, consistent with post–germinal center memory B-cell differentiation. Classical cytogenetic studies are often negative, due to the relatively low proliferation rate of the neoplasm, but interphase FISH studies are useful in detecting a variety of abnormalities in over 80% of cases (see Table 27).[234] Those cases with 13q14

Figure 134. Chronic lymphocytic leukemia/small lymphocytic lymphoma, CD5 stain. Note the two levels of staining, with scattered cells, presumably representing reactive T-cells, staining strongly for CD5, while the majority of the population, presumably the neoplastic B-cells, show a weaker level of positivity.

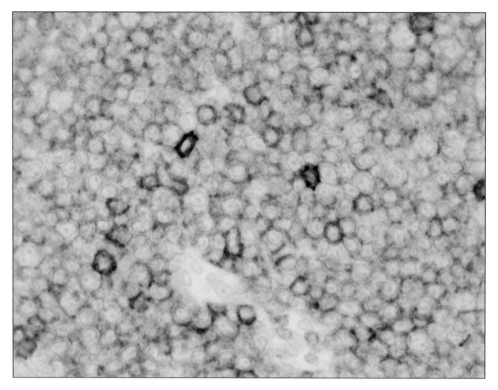

Figure 135. Chronic lymphocytic leukemia/small lymphocytic lymphoma, CD23 stain. At left is staining of a residual follicle, while most of the cells show weak expression of CD23, characteristic of this neoplasm.

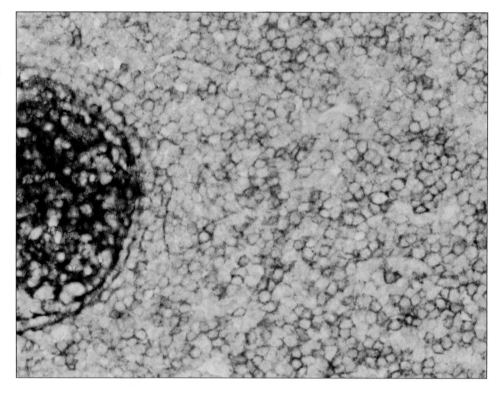

abnormalities are more likely to have somatic mutations, while those cases with deletions of 11q23 (ataxia telangiectasia–mutated [ATM] gene locus) and 17p (p53 gene locus) are more likely to show a naive phenotype. Deletions at 11q22–23 are associated with younger patients of male sex who often present with generalized lymphadenopathy.

The Rai and Binet systems are the most frequently used clinical staging systems (see Tables 28 and 29). The International Workshop on Chronic Lymphocytic Leukemia recommends a system that integrates the previous two systems, but this system is not popular and is most commonly used in reports of clinical trials. Additional adverse prognostic features include older age, male sex, a diffuse pattern of bone marrow infiltration, high Ki-67 index, high serum levels of thymidine kinase, β2-microglobulin, soluble CD23, and tumor necrosis-α, unmutated variable regions (indirectly reflected by expression of ZAP-70 and CD38), deletion of 11q23, and loss or mutation of the p53 gene. Determination of ZAP-70 and CD38 expression is difficult to determine in paraffin sections and can be even problematic by flow cytometry. The presence of a deletion at 13q14 or the absence of any cytogenetic abnormalities is associated with a good prognosis.

The differential diagnosis includes other B-cell lymphomas and Hodgkin lymphoma. Some cases of chronic lymphocytic leukemia/small lymphocytic lymphoma may have small lymphoid cells with some nuclear atypicality, and, conversely, some cases of mantle cell lymphoma may be composed of small lymphoid cells without evident nuclear irregularities. The presence of definite proliferation centers should exclude mantle cell lymphoma, which always lacks these structures. Immunophenotypically, these two lymphomas typically share CD5 and CD43 coexpression, and both typically lack CD10 expression. Over 95% of cases of mantle cell lymphoma are strongly cyclin D1 positive, and although some cases of chronic lymphocytic lymphoma/small lymphocytic lymphoma may show cyclin D1 positivity, the staining is usually weak. In addition, mantle cell lymphoma is typically CD23 negative, in contrast to chronic lymphocytic leukemia/small lymphocytic lymphoma. Almost all cases of mantle cell lymphoma carry the t(11;14) translocation, which although has been reported in the past in a small number of cases of chronic lymphocytic leukemia rules out that diagnosis at this point in time. Nodal marginal zone B-cell lymphoma usually consists of cells that have slightly larger nuclei and more abundant cleared cytoplasm than chronic lymphocytic leukemia/small lymphocytic lymphoma. Although scattered larger cells are typical of marginal zone lymphoma, they are not aggregated into proliferation centers. In addition, marginal zone lymphoma much more often shows plasmacytic differentiation. Marginal zone lymphoma may show coexpression of CD43 (about 50% of cases), and may even show CD5 coexpression (less than 10% of cases), but does not share the cytogenetic abnormalities typical of chronic lymphocytic leukemia/small lymphocytic lymphoma.

Approximately 3% of cases of chronic lymphocytic leukemia/small lymphocytic lymphoma undergo transformation to diffuse large B-cell lymphoma (Richter transformation). In a small subset of cases, one sees paraimmunoblastic features, in which the neoplastic cells have the appearance of paraimmunoblasts, cells with nuclei slightly smaller and more uniform than the cells of typical diffuse large B-cell lymphoma, with single moderately sized nucleoli (Figure 136). Occasionally, the lymphomas may show immunoblastic features, but most often the morphologic features are nonspecific. They may or may not share the same clone as the original neoplasm. The distinction between chronic

Table 27. CLL/SLL: Molecular Cytogenetics[231,234]

Deletions at 13q (up to 50%) (good prognosis)

Trisomy 12 (20%) (aggressive)

Deletions at 6q21 (5%) (aggressive)

Deletions at 11q22–23 (20%) (more aggressive)

Deletions at 17p13 (10%) (more aggressive)

Table 28. Rai Staging System for Chronic Lymphocytic Leukemia/ Small Lymphocytic Lymphoma[227]

Stage 0: Lymphocytosis

Stage I: Lymphadenopathy

Stage II: Hepatomegaly or splenomegaly

Stage III: Anemia

Stage IV: Thrombocytosis

Table 29. Binet Staging System for Chronic Lymphocytic Leukemia/ Small Lymphocytic Lymphoma[228]

Group A: <3 areas of lymphadenopathy

Group B: ≥3 areas of lymphadenopathy

Group C: Anemia <10 g/dL or thrombocytopenia <100,000/μL

Figure 136. Chronic lymphocytic leukemia/small lymphocytic lymphoma, with paraimmunoblastic transformation. The cells are intermediate in size, but have a vesicular chromatin pattern with distinct nucleoli. The prognosis of these cases is intermediate between chronic lymphocytic leukemia/small lymphocytic lymphoma and more typical cases of Richter transformation.

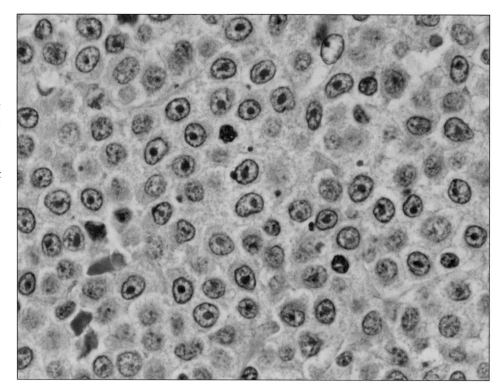

lymphocytic leukemia/small lymphocytic lymphoma and transformation to diffuse large B-cell lymphoma may be difficult. As long as the large cells are organized into proliferation centers, I do not diagnose transformation; I only diagnose transformation to diffuse large B-cell lymphoma when disorganized sheets of large cells are present.

Less frequently, probably occurring in less than 1% of cases, there is transformation of chronic lymphocytic leukemia/small lymphocytic lymphoma to classical Hodgkin lymphoma. Usually, this manifests as scattered Hodgkin cells arising within the B-cell proliferation, usually with an immediate rim of T-cells (Figure 137). The Hodgkin cells have the typical immunophenotype of classical Hodgkin lymphoma, and most of the cases are EBV associated. Studies of small number of cases have suggested that EBV-negative Hodgkin transformation represents a clonal transformation of the original neoplasm, while EBV-associated Hodgkin lymphoma represents a distinct clonal expansion unrelated to the original neoplasm.

LYMPHOPLASMACYTIC LYMPHOMA[235]

Lymphoplasmacytic lymphoma is a low-grade B-cell neoplasm with differentiation toward small lymphocytes, plasmacytoid lymphoid cells, and plasma cells. It represents the major subset of patients with the clinical syndrome of Waldenstrom macroglobulinemia, that is, the presence of a monoclonal IgM serum paraprotein greater than 3 g/dL, with a resulting hyperviscosity syndrome, cryoglobulinemia syndrome, and/or cold agglutinin anemia. However, it is not

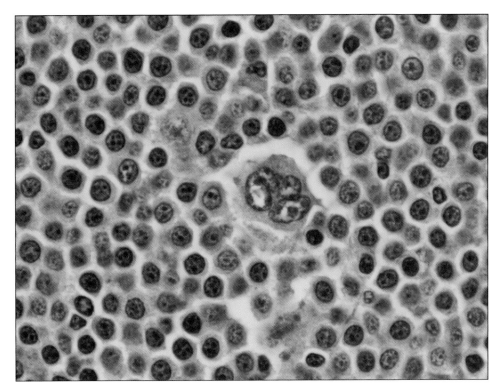

Figure 137. Chronic lymphocytic leukemia/small lymphocytic lymphoma, with transformation to Hodgkin lymphoma. A classical Reed-Sternberg cell is seen in a background of chronic lymphocytic leukemia/small lymphocytic lymphoma. The Hodgkin cells in this case were positive for CD30, CD15, and EBV-LMP, while the background lymphoid cells expressed B-lineage markers with coexpression of CD43 and CD5.

entirely synonymous with Waldenstrom macroglobulinemia, since this latter syndrome may be seen in several other malignant lymphomas associated with IgM paraproteinemia, including chronic lymphocytic leukemia/small lympho-cytic lymphoma and splenic marginal zone lymphoma. Conversely, some patients with lymphoplasmacytic lymphoma do not present with clinical fea-tures of Waldenstrom macroglobulinemia. These latter patients usually have generalized lymphadenopathy, often with splenomegaly. Lymphoplasmacytic lymphoma represents about 1% of lymphomas occurring in the lymph nodes. Patients are typically older adults, with a slight male predominance, and there may be an association with hepatitis C infection. The neoplasm is indolent but, as yet, incurable. Patients are typically treated with alkylating agents and, more recently, purine analogs, including fludarabine or cladribine. The hyperviscosity syndrome is treated symptomatically, often using plasmapheresis.

Histologically, one sees diffuse effacement of architecture or a preferentially paracortical process, occasionally with patent sinuses. At high magnification, there is a mixture of small, mature lymphoid cells, mature plasma cells, and cells with intermediate features (Figure 138). Dutcher bodies, intranuclear PAS-positive inclusions, are frequently seen (Figure 139). There are usually also variable numbers of immunoblasts, often with plasmacytoid features. There may also be scattered epithelioid histiocytes and mast cells. Immunophenotyping studies show expres-sion of pan-B-cell antigens and membrane and cytoplasmic expression of mono-typic immunoglobulin, most often (but not exclusively) of IgM type. The cells are CD5, CD10, cyclin D1, and CD23 negative, but they frequently aberrantly coexpress CD43 (Table 26). Molecular studies reveal monoclonal rearrangement of the immunoglobulin heavy and/or light chain genes, with somatic mutations in

Figure 138.
Lymphoplasmacytic
lymphoma/Waldenstrom
macroglobulinemia. There is
an intimate admixture of
lymphoid cells, plasma cells,
and intermediate forms.

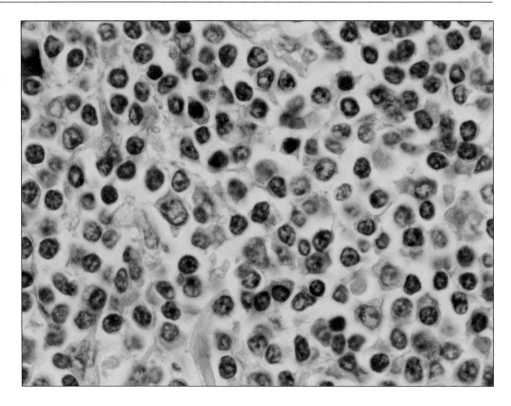

Figure 139.
Lymphoplasmacytic
lymphoma/Waldenstrom
macroglobulinemia. The cells
appear to be more lymphoid
than plasmacytic, but
numerous Dutcher bodies
are seen.

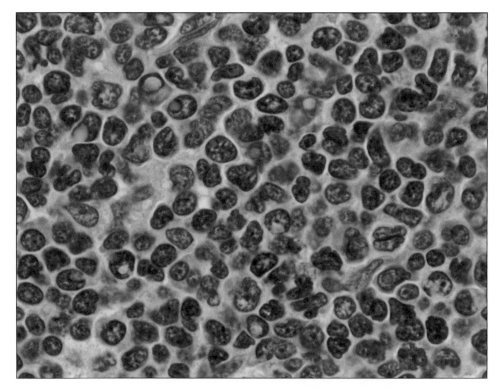

the variable region genes, consistent with post–germinal center differentiation. A subset of cases are associated with a t(9;14)(p13;q32), involving the PAX-5 gene.

The differential diagnosis includes any malignant lymphoma that can show lymphoplasmacytoid differentiation. Chronic lymphocytic leukemia/small lymphocytic lymphoma may show plasmacytoid differentiation, but it is usually subtle.

Lymphoplasmacytic lymphoma lacks proliferation centers, which are typically seen in chronic lymphocytic leukemia/small lymphocytic lymphoma. In addition, CD5 is almost always positive in chronic lymphocytic leukemia/small lymphocytic lymphoma and is consistently negative in lymphoplasmacytic lymphoma. Marginal zone B-cell lymphoma, of both nodal and extranodal type, may frequently show plasmacytic differentiation. In marginal zone lymphoma, a preferentially marginal zone pattern of infiltration is often seen. In addition, the plasmacytic differentiation is most often distinct from the lymphoid population, both architecturally and cytologically; that is, areas of plasma cells are often present compartmentalized from other areas showing lymphoid features and without a gradual admixture of intermediate cells. In addition, the small lymphoid cells usually show more nuclear irregularities and a greater amount of clear or pale cytoplasm. In a subset of cases of lymphoplasmacytic lymphoma, there is transformation to a diffuse large B-cell lymphoma, often of immunoblastic type. I do not diagnose large-cell transformation unless there are patternless sheets of large cells, without large numbers of intervening small lymphocytes and lymphoplasmcytoid forms.

PLASMACYTOMA[239–242]

Plasma cell neoplasms are clonal proliferations of mature immunoglobulin-secreting B-cells. The bone marrow–based plasma cell myeloma is by far the most common plasma cell neoplasm; however, it rarely if ever presents in lymph nodes, and any lymph node involvement is completely incidental to other more significant disease. Lymph node involvement may also occur as local spread from another extraosseus (extramedullary) plasmacytoma. Finally, and perhaps the rarest manifestation of plasma cell neoplasms involving the lymph node, primary plasmacytoma may occur within lymph nodes. These cases usually involve older adults, with no age predilection. Most patients do not progress after surgical excision, although a minority may show progression to a systemic plasma cell neoplasm.

Histologically, involved lymph nodes are typically enlarged, with an intact capsule. The cortical follicles are retained, but the remaining lymph node parenchyma shows sheets of plasma cells, with extension into the sinuses. The plasma cells are usually monotonous, without significant atypia, although some cases may show more enlarged nuclei, irregular nuclear contours, prominent nucleoli, and binuclear cells (Figures 140A and 140B). Dutcher bodies (intranuclear inclusions) and Russell bodies (intracytoplasmic inclusions) are usually readily identified in most cases. Occasional cases may show plasmablastic features (Figure 141), mimicking a plasmablastic or immunoblastic lymphoma, and requiring knowledge of the clinical and laboratory findings to make the distinctions. There is no evidence of a neoplastic lymphocytic infiltrate associated with the plasma cells or in other parts of the lymph nodes. Some cases may show associated amyloid deposition.

Immunophenotypic studies show the phenotype of mature plasma cells, with cytoplasmic immunoglobulin showing light chain restriction and expression of CD138, CD79a, CD38, CD43, and CD56 in most cases. There is usually no

Figure 140A. Plasmacytoma, involving lymph node. An extensive infiltrate of plasma cells is seen, essentially replacing the lymph node parenchyma.

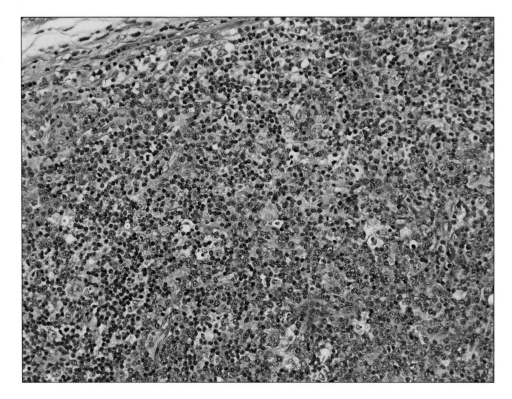

Figure 140B. Plasmacytoma, involving lymph node. The cells show obvious but somewhat atypical plasma cell differentiation. A Dutcher body is seen at the bottom.

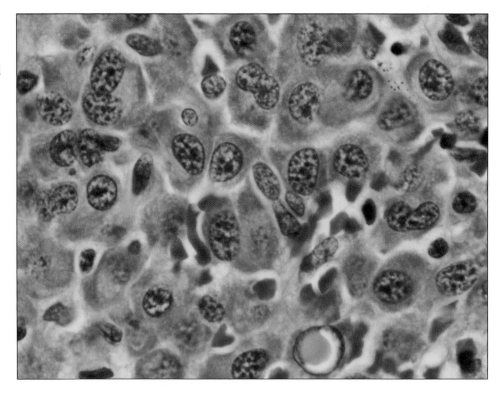

staining for CD45, CD20, CD19, or PAX-5. PCR studies show monoclonal (or occasionally multiclonal) rearrangements of the immunoglobulin heavy and/or light chain genes. FISH studies often demonstrate translocations involving the immunoglobulin heavy chain locus, as well as hyperdiploidy and other specific abnormalities (see Table 30). There is no evidence of EBV or HHV-8.

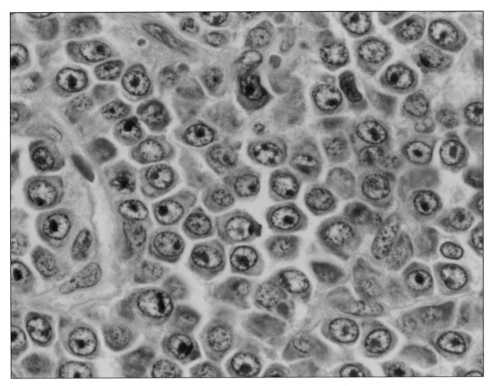

Figure 141. Plasmacytoma, involving lymph node. Plasmablastic features are seen. Immunostains for CD45, CD20, and CD138, as well as clinical information, would be useful in making the distinction with plasmablastic or immunoblastic lymphoma.

The differential diagnosis includes reactive plasma cell infiltrates, Castleman disease, or malignant lymphomas with a plasmacytic component. The demonstration of monotypic light chain restriction should eliminate the possibility of reactive plasma cell infiltrates. The plasma cell and multicentric variants of Castleman disease may show monocytic lambda (but not kappa) light chain restriction; however, these cases are usually associated with systemic symptoms typical of these variants of Castleman disease (fever, night sweats, malaise) and are usually associated with increased serum IL-6. Histologically, they usually also contain plasmacytoid immunoblasts or HHV-8–positive plasmablasts in addition to plasma cells. Lymphomas with a plasmacytic component, particularly nodal marginal zone B-cell lymphoma with extensive plasmacytic differentiation and lymphoplasmacytic lymphoma, are probably most easily confused with plasmacytoma of lymph nodes. Nodal marginal zone B-cell lymphoma may show areas with sheets of cells showing plasma cell differentiation, but at least some other areas of lymphoid cell differentiation should also be present. These areas are often highlighted by CD45, CD20, or PAX-5 stains. Lymphoplasmacytic lymphoma usually shows a more even admixture of lymphocytes, lymphoplasmacytic cells, and plasma cells, while plasmacytoma on the other hand consists of a relatively monotonous population of plasma cells.

Table 30. Plasma Cell Neoplasms: Molecular Genetics[241,242]

50% of MGUS and myeloma have IgH translocations

    11q13 (BCL1) (15%) (good prognosis)

    6p21 (CCND3) (5%) (good prognosis)

    4p16.3 (FGFR-3 and MMSET) (15%) (aggressive)

    16q23 (c-MAF) (5%) (aggressive)

    20q11 (MAFB) (2%) (aggressive)

50% associated with hyperdiploidy (good prognosis)

HAIRY CELL LEUKEMIA[243–245]

Hairy cell leukemia is a chronic lymphoproliferative disorder of small B-cells with distinctive *hairy* projections. It is uncommon, occurring in adults, with

Figure 142. Hairy cell leukemia. A paracortical distribution is seen. Incidental anthracotic pigment is also seen.

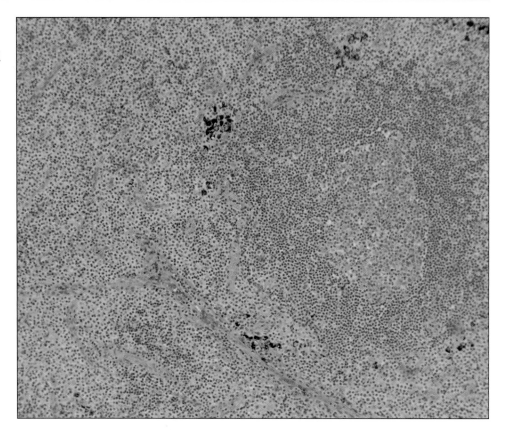

a distinct male predilection. Patients usually present with abdominal fullness due to splenomegaly, systemic symptoms, or complications of cytopenia. The disease manifests primarily in spleen and bone marrow, and most patients have pancytopenia at the time of diagnosis. Lymph node involvement other than splenic hilar lymph nodes is rare at diagnosis, but eventually occurs in about 15% of patients. It is usually of no clinical significance, with the exception of a syndrome of massive abdominal lymphadenopathy centered about the celiac axis. Although most patients with massive abdominal lymphadenopathy still respond to therapy, usually 2-chlorodeoxyadenosine, there is a relative resistance to treatment.

Involved lymph nodes typically show a marginal zone or paracortical pattern of infiltration, with sparing of follicles and nodal sinuses almost always preserved (Figure 142). Although blood lake formation is unusual, extravasated erythrocytes are common within and around the hairy cell infiltrate, and scattered plasma cells are also typically seen. At high magnification, the cells usually have small round, oval to reniform nuclei, with a relatively mature chromatin pattern and indistinct nucleoli (Figure 143). The cytoplasm is usually relatively abundant, with distinct cell membranes imparting a *fried-eggs* appearance. In some cases with massive abdominal lymphadenopathy, a more atypical appearance may be seen, with an admixed population of larger hyperchromatic cells with oval or reniform nuclei and prominent nucleoli, consistent with blastically transformed hairy cells.

Immunophenotypic studies show a mature B-cell phenotype, with expression of CD45, multiple B-lineage antigens, and surface immunoglobulin. CD20

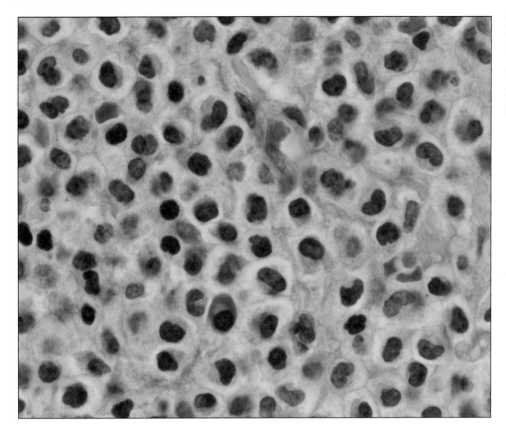

Figure 143. Hairy cell leukemia. The nuclei are bland and often reniform. The moderate cytoplasm shows a fried-eggs appearance with a zone of peripheral clearing.

staining often shows a distinctive thick granular membrane pattern of staining. In addition, hairy cells are positive for CD11a, CD25, FMC-7, CD103, DBA.44, and tartrate-resistant acid phosphatase and are negative for CD5, CD10, and CD23. A subset of the hairy cells often show a dim nuclear positivity for cyclin D1. The Ki-67 index is usually below 10%. Molecular studies show clonal rearrangements of the immunoglobulin heavy and/or light chain genes. There are no recurrent chromosomal abnormalities. Despite the frequent staining for cyclin D1, there is no t(11;14).

The differential diagnosis is usually not a problem when there is adequate clinical history available. Involvement of splenic hilar lymph nodes does not occur without spleen involvement, and abdominal lymphadenopathy usually only occurs in patients with longstanding disease. Nodal marginal zone B-cell lymphoma, splenic marginal zone B-cell lymphoma, mast cell disease, and even metastatic lobular carcinoma of the breast may all be confused with hairy cell leukemia without an adequate history. The marginal zone lymphomas can all be virtually indistinguishable from hairy cell leukemia involving lymph node, requiring immunohistochemical analysis. Both CD103 and tartrate-resistant acid phosphatase stains may be helpful, although neither antibody alone has a high specificity. Cyclin D1 stains may also be useful, as this antibody is consistently negative in the marginal zone lymphomas. Although cyclin D1 positivity may raise consideration of mantle cell lymphoma, the staining is usually much weaker and is only present in a subset of the cells. Mast cell disease usually has admixed eosinophils and is CD117 and tryptase positive.

Figure 144. Nodal marginal zone B-cell lymphoma. There is an interfollicular pattern of involvement, with sparing of the follicle with both its mantle and germinal center.

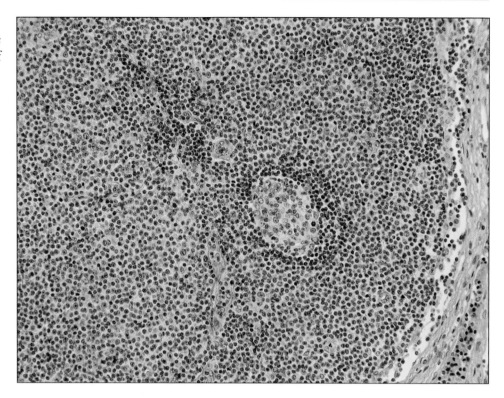

Metastatic lobular carcinoma of the breast may be easily evaluated by keratin stain.

NODAL MARGINAL ZONE B-CELL LYMPHOMA[246–253]

Primary nodal marginal zone B-cell lymphoma, also known as monocytoid B-cell lymphoma, is defined as a lymphoma derived from marginal zone B-cells, occurring in patients without evidence of Sjogren syndrome, Hashimoto thyroiditis, or extranodal lymphoma. It is uncommon, accounting for less than 2% of all cases of malignant lymphoma. Most, but not all patients, are adults, with a median age of about 55, and a female predilection. Most patients present with lymphadenopathy, particularly of the neck or para-aortic region. About two-thirds of patients present in stage III or IV, with frequent involvement of bone marrow. Involvement of peripheral blood may also be seen. Treatment consists of single- or multiagent chemotherapy, often combined with rituxan. Although a complete response is seen in about 50% of patients, relapses are common. Most relapses occur in lymph nodes and show a similar histologic appearance; however, progressive to diffuse large B-cell lymphoma may occur over time. The overall median survival is about 5 years.

A variety of architectural patterns may be seen. There may be either diffuse effacement of architecture or only partial involvement. Some cases showing diffuse effacement may have extension of the process beyond the lymph node capsule. Cases of partial involvement may show preferential involvement of the perisinusoidal area, parafollicular area, or paracortical regions or may show a preferential perivascular pattern of involvement (Figure 144). Occasionally,

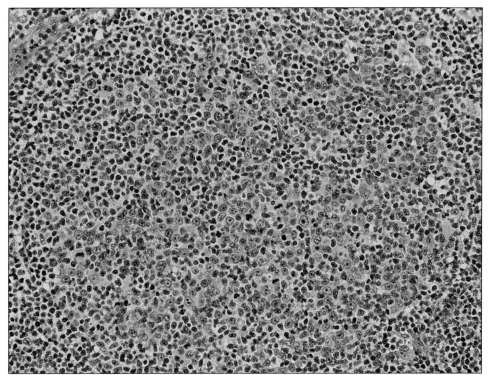

Figure 145. Primary nodal marginal zone B-cell lymphoma. There is a germinal center, which has been colonized by the lymphoma. Note the population of lymphoma cells at the edge of the germinal center.

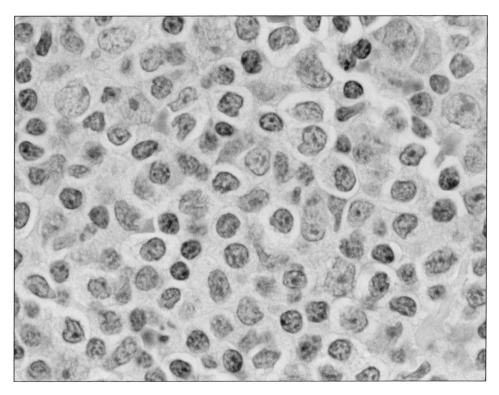

Figure 146. Nodal marginal zone B-cell lymphoma. The nuclei are small to medium sized, with somewhat irregular nuclear outlines, and the cytoplasm is moderate in amount and pale to clear.

there may be colonization of germinal centers, but more often residual follicles are normal or atrophic, with a relatively well-preserved mantle cuff (Figure 145). At high magnification, a variety of cell types may be seen. Most often, one sees small- to intermediate-sized cells with a moderate amount of pale to clear cytoplasm, so-called monocytoid cells (Figure 146). The nuclei generally have

Figure 147. Nodal marginal zone B-cell lymphoma. The right half of the picture shows distinct plasma cell differentiation, while the left half shows *monocytoid* features.

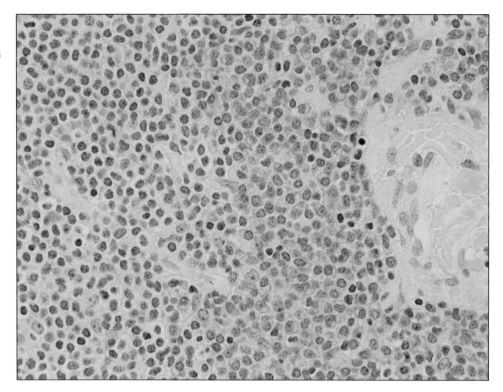

a mature chromatin pattern, but may show abnormalities of the nuclear membranes. In addition, similar cells with plasmacytoid features are common, as are plasma cells, which may form sheets and may show Dutcher bodies (Figure 147). Occasionally, scattered neutrophils may also be seen. Finally, scattered large cells with large nuclei and more prominent nucleoli are typically found admixed among the small cells.

Immunophenotypic studies show a B-cell lineage with expression of CD45, multiple B-lineage antigens, and surface immunoglobulin, usually of IgM type. Light chain restriction is usually readily identified when plasmacytoid features are seen, although occasionally reactive polyclonal plasma cells may be present. CD43 is aberrantly coexpressed in about one-third to one-half of cases, and CD5 may be aberrantly coexpressed in about 5–10% of cases (Table 26). CD10, CD23, bcl-6, and cyclin D1 are usually negative, but each may be expressed in rare cases. The bcl-2 stain is positive in most cases. The Ki-67 index is variable, but averages about 10–20%. IRTA-1 antibody is a recently described antibody that may be relatively specific for this lymphoma type. Gene rearrangement studies show clonal rearrangements of the immunoglobulin heavy and/or light chain genes. No recurrent chromosomal abnormalities have been consistently reported in multiple studies; specifically, this neoplasm usually lacks the translocations reported for extranodal (MALT) marginal zone B-cell lymphoma.

The differential diagnosis includes reactive monocytoid B-cell proliferations, extranodal marginal zone B-cell lymphoma involving lymph nodes, splenic and splenic-type marginal zone lymphoma, other small-cell lymphomas, follicular lymphoma, plasmacytic neoplasms, and diffuse large B-cell lymphoma. Reactive monocytoid B-cell proliferations may mimic partial involvement by nodal marginal B-cell lymphoma. Reactive monocytoid B-cell proliferations are usually associated with other reactive changes such as reactive follicular hyperplasia, more consistently show an admixture of neutrophils, and usually comprise less than 50% of the lymph node cross-sectional area, while nodal marginal B-cell lymphoma only rarely is associated with reactive follicles, frequently shows an admixture of plasma cells and large cells, and comprises greater than 50% of the lymph node cross-sectional area. In addition, bcl-2 is consistently negative in reactive monocytoid B-cells, but is almost always expressed in nodal marginal zone B-cell lymphoma.

Extranodal marginal zone B-cell lymphoma typically shows identical morphologic and immunophenotypic features to nodal marginal zone B-cell lymphoma. As discussed above, by definition, the presence of extranodal lymphoma, Sjogren syndrome, or Hashimoto syndrome should rule out a diagnosis of nodal marginal zone B-cell lymphoma, although occasionally these findings may only become evident upon follow-up of the patient. Nodal marginal zone B-cell lymphoma does not have the specific translocations of MALT lymphomas, so their identification would also rule out the former. Splenic and splenic-type marginal zone lymphomas are discussed in the section Splenic Marginal Zone Lymphoma Involving Lymph Nodes and Primary Nodal Marginal Zone Lymphoma of Splenic Type. Briefly, these lymphomas efface rather than preserve the mantle cuffs and consistently express IgD.

Lymph node involvement by chronic lymphocytic leukemia/small lymphocytic lymphoma may be distinguished by the presence of proliferation centers; the usual lack of plasmacytoid features; and its consistent expression of CD5, CD43, and CD23. Mantle cell lymphoma may be distinguished by its monomorphic cytologic appearance, without plasmacytoid differentiation or scattered large cells, and by its consistent strong expression of cyclin D1. Nodal marginal zone B-cell lymphoma may mimic follicular lymphoma when there is colonization of the follicles. However, the cytologic features of the B-cells within the follicles are not those of follicular center cells, and the extranodal proliferation is dominant. In addition, there may be aberrant coexpression of CD43 and CD10 is usually negative (although CD10 may be negative in the interfollicular involvement by follicular lymphoma).

The extensive plasma cell proliferation in nodal marginal zone B-cell lymphoma raises consideration of lymphoplasmacytic lymphoma and plasmacytoma involving lymph nodes. The distinction with lymphoplasmacytic lymphoma may be very difficult and require clinical findings, such as the absence of Waldenstrom macroglobulinemia. However, lymphoplasmacytic lymphoma generally shows a more diffuse and dispersed lymphoplasmacytic infiltrate, while the plasmacytic differentiation in nodal marginal zone B-cell lymphoma is usually more focal or compartmentalized. The distinction with plasmacytoma rests on the identification of the more lymphocytic nonplasma cell areas, with expression of CD45 and multiple B-lineage antigens. Finally, I do not diagnose transformation to large-cell lymphoma, until I see patternless sheets of large cells effacing architecture.

EXTRANODAL MARGINAL ZONE B-CELL LYMPHOMA OF MUCOSA-ASSOCIATED LYMPHOID TISSUE (MALT) INVOLVING LYMPH NODES[246,251,253-260]

Extranodal marginal zone B-cell lymphoma of MALT type is a primary malignant lymphoma derived from the marginal zone B-cell of extranodal tissues. It usually occurs in adults, although children may also be affected; there is slight female predilection. In descending order, the most frequently involved primary sites are stomach, lungs, head and neck, ocular adnexa, skin, and thyroid, although it may occur in virtually any site. Regional lymph nodes are frequently involved, and in about 10% of the time, there may be involvement of lymph nodes from multiple regions. Occasionally, there may be lymph node involvement by marginal zone B-cell lymphoma in which the patient only shows Sjogren syndrome or Hashimoto syndrome; these cases should also be considered to represent extranodal marginal zone B-cell lymphoma. It is not infrequent for a diagnosis of nodal marginal zone B-cell lymphoma to be made only to have the patient later develop a similar lesion at an extranodal site; these cases should be reassessed as extranodal marginal zone B-cell lymphoma secondarily involving the lymph node, even though the presentation is reversed.

Histologically, involved lymph nodes show histologic findings very similar if not identical to primary nodal marginal zone B-cell lymphoma. There is typically partial involvement, with preferential infiltration of the perisinusoidal, parafollicular, or perivascular regions. A polymorphous infiltrate of monocytoid B-cells, lymphoplasmacytic cells (sometimes with Dutcher bodies), plasma cells, and larger cells with large nuclei and more prominent nucleoli are usually seen; often there is architectural segregation of the plasmacytic component. Monocytoid B-cells are small to intermediate in size, with a mature chromatin pattern, slightly irregular nuclear outlines, and pale to clear cytoplasm showing a distinct cell membrane. The immunophenotypic findings are also identical to those seen in nodal marginal zone B-cell lymphoma, with expression of CD45, multiple B-lineage antigens, and bcl-2. CD10, CD23, and CD5 are usually negative, but aberrant coexpression of CD43 is seen in about 50% of cases (Table 26). Cases with plasmacytoid features usually show light chain restriction, although occasionally the plasma cells turn out to be polyclonal and apparently not part of the neoplastic clone. The one distinguishing feature from nodal marginal zone B-cell lymphoma is the presence of specific translocations that have been described in extranodal marginal zone B-cell lymphoma (see Table 31).[261,262] The histologic and immunophenotypic differential diagnosis has been discussed in the section Nodal Marginal Zone B-cell Lymphoma.

Table 31. MALT Lymphoma: Molecular Cytogenetics[261,262]

Trisomy 3, 30%, including 53% of salivary gland

Trisomy 18, 10%, including 25% of intestine and 15% of salivary gland

t(11;18)(q21;21) (ASP12/MALT1), 15% – including 25% of gastric and 50% of lung

t(14;18)(q32;q21) (IgH/MALT1), 10% – including 25% of ocular and 15% of skin

t(1;14)(p22;q32) (BCL10/IgH), 2% – including 15% of intestinal

t(1;2) (BCL10/IgK) 1%

t(3;14) (FOXP1/IgH) 1%

SPLENIC MARGINAL ZONE LYMPHOMA INVOLVING LYMPH NODES AND PRIMARY NODAL MARGINAL ZONE LYMPHOMA OF SPLENIC TYPE[247,254,255,263]

Splenic marginal zone lymphoma is a B-cell lymphoma theoretically derived from a marginal zone splenic B-cell. It is rare, occurring primarily in older adults, with no sex predilection. It involves the spleen, with frequent spread to splenic hilar and less frequently other abdominal or peripheral lymph nodes, the bone marrow, and the blood, in which circulating villous lymphocytes may be found. Patients typically present with splenomegaly or a picture simulating chronic lymphocytic leukemia. There may be autoimmune thrombocytopenia or anemia, and a small monoclonal serum protein may be present in a subset of patients. Rarely, patients may develop solitary lymphadenopathy in which the pathologic findings are very similar to those of splenic marginal zone lymphoma involving lymph nodes; these cases have been called primary nodal marginal zone lymphoma of splenic type. The reported cases have all occurred in adults, with neck, axillary, or inguinal lymphadenopathy. Most patients have presented in stage I, although some patients have had multiple lymph node groups involved. By definition, splenomegaly was absent in all cases, and there was no evidence of involvement of the bone marrow or peripheral blood.

Histologically, a slightly different low-magnification appearance is seen, depending on whether the lymph node is derived from the splenic hilum vs. other sites. Lymph nodes taken from the splenic hilum typically show preservation of the sinuses, which are often dilated and may contain histiocytes with erythrophagocytosis (Figure 148). A vague nodular appearance is seen, with the centers comprising nonneoplastic follicles varying from containing residual germinal centers to completely atrophic, without a surrounding mantle zone. Lymph nodes from peripheral sites show effacement of the sinuses, often with extension of the lymphoma into the pericapsular soft tissues. In addition, a more conspicuous nodular pattern is seen. On high magnification, the cytologic appearance is similar in both splenic hilar and other lymph node sites. There is a polymorphous infiltrate, with small- to intermediate-sized lymphocytes with a mature chromatin pattern and somewhat irregular nuclear membranes admixed with scattered larger cells, with larger nuclei and more prominent

Figure 148. Splenic marginal zone lymphoma, involving a splenic hilar lymph node. A somewhat nodular appearance is seen, along with patent medullary sinuses.

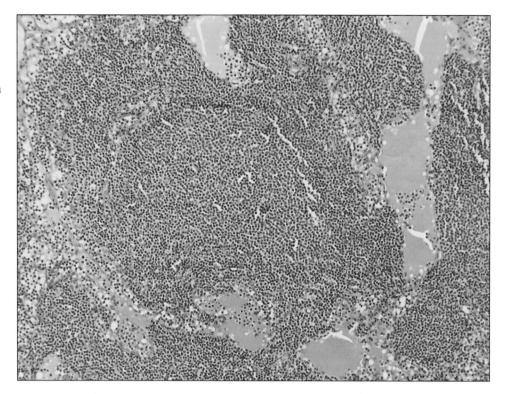

Figure 149. Splenic marginal zone B-cell lymphoma, involving a lymph node. Most of the cells are small, with a mature chromatin pattern, although there is a second population of cells with larger nuclei, with a more vesicular chromatin pattern and larger nucleoli.

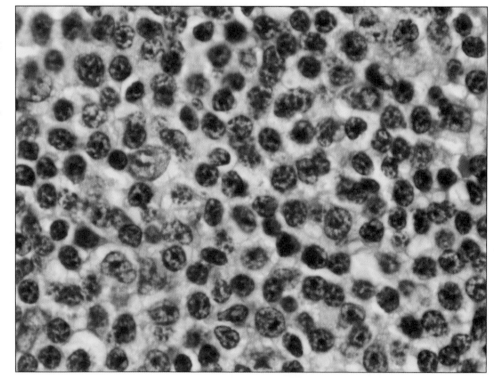

nucleoli (Figure 149). Occasional epithelioid histiocytes may be seen, singly or in small clusters, in the nodules. The bizonal growth pattern seen in the spleen in which the tumor mimics mantle and marginal zone differentiation is not generally seen in lymph nodes. Some cases may show sheets of large cells, indicative of large-cell transformation.

Immunophenotypic studies show the tumor cells to express CD45, multiple B-lineage antigens, bcl-2 protein, and surface IgM and IgD. CD5, CD43, CD10, CD23, and cyclin D1 are negative. Stains for follicular dendritic cells demonstrate that the centers of the nodules contain residual follicles that often contain a bcl-2–negative reactive germinal center. Molecular studies show clonal rearrangements of the immunoglobulin heavy and/or light genes. About 40% of cases of splenic marginal zone B-cell lymphoma have allelic loss of chromosome 7q21-32, and trisomy 3 may be present in a small subset of cases.

The differential diagnosis includes primary nodal marginal zone B-cell lymphoma, follicular lymphoma, and mantle cell lymphoma. Obviously, the diagnosis is easier to establish with a history of splenic marginal zone B-cell lymphoma or even a history of splenomegaly. Cases of primary nodal marginal zone B-cell lymphoma tend to have a predominantly perisinusoidal, parafollicular, or perivascular distribution; often show plasmacytoid differentiation; are IgD negative; and show a preserved cuff of mantle cells. In contrast, cases of splenic or splenic-type marginal zone B-cell lymphoma tend to show a nodular distribution, rarely show plasmacytoid differentiation, are IgD positive, and usually do not show a preserved cuff of mantle cells. The nodular pattern and irregular nuclear membranes may raise consideration of follicular lymphoma, but the presence of bcl-2–negative remnants of reactive germinal centers, along with negativity for CD10, should eliminate that diagnosis. Mantle cell lymphoma may be considered due to the superficial mantle zone appearance; however, the polymorphic infiltrate and negativity for cyclin D1 should eliminate that possibility.

FOLLICULAR LYMPHOMA[16,264–278]

Follicular lymphoma is defined by the WHO Classification as a lymphoma of follicle center B-cells that has at least a focally follicular pattern. It accounts for about one-third of all malignant lymphomas in the United States (excluding chronic lymphocytic leukemia), but has a lower incidence outside of Western countries. In contrast to most other lymphomas, there is a female predominance, with about a 1:1.5 M:F ratio. There is a higher incidence in whites than blacks, and a low incidence in Asian populations. It is usually a neoplasm of older adults, with a median age around 60. It is rare in patients under the age of 40, but may still occur in children. These latter cases show a male predominance, with a predilection for the head and neck, and may have a different pathogenesis than adult cases. Patients usually present with slowly progressive lymphadenopathy, often generalized, but without other symptoms. Staging studies usually demonstrate stage III or IV disease, with involvement of bone marrow, liver, and spleen each seen in about one-half of cases. There is some association with smoking. The pathogenesis probably involves deregulation of the bcl-2 gene as a result of a t(14;18), although this mechanism may be less common in Asians or in the pediatric age group.

Involved lymph nodes are usually but not always enlarged. A distinct nodularity can often be appreciated on gross examination of the cut surface of the

Figure 150. Follicular lymphoma. Numerous relatively evenly sized follicles are seen, with little interfollicular space.

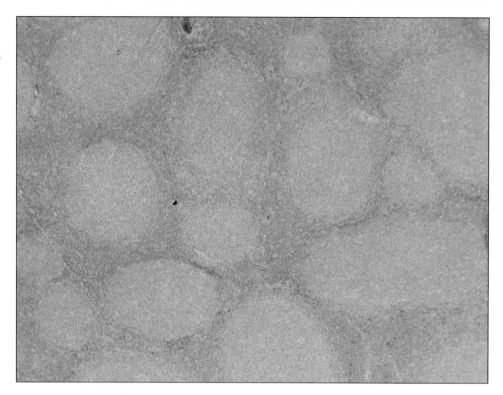

Figure 151. Follicular lymphoma. The centers of the follicles are composed of small and large cleaved cells, with few, if any, tingible-body macrophages and a low mitotic count.

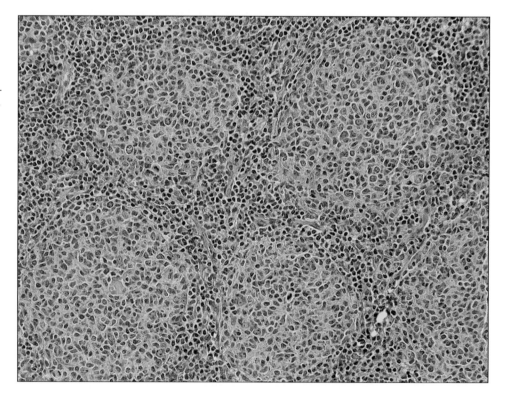

lymph node. At low magnification, there is usually a high density of follicles, often with follicles distributed evenly through the nodal parenchyma (Figures 150 and 151). Often, but not always, the follicles are of similar size and shape from one to another. Follicles may also be present outside the capsule and usually resemble those within the lymph node proper. The interfollicular areas are usually

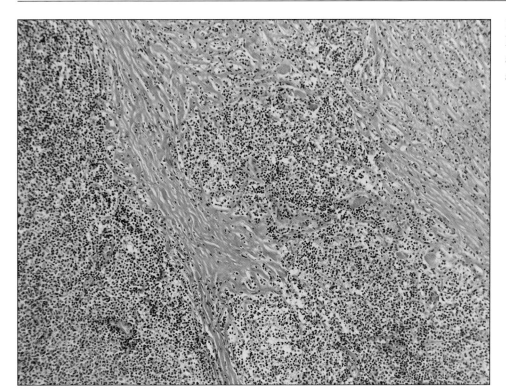

Figure 152. Follicular lymphoma. This lymphoma shows a typical pattern of sclerosis.

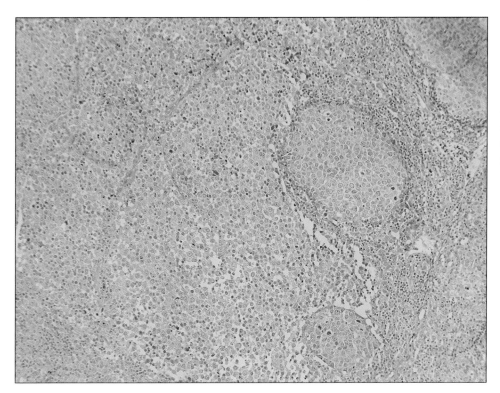

Figure 153. Follicular lymphoma, follicular and diffuse. One should see areas of architectural effacement, such as seen at left, and not merely expanded interfollicular areas, to diagnose a diffuse component in a follicular lymphoma.

compressed. In some cases, particularly those with a predominance of large cells, there may be significant areas of diffuse effacement, often showing significant sclerosis (Figure 152), although, by definition, at least focal areas of follicularity must be present (Figure 153). Cases with areas of diffuse effacement (and not considering merely enlarged interfollicular areas) are reported as follicular

Figure 154. Follicular lymphoma with marginal zone differentiation. This neoplastic follicle is surrounded by a rim of marginal zone B-cells, which represents part of the neoplastic clone.

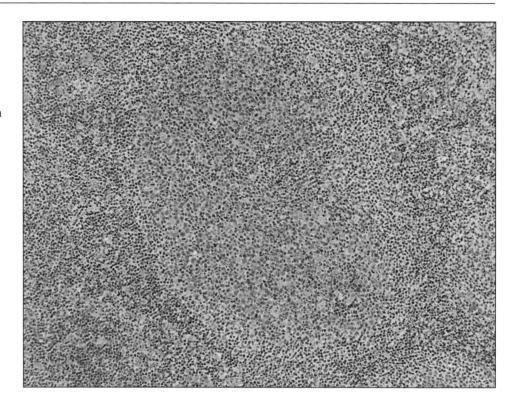

(>75% follicular), follicular and diffuse (25–75% follicular), or minimally follicular (<25% diffuse). Mantle zones may be present, but are frequently attenuated or may even be completely absent. Occasionally, one can see a rim of marginal zone B-cells surrounding the follicles; this represents part of the neoplastic process (Figure 154).

At high magnification, either a monomorphic or polymorphic population may be present within the follicles (Figures 155, 156, 157, and 158). Cell polarization (light and dark zones) is almost always absent. The cells consist of varying numbers of centrocytes and centroblasts. Centrocytes are cells with small (or sometimes large) nuclei with condensed chromatin, irregular nuclear outlines, and inconspicuous nuclei. Centroblasts are cells with large (and sometimes small) nuclei with a vesicular chromatin pattern, usually round nuclear outlines, and one to three peripheral nucleoli. Cytoplasm is scanty in both cell types, but is more basophilic in centroblasts. Centrocytes usually predominate, but at least some centroblasts are always present. Rarely, the cells in the follicles may show plasmacytoid features; small, round cells resembling the cells of small lymphocytic lymphoma; and signet-ring features, either with an eosinophilic inclusion (immunoglobulin) or with a clear inclusion (Figure 159). Mitoses are usually less numerous than seen in reactive follicular hyperplasia, although significant numbers may be seen in cases with large numbers of centroblasts. Scattered follicular dendritic cells may be seen. Similarly, tingible-body macrophages may be present, but are usually fewer than those seen in reactive follicular hyperplasia. The 2001 WHO Classification recommends grading cases of follicular lymphoma by the number of centroblasts in the follicles, given in Table 32. The interfollicular areas may show normal paracortex or may show involvement by follicular lymphoma. In the

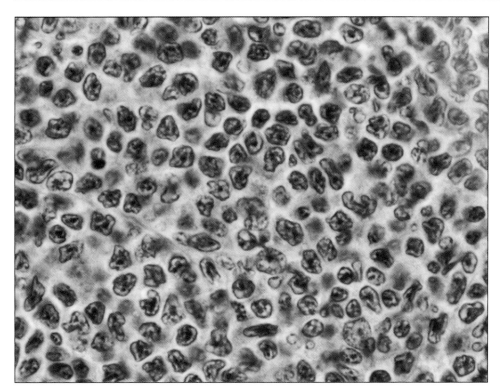

Figure 155. Follicular lymphoma, grade 1. A marked predominance of small cleaved cells is seen, consistent with cytologic grade 1.

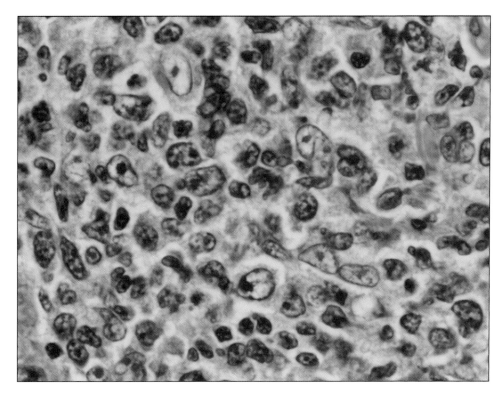

Figure 156. Follicular lymphoma, grade 2. Scattered large noncleaved cells between five and fifteen per high-power field area are seen, consistent with cytologic grade 2. Note that follicular dendritic cells (of which there are three in this picture [one uninucleate cell at the top left, one multilobated cell near the middle upper left, and one binucleate cell at the middle lower left]) should be avoided when making the count.

latter case, a mixture of centrocytes and centroblasts is seen, often with a greater percentage of centrocytes than seen within the follicles.

The neoplastic cells of follicular lymphoma show a phenotype similar to that of normal germinal center cells, expressing all pan-B-cell markers, including CD20, CD79a, PAX-5, as well as the B-cell transcription factors BOB.1 and

Figure 157. Follicular lymphoma, grade 3a. There are numerous large noncleaved cells greater than fifteen per high-power field.

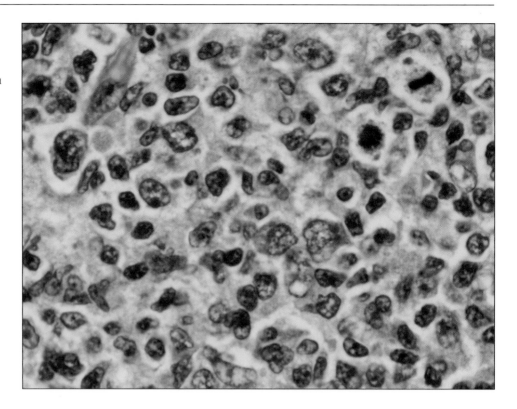

Figure 158. Follicular lymphoma, grade 3b. There is a nearly pure population of large noncleaved cells within the follicle.

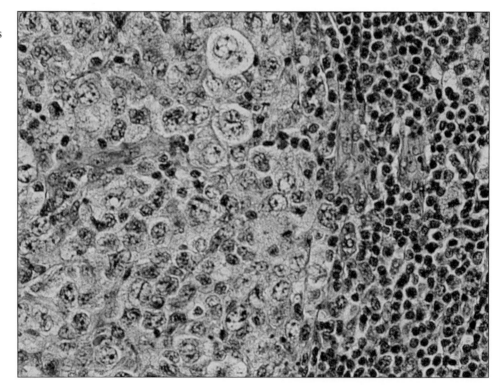

OCT-2 (Figure 160). They also show consistent expression of the germinal center markers CD10 and bcl-6 (Figure 161) and negativity for CD5 and CD43 (Table 26). They usually show expression of surface immunoglobulin, IgM more often than IgG. In contrast to reactive germinal center cells, the neoplastic cells of follicular lymphoma exhibit monotypic light chain expression

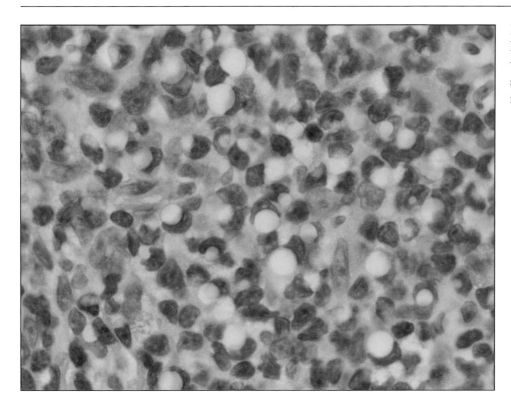

Figure 159. Follicular lymphoma, signet-ring cell variant. This unusual variant should not be mistaken for metastatic carcinoma.

Table 32. Follicular Lymphoma Grading[279]

	Grade 1	Grade 2	Grade 3[a]
American Optical (40×, 10×)	0–5	6–15	>15
American Optical (40×, 15×)	0–4	5–12	>12
Olympus (40×, 10×)	0–7	8–20	>20
Olympus (40×, 15×)	0–3	4–9	>9
Nikon (40×, 10×)	0–7	8–20	>20
Nikon (40×, 15×)	0–4	5–12	>12

[a]3a, with centrocytes; 3b, without centrocytes.

and usually show positivity for bcl-2 (Figure 162). Grade 3 follicular lymphoma may show alternative phenotypes, including a higher incidence of bcl-2 negativity (about 25%), immunoglobulin negativity (about 20%), and aberrant expression of CD43 (about 5%) than other grades of follicular lymphoma (Figure 163). In addition, cases of pediatric follicular lymphoma may show high rates of bcl-2 negativity, with as many as two-thirds of cases bcl-2 negative.

The neoplastic cells of follicular lymphoma undergo consistent monoclonal heavy and light chain gene rearrangement, although, from a practical standpoint, this is only detectable about 80% of the time when PCR technology is employed, due to the presence of somatic mutations which impede recognition by the commonly used primer sets. A t(14;18)(q32;21) involving translocation of the immunoglobulin heavy chain gene and the bcl-2 gene occurs in about 85% of cases. The translocation occurs least frequently in grade 3 follicular lymphoma (about 75% positive) and pediatric follicular lymphoma (10–20% positive), in

Figure 160. Follicular
lymphoma, CD20 stain. Both
the follicular and
interfollicular cells mark as
B-cells in this case. In reactive
follicular hyperplasia, one
would not expect to see such
a large population of B-cells
in the interfollicular region.

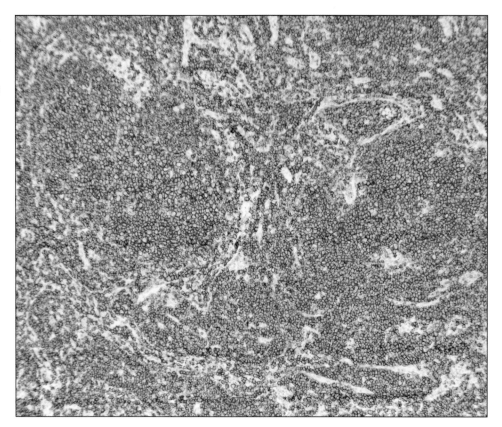

Figure 161. Follicular
lymphoma, CD10 stain. The
intrafollicular cells of
follicular lymphoma
consistently stain for CD10,
but the interfollicular
neoplastic B-cells may or may
not be positive.

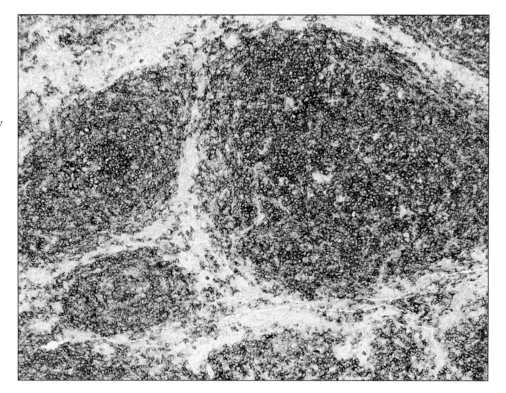

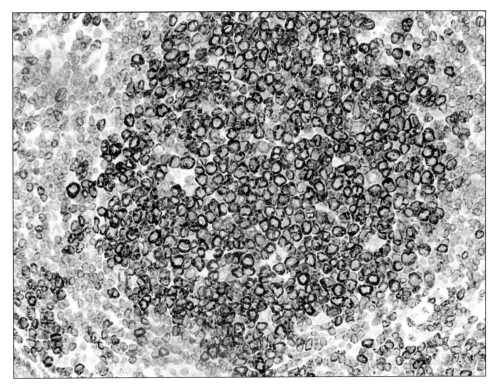

Figure 162. Follicular lymphoma, bcl-2 stain. Note that both small and large cells are positive in the follicles. In this case, the staining is strong than the adjacent cells, but may be similar in intensity or even weaker. Bcl-2 staining in follicles should always be compared to T-cell stains to rule out the possibility of bcl-2 staining of intrafollicular T-cells being mistaken for staining of neoplastic follicular B-cells.

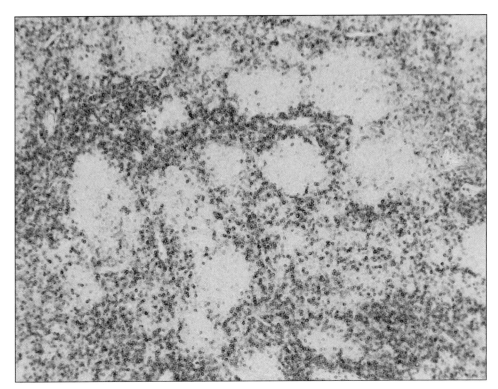

Figure 163. Follicular lymphoma, bcl-2 stain. This follicular lymphoma is negative for bcl-2. Negative staining for bcl-2 is seen in about one-third of cases of follicular lymphoma, grade 3, and does not rule out the diagnosis. In this picture, one can see the outlines of relatively even, closely packed follicles typical of follicular lymphoma.

which the pathogenesis may differ from t(14;18)-positive cases. The t(14;18) may also be detected by PCR studies, although the incidence is somewhat lower, due in this case to the presence of alternative breakpoints on a subgene level. A wide variety of other abnormalities are present in about 90% of cases, including gains of chromosome 7 (the p or q arm), 18q, 12q, and Xq, as well

Table 33. International Prognostic Index for Follicular Lymphoma[275]

1. Age >60 years
2. Stage III or IV
3. Hemoglobin <120 g/L
4. Nodal areas >4
5. Serum lactate dehydrogenase elevated

Low risk	0–1 factors
Intermediate	2 factors
Poor risk	3–5 factors

as deletions at 6q23–26 and 17p (the site of the p53 gene), each seen in about 10–20% of cases.

Clinical prognostic factors include the classical determinants of prognosis in malignant lymphoma, including age, stage, B symptoms, performance status, serum lactate dehydrogenase, hemoglobulin, bulky disease, and extranodal involvement. Five of these factors have been combined to create a Follicular Lymphoma International Prognostic Index (see Table 33).[279] In addition to clinical factors, the cytologic grade 3 also predicts for poor outcome and the need for more aggressive therapy with adriamycin-containing regimens. In one study, the presence of focal marginal zone differentiation also had an adverse impact on survival, and some studies have suggested that the percentage of follicular architecture may have prognostic significance as well.

The primary differential diagnosis of follicular lymphoma is reactive follicular hyperplasia. The key distinguishing features are given in Tables 4 and 5. No one criterion is pathognonomic for one diagnosis or the other. One must weigh a constellation of factors, optimally supported by immunohistochemical and even molecular studies, if the former do not resolve the dilemma. In regard to immunohistochemical studies, the demonstration of light chain restriction, while uncommonly seen in paraffin sections, is virtually diagnostic of lymphoma, seen only rarely as light chain restriction in highly reactive follicular hyperplasia in children. More useful in daily practice, bcl-2 positivity of the neoplastic follicular center cells is virtually diagnostic of follicular lymphoma, although one must be careful to distinguish this from bcl-2 staining of reactive intrafollicular T-helper cells that are bcl-2 positive, bcl-2 staining of primary follicles, and bcl-2 staining of other lymphomas (such as marginal zone B-cell lymphoma) that are merely colonizing the follicles. One as yet unresolved area is the presence of scattered bcl-2–positive follicular center cells in a few follicles (Figure 164). Often, the staining for bcl-2 is more intense than adjacent normal bcl-2–positive lymphoid cells. This phenomenon has been termed in situ follicular lymphoma. However, when the staining is truly confined to only a few follicles, it is not clear whether this represents an early form of follicular lymphoma or a nonprogressive finding similar to (or even a tissue manifestation of) the circulating t(14;18)-carrying B-cells that may occur in the peripheral blood of some adults that do not progress to follicular lymphoma.

One histologic variant of follicular lymphoma that may be difficult to distinguish from progressive transformation of germinal centers or nodular lymphocyte–predominant Hodgkin lymphoma is the floral variant of follicular lymphoma.[280] Two variants have been described, both with a superficial resemblance to floral designs, hence the name. In the more common variant, a macrogerminal center pattern is seen in which mantle zone lymphocytes are invaginated into the neoplastic germinal center, with large clusters of neoplastic cells. This variant may closely mimic progressive transformation of germinal centers. In the second variant, a microgerminal center pattern is seen in which massive invasion of mantle zone lymphocytes isolates the neoplastic cells into isolated tumor cells or small clusters up to twenty cells. This latter variant may closely mimic nodular lymphocyte

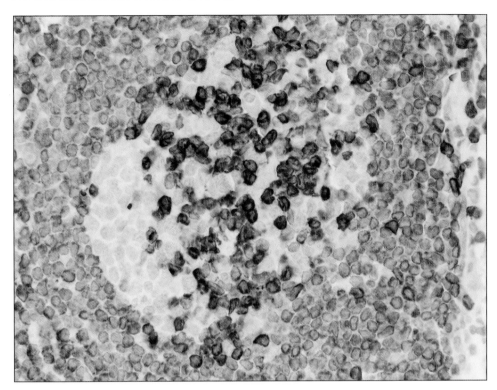

Figure 164. Follicular lymphoma, bcl-2 stain. Only a few follicles in this biopsy showed bcl-2–positive B-cells in the follicles. Note the strong staining as compared to the adjacent cells, a helpful finding in ruling out bcl-2 staining of reactive intrafollicular T-cells.

predominance. Despite the morphologic similarities, immunostains, particularly bcl-2 staining, should resolve the diagnostic problem.

Another diagnostic dilemma may arise when one observes a diffuse neoplasm with the same cytologic features as grade 1 or 2 follicular lymphoma; however, no clear follicular structures can be discerned. Since the presence of follicular structures is part of the WHO Classification definition of follicular lymphoma, that diagnosis is not appropriate. These cases are termed diffuse follicle center lymphoma. Before making that diagnosis, one must perform immunostains to ensure that the small atypical cells have the typical immunoprofile of neoplastic follicular center cells described above and are not T-cells. If the small cells are T-cells, then the appropriate diagnosis is that of a T-cell/histiocyte-rich B-cell lymphoma. In addition, if there are greater than 15 centroblasts/hpf, then the appropriate diagnosis is that of diffuse large B-cell lymphoma, regardless of whether the cells have a follicular center cell phenotype or not.

Follicular lymphoma may be associated with or transform to diffuse large B-cell lymphoma. Coexisting diffuse large B-cell lymphoma is diagnosed whenever there are diffuse areas of effacement in which grade 3 (>15 centroblasts/hpf) cytology is present. This is seen most often in association with grade 3 follicular lymphoma, but may also be found in grade 1 or 2 follicular lymphoma, in which a discordant higher grade (3) is seen in the diffuse areas. Transformation of a known follicular lymphoma to a diffuse large B-cell lymphoma of germinal center B-cell phenotype occurs at a rate of about 5–10% per year, independent of the type of treatment, occurring more frequently in those patients with higher cytologic grade as well as in those neoplasms with a 6q23–26 or 17p abnormality. Virtually, all patients with follicular lymphoma who die of disease have areas of diffuse large B-cell lymphoma at autopsy. Rarely, transformation may manifest as a blastic transformation, closely resembling a lymphoblastic neoplasm. Transformation of follicular lymphoma to diffuse large-cell lymphoma occurs by at least two different molecular mechanisms, one characterized by high proliferation and the presence of recurrent oncogenic abnormalities and the other in which the proliferation rate is not increased.

One final entity that must be distinguished from follicular lymphoma is KSHV- and EBV-associated germinotropic lymphoproliferative disorder.[281] This is a rare disease that presents as localized lymphadenopathy in immuno-competent patients. Involved lymph nodes show a proliferation of plasmablasts that preferentially involve germinal center, forming confluent aggregates. They lack CD20, CD79a, CD10, CD138, or bcl-2 expression, but show monotypic light chain (kappa or lambda), and are positive for both EBV and KSHV. Molecular studies show a polyclonal or oligoclonal pattern of immunoglobulin gene rearrangement, suggesting that this may not represent a true malignant lymphoma. Clinically, it responds favorably to conventional therapy.

MANTLE CELL LYMPHOMA[251,282–293]

Mantle cell lymphoma is a non-Hodgkin lymphoma in which the neoplastic cells differentiate toward inner zone mantle zone B-cells. It is a relatively common lymphoma, accounting for about 5–10% of cases of non-Hodgkin lymphoma. There is a male predominance, with an M:F ratio of about 3:1 and a median age of about 65 years, predominantly occurring in older adults and rare in children.

There is no known etiology. The neoplasm is a neoplastic B-cell prolifera-tion, with clonal rearrangements of the immunoglobulin genes. Virtually, all cases possess a t(11;14)(q13;q32), involving the cyclin D1 (BCL1) and immu-noglobulin heavy chain genes. These cases show overexpression of cyclin D1 mRNA and overexpression of the cyclin D1 protein. About 1% of cases lack cyclin D1 overexpression, but may have overexpression of cyclin D2 and D3. Gene expression profiling studies have shown that mantle cell lymphoma rep-resents a homogeneous entity with the presence of multiple concurrent alter-ations in the proliferation, apoptosis, tumor necrosis factor, and NF-κB pathways, with upregulation of the IL-10 receptor (IL-10R) and SPARC genes. Mutations in the ATM gene are found in about 40% of cases. Blastoid cases are associated with increased expression of proliferation genes, decreased expression of apoptosis genes, and increased expression of the oncoproteins CDK4 and p53.

Patients usually present with generalized lymphadenopathy and are most often found to be in stage III or IV at presentation. There is a high incidence of involvement of bone marrow and the gastrointestinal tract, particularly if screen-ing biopsies are taken. In a significant subset of patients, there is also involvement of the peripheral blood. There is not yet optimal treatment for mantle cell lym-phoma. Typical therapies include anthracycline-containing regimens with ritux-imab, high-dose chemotherapy followed by autologous stem cell transplantation, or fludarabine-containing regimens. Allogenic transplantation may represent

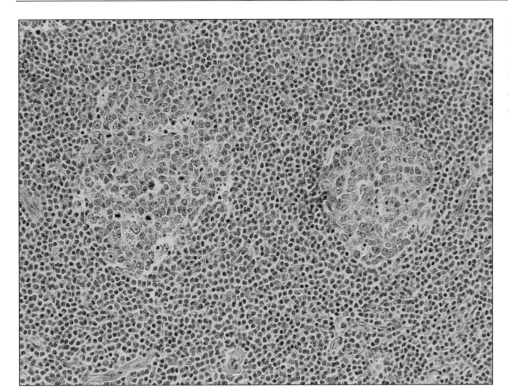

Figure 165. Mantle cell lymphoma. A mantle zone pattern is seen, with neoplastic cells arranged around bare reactive germinal centers.

the only potentially curative therapy, but is experimental at present. Adverse pathologic prognostic factors include the proliferation rate, blastoid morphology, peripheral blood involvement, karyotypic complexity, p53 mutation and/or over-expression, and loss of p53 gene expression. Adverse clinical prognostic factors include age, performance status, and the presence of splenomegaly.

At low magnification, mantle cell lymphoma may show three architectural patterns. In the classic (although not the most common) mantle cell zone pattern, the neoplastic proliferation surrounds reactive germinal centers, forming an expanded mantle zone (Figure 165). This progresses to the nodular pattern, in which the neoplastic cells overrun the germinal centers, occasionally leaving remnants of a germinal center with residual centrocytes and centroblasts (Figure 166). The most common pattern is the diffuse pattern, in which there is diffuse effacement of the lymph node architecture, without proliferation centers (Figure 167). The capsule is usually intact, and fibrosis is not seen. At high magnifications, one sees a homogeneous lymphoid population, although scattered epithelioid histiocytes are often seen. The lymphoid cells are usually small to medium sized, even in size within a given case. The nuclei generally have a mature chromatin pattern, with inconspicuous nucleoli, but show nuclear irregularities approaching those of a centrocyte (Figure 168). Admixed large lymphoid cells, paraimmunoblasts, or immunoblasts are not seen. In some cases, the cytologic features of the proliferating mantle cells may mimic those of chronic lymphocytic leukemia or marginal zone B-cell lymphoma, but an admixture of larger cells is never seen. In about 10–20% of cases, a blastoid cytology is seen. In the more common classic blastoid type, the cells have a fine blastic chromatin appearance closely resembling lymphoblastic leukemia

Figure 166. Mantle cell lymphoma. A follicular pattern is seen, in which the follicles are completely replaced by neoplastic mantle cells. Note the scattered epithelioid histiocytes.

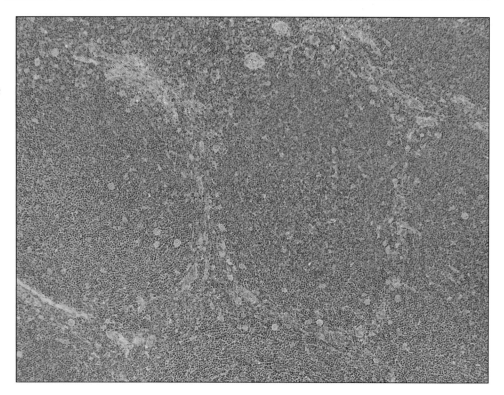

Figure 167. Mantle cell lymphoma. A diffuse architecture is seen, with a uniform proliferation of neoplastic mantle cells along with scattered epithelioid histiocytes.

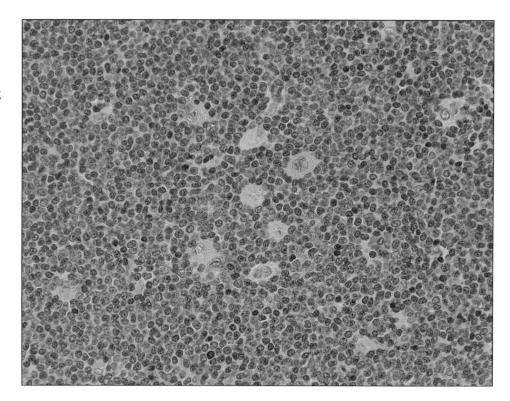

(Figure 169). The mitotic rate is high, usually at least 20/10 hpf. In the pleomorphic blastoid variant, the cells are more pleomorphic and much larger in size, approaching the size of the neoplastic cells of diffuse large B-cell lymphoma (Figure 170). The cells still have a fine blastic chromatin appearance, but may have large nucleoli.

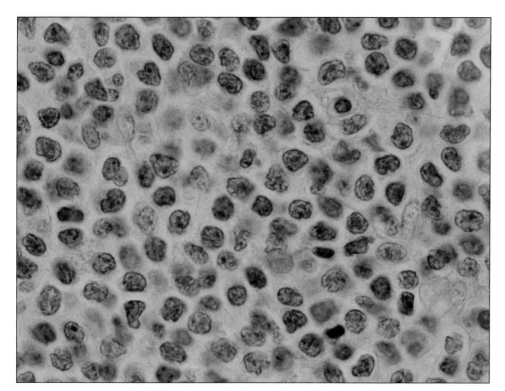

Figure 168. Mantle cell lymphoma. The cells are uniform, with an irregular nuclear outline and small to unrecognizable nucleoli.

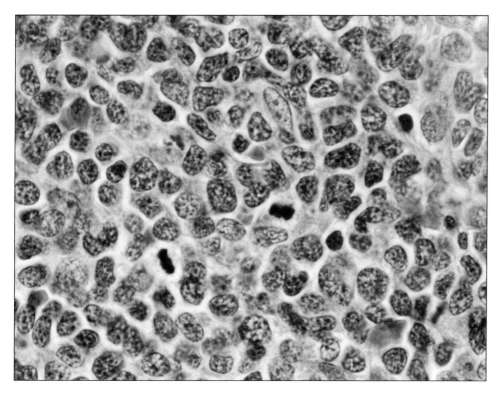

Figure 169. Mantle cell lymphoma, blastoid type. A uniform population of intermediate cells with a fine granular chromatin pattern is seen, indistinguishable from a lymphoblastic neoplasm. Note the high mitotic rate.

The immunophenotype of mantle cell lymphoma is summarized in Table 26. Mantle cell lymphoma expresses all pan-B-markers. Bcl-2 is consistently positive and, since it is a cytoplasmic marker, may show the irregular nuclear membranes to advantage when morphology is not adequate. The hallmark of mantle cell lymphoma is consistent expression of cyclin D1, seen in about 98% of cases

Figure 170. Mantle cell lymphoma, pleomorphic blastic type. The cells are intermediate to large in size and have a more vesicular chromatin pattern than typical cases of mantle cell lymphoma, although there is still some granularity to the chromatin. Some cells have prominent nucleoli. This case coexpressed CD5 and had overexpression of cyclin D1.

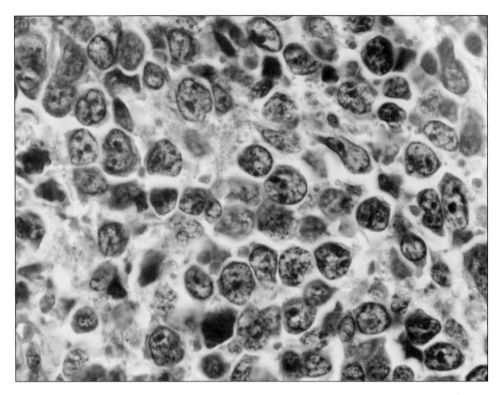

Figure 171. Mantle cell lymphoma, cyclin D1 staining. Note the variation in the level of positivity from cell to cell. This is a reproducible finding that is helpful in assessing the veracity of the stain.

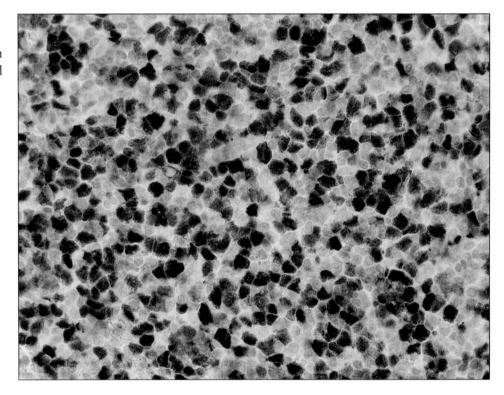

(Figure 171). Usually, there is some variability in the staining from cell to cell, dependent on the point in the cell cycle that the individual cells are in. Cases that are negative for cyclin D1 may show overexpression of cyclin D2 or cyclin D3. Mantle cell lymphoma usually shows coexpression of CD5 and CD43, although the rates of positivity are somewhat less than chronic lymphocytic leukemia. Most cases are negative for CD10, bcl-6, and CD23. FMC-7 staining is usually present, reflecting a high level of CD20 expression, but requires flow cytometry studies. Blastoid cases have a high Ki-67 index and often show strong nuclear positivity for p53 protein. Clonal immunoglobulin gene rearrangements are seen in all cases of mantle cell lymphoma. Most, but not all, cases have unmutated immunoglobulin genes, consistent with a pre–germinal center derivation. As mentioned above, almost all cases possess a t(11;14). This may be most reliably detected in FISH studies, with conventional cytogenetics or PCR positive in only about 75% of cases.

The differential diagnosis of mantle cell lymphoma includes both low-grade and high-grade non-Hodgkin lymphomas. Fortunately, application of cyclin D1 immunostains should resolve most cases. One must keep in mind that rare cases of mantle cell lymphoma may lack cyclin D1 expression. Staining with cyclin D2 or cyclin D3, if this is available, may resolve the diagnostic dilemma. In the absence of these stains, it is still legitimate to consider a diagnosis of mantle cell lymphoma in the face of cyclin D1–negative immunoreactivity if all other features are classic for the lymphoma. Lymphoid neoplasms other than mantle cell lymphoma that may show cyclin D1 staining include multiple myeloma (those cases with a t(11;14)), hairy cell leukemia, and a small subset of cases of chronic lymphocytic leukemia. Of these, only chronic lymphocytic leukemia should really come up in the morphologic differential diagnosis. Although chronic lymphocytic leukemia shares CD5 and CD43 coexpression with mantle cell lymphoma, chronic lymphocytic leukemia is usually CD23 positive and FMC-7 negative. In addition, chronic lymphocytic leukemia always has an admixture of larger cells with relatively prominent nucleoli, either scattered singly or organized into proliferation centers.

To distinguish an ordinary case of mantle cell lymphoma from a classic blastoid variant, one should pay close attention to the fine chromatin pattern and the high mitotic rate in the blastoid variant. In difficult cases, the identification of strong overexpression of p53 protein would strongly favor a blastoid variant. The classic blastoid variant can be distinguished from lymphoblastic neoplasms by a combination of cyclin D1 and terminal deoxyribonucleotidyl transferase staining (Table 34). The pleomorphic blastic variant may be difficult to distinguish from a diffuse large B-cell lymphoma. Cyclin D1 staining should resolve the problem if the diagnosis of mantle cell lymphoma is considered, but often one does not think of mantle cell lymphoma in the differential diagnosis of large-cell lymphoma. CD5 coexpression in a case in which the diagnosis of diffuse large B-cell lymphoma is being considered should raise concern for mantle cell lymphoma and prompt cyclin D1 testing to rule out that diagnosis, although a subset of diffuse large B-cell lymphoma may truly coexpress CD5.

DIFFUSE LARGE B-CELL LYMPHOMA[294–307]

Diffuse large B-cell lymphoma is a major category of non-Hodgkin lymphoma, representing the most common lymphoma subtype in both Western and

Table 34. Differential Diagnosis of Blastic Neoplasms

	PAX-5	Pan-T-Cell Markers	TdT	Cyclin D1	CD56	CD10	Bcl-6	C-myc Translocation	Myeloperoxidase
T-precursor lymphoblastic	−	+	+	−	−	−/+	−	−	−
B-precursor lymphoblastic	+	−	+	−	−	+/−	−	−	−
Burkitt	+	−	−	−	−	+	+	+	−
Blastic mantle cell	+	−	−	+	−	−	−	−	−
Blastic transformation of follicular lymphoma	+	−	−	−	−	+	+	+/−	−
Acute myeloid leukemia	−/+	−/+	−/+	−	−	−	−	−	+
Precursor plasmacytoid dendritic cell neoplasm	−	−/+	+/−	−	+	−	−	−	−

developing countries. Although the age range affected is wide, including children, in general, it is a lymphoma of older adults, with a slight predominance in males. It occurs with increased frequency in those patients with immunosuppression, from whatever cause, including aging, in which there is a strong association with EBV. These lymphomas are discussed in Chapter 9. Patients usually present with rapidly enlarging lymphadenopathy, although one-third may present with a mass in an extranodal site. About one-third of patients have B symptoms. About 25% present in stage I, 25% present in stage II, and one-half present in higher stage. The pathogenesis of diffuse large B-cell lymphoma is complex, reflecting the fact that it actually represents a heterogeneous group of neoplasms, each probably with its own molecular profile. Recently, cDNA microarray studies have separated large B-cell lymphoma into at least three major groups: germinal center B-cell–like, activated B-cell–like and type 3. Although most neoplasms develop de novo, a significant percentage of cases occur as a transformation of a low-grade B-cell lymphoma.

Lymph nodes involved by diffuse large B-cell lymphoma are typically enlarged and show a soft tan fleshy mass on cut section, sometimes with areas of necrosis or hemorrhage. At low magnification, diffuse effacement of architecture is usually seen, although preferential involvement of the paracortical region and/or sinusoids may be present in some cases. The capsule is often infiltrated, with extension to the pericapsular soft tissues, and there may be fine to thick bands of fibrous tissue. At high magnification, the neoplastic cells are uniformly large, but the nuclei may take on a number of different appearances. Most often, most of the nuclei resemble centroblasts, with large vesicular nuclei and one to three peripherally arranged nuclei, known as the centroblastic variant. The nuclear membranes may be round, but more often have, varying from minor *cleaves* to frankly hyperlobated cells (Figures 172 and 173). Other cells may resemble immunoblasts, with large vesicular nuclei with one centrally located prominent nucleolus and often showing plasmacytoid cytoplasmic features (Figure 174). When immunoblasts are in the

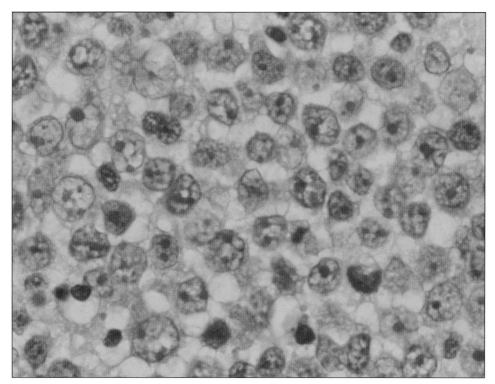

Figure 172. Diffuse large B-cell lymphoma, centroblastic variant. The neoplastic cells have a close resemblance to the large noncleaved cells of the normal germinal center, with a vesicular chromatin pattern and several nucleoli often found at the edge of the nuclear membrane.

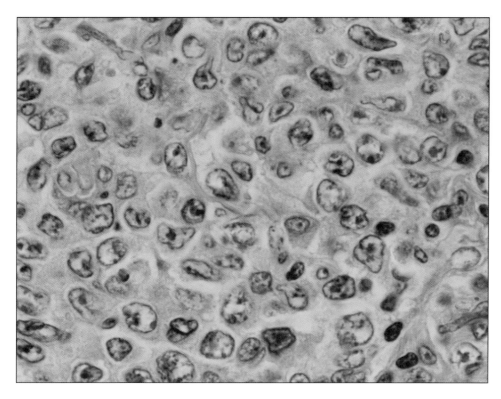

Figure 173. Diffuse large B-cell lymphoma, centroblastic variant. This case has marked irregularities of the nuclear membranes.

distinct majority (defined as high as >90% of the cells in the 2001 WHO Classi-fication), the term immunoblastic variant may be used. Other cases may contain numerous cells with large, bizarre, and pleomorphic nuclei, the so-called anaplastic variant (Figure 175). These cases may even show a sinusoidal pattern involvement, closely mimicking non–ALK-expressing anaplastic large-cell lymphoma.

Figure 174. Diffuse large B-cell lymphoma, immunoblastic variant. The neoplastic cells have large nuclei, with large, centrally placed nucleoli, and a moderate amount of amphophilic to basophilic cytoplasm.

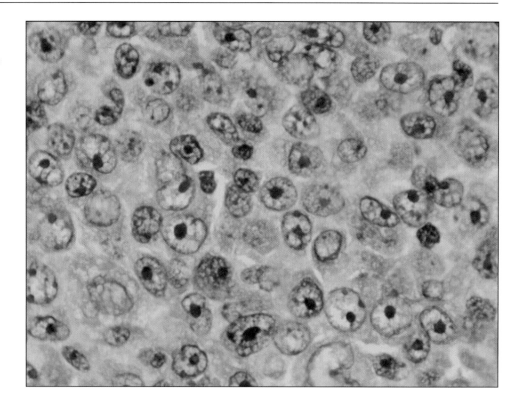

Figure 175. Diffuse large B-cell lymphoma. This anaplastic variant could easily be mistaken for anaplastic large-cell lymphoma if not for the identification of multiple B-lineage markers on the atypical cells.

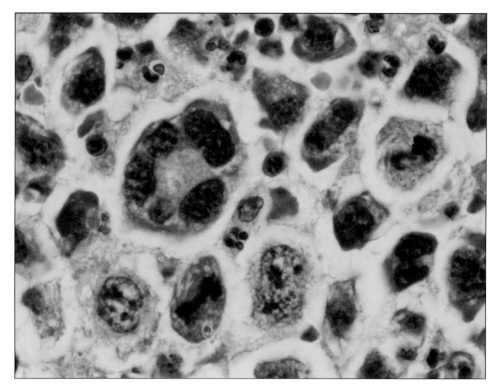

Nonetheless, if a B-lineage can be demonstrated, these cases probably just represent a peculiar morphologic variant of diffuse large B-cell lymphoma. Other unusual variants of diffuse large-cell lymphoma include the spindle-cell variant of diffuse large-cell lymphoma, large-cell lymphoma forming rosettes, and diffuse large-cell lymphoma with anemonelike projections (Figures 176, 177, 178, and 179).

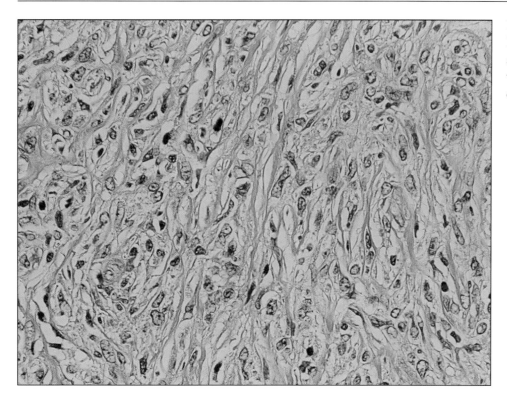

Figure 176. Diffuse large B-cell lymphoma, with spindle-cell features. This variant could easily be confused with a sarcoma.

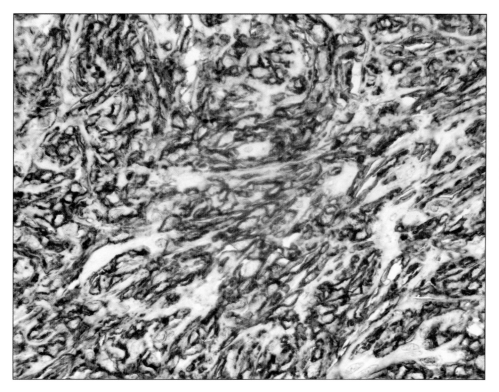

Figure 177. Diffuse large B-cell lymphoma, with spindle-cell features (same case as previous figure), CD20 stain. The expression of CD20 and other B-cell markers establishes this case as an unusual variant of diffuse large B-cell lymphoma.

T-cell/histiocyte-rich B-cell lymphoma represents a variant of diffuse large B-cell lymphoma in which the majority of cells are non-neoplastic T-cells with or without large numbers of histiocytes, and fewer than 10% large neoplastic B-cells are present.[244,308,309] It encompasses both of the formerly recognized entities of T-cell–rich B-cell lymphoma and histiocyte-rich B-cell lymphoma. The large

Figure 178. Diffuse large B-cell lymphoma, with rosettes. The presence of rosettes raises a differential diagnosis with several other types of neoplasms, but the cytologic features are still those of a lymphoid neoplasm.

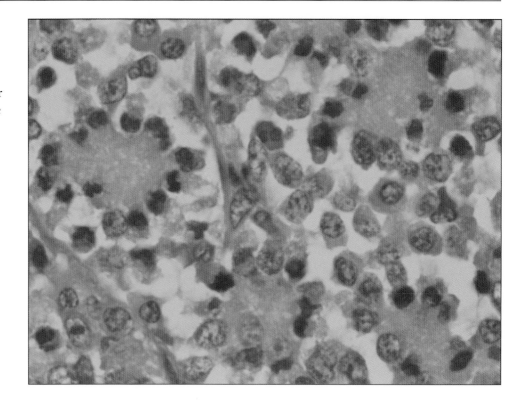

Figure 179. Diffuse large B-cell lymphoma, with fibrillar projections. This rare anaplastic variant of diffuse large B-cell lymphoma has been called anemone lymphoma; it often shows a sinusoidal pattern of infiltration.

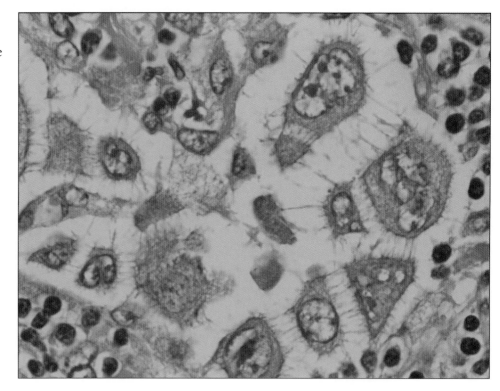

cells may have the morphologic appearance of centroblasts, immunoblasts, L&H cells, or even Hodgkin cells (Figures 180, 181, and 182). The background consists of small T-cells and varying numbers of histiocytes (which may or may not be epithelioid), usually without large numbers of eosinophils or plasma cells. Clinically, some differences have been noted between T-cell/histiocyte-rich B-cell

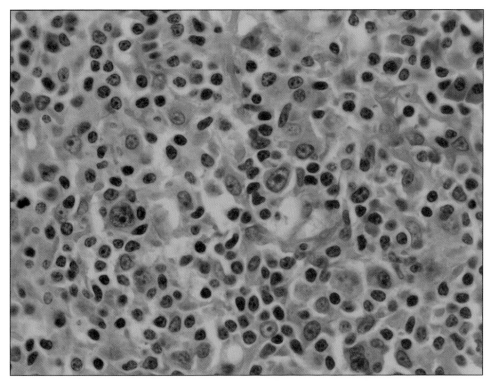

Figure 180. Diffuse large B-cell lymphoma, T-cell/histiocyte-rich variant. Only a few neoplastic cells are seen, in a background that includes large numbers of histiocytes and lymphocytes marking as T-cells. The presence of prominent nucleoli in the large cells raises a differential diagnosis with Hodgkin cells.

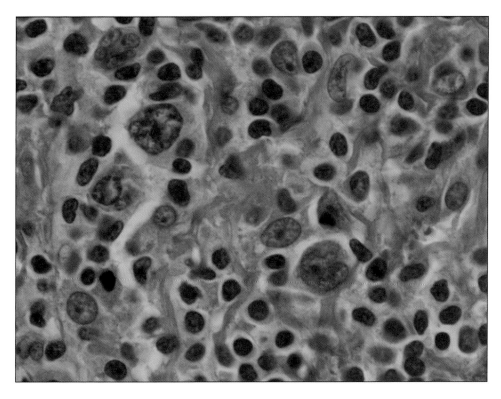

Figure 181. Diffuse large B-cell lymphoma, T-cell/histiocyte-rich variant. In this case, the large cells have a resemblance to L&H cells, raising the differential diagnosis with nodular lymphocyte–predominant Hodgkin lymphoma.

lymphoma and other cases of diffuse large B-cell lymphoma, with a younger age at presentation (median in the 40s) and a marked male predominance (about a 2:1 M:F ratio). In addition, there is a higher incidence of involvement of the bone marrow (about 33%), spleen (about 50%), and liver (about 33%) and a higher incidence of B symptoms.

Figure 182. Diffuse large B-cell lymphoma, T-cell/ histiocyte-rich variant, CD20 stain. The large lymphoid cells show consistent expression of CD20, while virtually all of the small cells are negative.

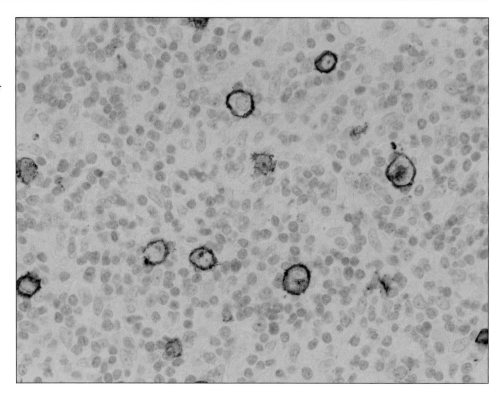

Table 35. Algorithm for Assigning DLBCL Cases to Germinal Center vs. Non–Germinal Center[294]

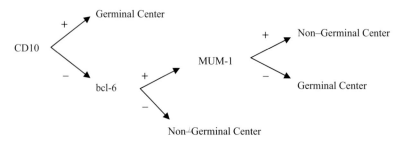

Immunohistochemically, the cells of diffuse large B-cell lymphoma, by definition, express a B-lineage. The pan-B-cells markers CD20, CD79a, CD19, CD22, and PAX-5 as well as the B-cell transcription markers BOB.1 and OCT-2 are each expressed in greater than 95% of cases. Cases most likely to lack expression of one or more pan-B-cell markers are those with plasmacytoid differentiation. Surface immunoglobulin is present in a majority of cases, and cytoplasmic immunoglobulin may be present in cases showing plasmacytoid differentiation. Immunostains may be used to separate the germinal center B-cell–like subset of diffuse large B-cell lymphoma from other subsets; a proposal algorithm employing the germinal center cell markers CD10 and bcl-6, and the B-cell activation marker MUM-1 is given in Table 35. About 50% of diffuse large B-cell lymphomas may express bcl-2, about 10% of cases express CD5, and about 5% of cases express p53 protein. CD138 is uncommonly seen, found in cases with plasmacytoid features. Ki-67 staining is quite variable, generally from 30 to virtually 100%.[294]

As most mature B-cell lymphoma, diffuse large B-cell lymphoma shows consistent clonal rearrangement of the immunoglobulin heavy and light chain genes. Bcl-6 gene rearrangements are seen in about one-third of cases, and, in addition, the bcl-6 gene contains mutations in the 5′ noncoding region in about two-thirds of cases, with neither finding correlated with bcl-6 protein expression. Bcl-2 gene rearrangements are seen in about 25% of cases, restricted to those cases of germinal center B-cell type. C-myc translocations are found in about 10% of cases. In contrast to its occurrence in Burkitt lymphoma, in which the translocation is usually the only major cytogenetic abnormality present, in diffuse large B-cell lymphoma, the c-myc translocations are usually found in the context of a complex karyotype with many other cytogenetic abnormalities.

Major clinical prognostic factors in diffuse large B-cell lymphoma include age, stage, serum lactate dehydrogenase, performance status, and extranodal involvement. These factors have been combined into an International Prognostic Index and an Age-Adjusted International Prognostic Index (Table 24). Despite many attempts, there are as yet no good histologic prognostic factors. Individually, several immunomarkers have been used to determine poor prognosis, including bcl-2 expression, p53 overexpression, high K-67 fraction, and absence of bcl-6 expression. In addition, some studies have shown that expression of bcl-2 or absence of bcl-6 expression has predicted a positive response to rituxan therapy. More recently, separation of cases into germinal center B-cell–like vs. other groups, either by microarrays or by CD10/bcl-6/MUM-1 immunohistochemistry, has been effective in separating two major subgroups having a significantly different prognosis, particularly in the pre-rituximab era (Table 35). Cases determined to be of germinal center B-cell type have a 5-year overall survival of about 75% compared to about 33% for the non–germinal center B-cell type (using non-rituximab regimens). Conflicting results have been obtained for the significance of bcl-2 expression within these two categories, with some studies suggesting adverse prognosis for bcl-2 expression within the germinal center B-cell–like category only and another group suggesting an adverse prognosis for bcl-2 expression within the non–germinal center B-cell–like but not the germinal center B-cell–like category. Use of modern rituximab-including regimens have blunted the significance of these differences.

The WHO recognizes several additional categories of diffuse large B-cell lymphoma, including mediastinal (thymic) large B-cell lymphoma, plasmablastic, ALK-positive diffuse large B-cell lymphoma, intravascular large B-cell lymphoma, primary diffuse large B-cell lymphomas of the central nervous system, leg type diffuse large B-cell lymphoma, diffuse large B-cell lymphoma associated with chronic inflammation, primary effusion lymphoma, and lymphoma associated with HHV-8–associated multicentric Castleman disease (Figures 183 and 184).[310–314] Primary effusion lymphoma is covered in the section HIV-Associated Malignant Lymphomas and lymphoma associated HHV-8–associated multicentric Castleman disease is covered in the section Castleman Disease. With the exception of the latter lymphoma, all of these lymphomas either rarely present in or even involve lymph nodes. Plasmablastic lymphomas are

Figure 183. Diffuse large B-cell lymphoma, intravascular variant. This case, which came from a soft tissue biopsy (and not a lymph node), showed an exclusively intravascular distribution.

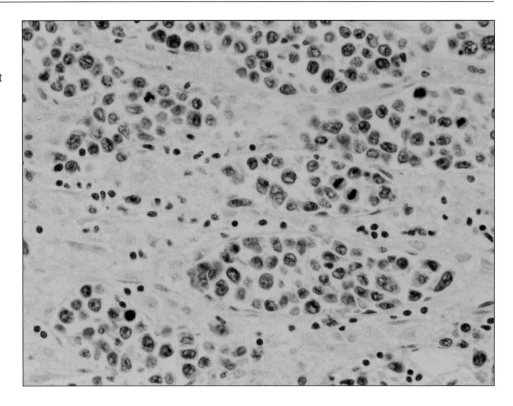

Figure 184. Diffuse large B-cell lymphoma, intravascular variant, CD20 stain. This case was also weakly positive for CD5, which is characteristic of these tumors.

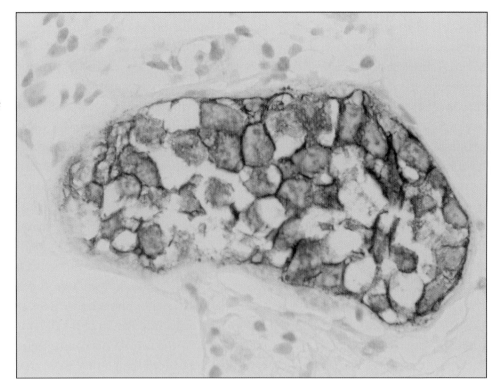

composed of cells resembling immunoblasts that typically lack CD45 and CD20, but show other markers indicative of a B-cell lineage, such as PAX-5, CD79a, BOB.1, or OCT-2 expression, and usually express the plasmacytic marker CD138 (Figure 185). While rare, ALK-positive diffuse large B-cell lymphoma does often involve lymph nodes. Involved lymph nodes show

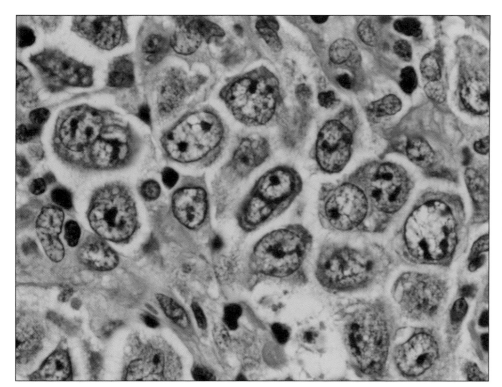

Figure 185. Diffuse large B-cell lymphoma, plasmablastic variant. This case was negative for CD45 and CD20, distinguishing it from immunoblastic lymphoma. The cells are anaplastic, yet are still somewhat reminiscent of plasma cells and need to be distinguished from an anaplastic variant of plasma cell myeloma clinically.

preferential involvement of sinuses by monomorphic immunoblast-like cells showing granular cytoplasmic and dotlike paranuclear positivity for ALK protein, due to a t(2;17) involving the ALK and clathrin genes. While the B-lineage of these cases can be proved by the presence of monoclonal heavy and light chain gene rearrangements, these cases typically lack pan-B-cell markers and CD30 and are weakly positive for CD45, but show light chain restriction with intracytoplasmic IgA and aberrant expression of CD4 and CD57.

Strictly speaking, mediastinal large B-cell lymphoma usually involves the soft tissue of the mediastinum, either arising from or directly adjacent to the thymus, and does not usually involve lymph nodes.[315–321] However, practically speaking, the tumor mass is easily mistaken for involvement of mediastinal lymph nodes, and the distinction is usually moot in the small mediastinal biopsies usually employed to make a diagnosis. Most patients are young adults, with a predilection for females. Patients present with a mediastinal mass that may cause superior mediastinal syndrome. The lymphoma usually does not spread to lymph nodes or bone marrow, but commonly involves extranodal sites. Clinical prognostic factors include performance status, pericardial effusion, bulk of disease, and lactate dehydrogenase (and not the International Prognostic Index). Patients are treated with regimens useful in diffuse large-cell lymphoma, with generally favorable results. At low magnification, a diffuse process is seen, often with a compartmentalizing fibrosis that typically encloses nests of 20–100 cells (Figure 186). At high magnification, a diffuse large lymphoid proliferation is seen. The cells are typically round to oval, often with irregularities of the nuclear membranes, a vesicular chromatin pattern, and one to several nucleoli. Cytoplasm is often abundant and may be pale to clear.

Figure 186. Mediastinal large B-cell lymphoma. Note the pattern of fibrosis, compartmentalizing the neoplastic large B-cells into discrete nests.

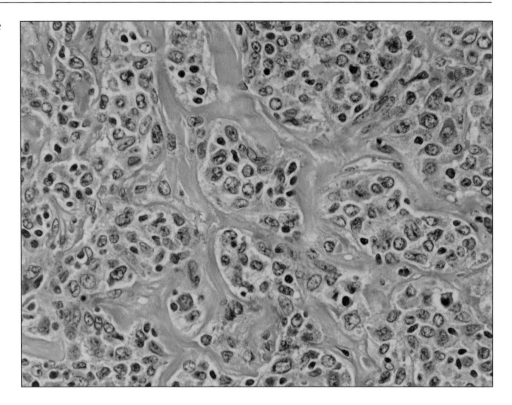

Usually, there is not a significant accompanying reactive infiltrate, but exceptions may occur. Immunohistochemical studies demonstrate CD45 expression as well as consistent expression of multiple pan-B-cell antigens, but immunoglobulin expression is most often absent. There is usually no aberrant coexpression of CD43 or CD5, and CD138 is also negative. CD10 and/or bcl-6 are usually negative and CD30 is often focally positive, and occasionally is diffusely positive. Coexpression of TRAF1 and nuclear c-rel may be a specific means to distinguish this neoplasm from other types of diffuse large B-cell lymphoma, as it occurs in about one-half of cases, as compared to 3% of other diffuse large B-cell lymphomas. Clonal gene rearrangements of the immunoglobulin heavy and/or light chain genes are found and bcl-2, bcl-6, and c-myc translocations are not seen, although bcl-6 point mutations are common. cDNA microarrays studies have shown a closer relationship to Hodgkin lymphoma than other B-cell lymphomas, but this does not yet have practical significance.

The differential diagnosis of diffuse large B-cell lymphoma is extremely wide. On the one hand, one must distinguish it from nonlymphoid neoplasms, and on the other hand, one must distinguish it from reactive hyperplasia, Hodgkin lymphoma, or other types of non-Hodgkin lymphoma. Carcinoma and malignant melanoma are the nonlymphoid neoplasms most often confused with diffuse large B-cell lymphoma. The most important factor in establishing the correct diagnosis is to consider these other neoplasms in the differential diagnosis. Fortunately, the inclusion of keratin and S-100 protein should provide easy separation of these entities. Acute leukemia may also be confused with diffuse large B-cell lymphoma. The uniformity of the proliferation, the presence of granular cytoplasm, or the admixture of eosinophils may all suggest the correct diagnosis. One must also keep in mind that acute myeloid leukemia with t(8;21) frequently shows expression of CD19, and promyelocytic leukemia may show aberrant expression of PAX-5. The addition of myeloperoxidase along with other immature myeloid markers such as CD34 and CD117 along with absence of CD20 staining allow for the correct diagnosis in most cases.

Reactive paracortical hyperplasia is the pattern of hyperplasia most easily confused with diffuse large B-cell lymphoma. Reactive paracortical hyperplasia is usually associated with an accompanying reactive follicular hyperplasia. Although the proliferating immunoblasts in reactive paracortical hyperplasia can closely resemble the cells of diffuse large B-cell lymphoma, they rarely form true sheets of cells with architectural effacement. EBV studies may be helpful if EBV-associated infectious mononucleosis is considered in the differential diagnosis, particularly in children and young adults. Immunohistochemical studies of reactive paracortical hyperplasia often show that there is a mixture of B- and T-cells, including the large cells. Kikuchi necrotizing histiocytic lymphadenitis may also show a close resemblance to diffuse large B-cell lymphoma. Identification of the large cells as histiocytes along with the demonstration of large numbers of CD8-positive cells maybe helpful in this distinction.

The distinction between diffuse large B-cell lymphoma and Hodgkin lymphoma may be difficult. Patients with classical Hodgkin lymphoma are usually younger than those with diffuse large B-cell lymphoma. Cases of nodular sclerosis may contain numerous Hodgkin cells, but these tend to cluster in aggregates rather than disperse evenly throughout the lymph node. The most difficult cases are those in which a diagnosis of lymphocyte depletion is being considered. Classical Hodgkin lymphoma may show CD20 positivity in a significant subset of cases, and expression of PAX-5 is seen in a large majority of cases. CD79a is usually negative in Hodgkin lymphoma, as are the B-cell transcription factors BOB.1 and OCT-2, although exceptions are not uncommon. Diffuse large B-cell lymphoma may show CD30 positivity, particularly anaplastic variants; however, CD15 staining would be most unusual. Sometimes, the distinction cannot be made even by experienced hematopathologists (so-called gray-zone lymphomas). In these unusual cases, the difficulty should be clearly documented in the report; often, clinicians will choose to treat for the more aggressive diffuse large B-cell lymphoma rather than for the more easily curable Hodgkin lymphoma. The differential diagnosis between lymphocyte predominance and transformation to diffuse large B-cell lymphoma has already been discussed in the section Nodular Lymphocyte–Predominant Hodgkin Lymphoma.

Diffuse low-grade B-cell lymphomas may contain significant numbers of large B-cells, raising the question of possible transformation to diffuse large B-cell lymphoma. I do not diagnose transformation to diffuse large B-cell lymphoma unless I see areas of complete architectural effacement by sheets of large cells. One must remember that significant numbers of large cells may be present in chronic lymphocytic leukemia/small lymphocytic lymphoma, and are within the spectrum of that lymphoma as long as they are contained within the proliferation centers, or present within the background of a small lymphocytic proliferation. Similarly, I diagnose diffuse large B-cell lymphoma transformation from follicular lymphoma, when there are diffuse areas of effacement showing grade 3 cytology. The presence of grade 3 cytology within follicles or confined to the interfollicular areas does not denote transformation.

Large-cell blastoid variants of mantle cell lymphoma may be easily confused for diffuse large B-cell lymphoma. A previous history of mantle cell lymphoma should suggest the correct diagnosis, but this history is often absent. The presence of a fine chromatin pattern or aberrant CD5 expression should raise the possibility of mantle cell lymphoma, prompting the performance of cyclin D1 staining, even though aberrant CD5 expression can be seen in about 10% of cases of diffuse large B-cell lymphoma. Strong expression of cyclin D1 has not been reported in diffuse large B-cell lymphoma and should be considered definitive evidence for mantle cell lymphoma.

Lymphoblastic lymphoma usually has a more monomorphic appearance, featuring intermediately sized cells with a finer, more blastic-appearing chromatin pattern than that seen in diffuse large B-cell lymphoma. In difficult cases, staining for terminal deoxyribonucleotidyl transferase should prove definitive. The differential diagnosis of diffuse large B-cell lymphoma and Burkitt lymphoma is discussed in the section Burkitt Lymphoma. Some cases of peripheral T-cell lymphoma may also show a close resemblance to diffuse large B-cell lymphoma. Paraffin section immunohistochemical studies should be performed in all cases of suspected diffuse large B-cell lymphoma to rule out this possibility, since prognosis and treatment is different for these two neoplasms.

The differential diagnosis of T-cell/histiocyte-rich B-cell lymphoma is particularly difficult and includes diffuse follicle center lymphoma, peripheral T-cell lymphoma, classical Hodgkin lymphoma, and lymphocyte predominance Hodgkin lymphoma. Patients with diffuse follicle center are typically older than those with T-cell/histiocyte-rich B-cell lymphoma and are the same age as patients with other types of follicular lymphoma. Similar to T-cell/histiocyte-rich B-cell lymphoma, diffuse follicle center lymphoma also has a population of large atypical cells, with the large cells usually resembling centroblasts and centrocytes. These cells also express CD45 and pan-B-cell markers. The large cells express markers of germinal centers, including CD10, bcl-6, and bcl-2. However, the most important distinction is in the character of the small cells. In diffuse follicle center lymphoma, the majority of these cells are centrocytes carrying the same phenotype as the large cells – expressing pan-B-cell markers, CD10, bcl-6, and bcl-2. This is in contrast to the small cells in T-cell/histiocyte-rich B-cell lymphoma, in which the small cells are almost all T-cells, with very few B-cells.

Peripheral T-cell lymphoma may be easily confused with T-cell/histiocyte-rich B-cell lymphoma, as several types of peripheral T-cell lymphoma may contain scattered reactive large B-cells/immunoblasts. Patients with peripheral T-cell lymphoma are, again, usually older than patients with T-cell/histiocyte-rich B-cell lymphoma. Morphologically, the key to the identification of peripheral T-cell lymphoma is noting that not only the large cells have atypical features but also there is a population of small- to medium-sized cells with cytologic atypia. These cells will have the phenotype of T-cells and may show aberrant patterns of expression, including loss of pan-T-cell antigens (such as CD7, CD5, CD3, or CD2) or gain of inappropriate antigens (such as CD10 and/or bcl-6). The large cells may or may not have a B-cell phenotype. If they have a B-cell phenotype, they may also be positive for CD30 and/or EBV, tip-offs that they may represent a reactive B-cell proliferation in a T-cell lymphoma. Gene rearrangement studies may be very helpful, with the demonstration of monoclonal T-cell receptor gene rearrangements. However, there may also be mono- or oligoclonal immunoglobulin heavy and/or light chain gene rearrangements.

Classical Hodgkin lymphoma, particularly of mixed cellularity subtype, can also be easily confused with T-cell/histiocyte-rich B-cell lymphoma. In fact, some pathologists have suggested that all cases with a presumptive diagnosis of mixed cellularity Hodgkin lymphoma be phenotyped, to rule out the possibility of T-cell/histiocyte-rich B-cell lymphoma. The large atypical cells of T-cell/histiocyte-rich B-cell lymphoma may be morphologically virtually identical to Hodgkin cells, although mixed cellularity Hodgkin lymphoma usually has a greater admixture of eosinophils and plasma cells. The immunohistochemical differences are outlined in Table 20.

Lymphocyte-predominant Hodgkin lymphoma probably represents the entity most easily confused with T-cell/histiocyte-rich B-cell lymphoma. Clinically, T-cell/histiocyte-rich B-cell lymphoma is more likely to present at higher stage, particularly with involvement of bone marrow, spleen, and/or liver. However, the morphologic appearance may be very similar, particularly in recurrences of lymphocyte predominance, in which a nodular architecture may not be well developed. The staining profile of the large cells is quite similar in both neoplasms, with positivity for CD45; CD20; and other major pan-B-cell markers, BOB.1 and OCT-2; and frequent positivity for bcl-6, as both neoplasms appear to differentiate toward germinal center B-cells. The presence of true follicular structures, whether seen as nodules morphologically or identified immunophenotypically (as nodules of small B-cells or networks of follicular dendritic cells), would favor lymphocyte predominance. Similarly, the presence of increased numbers of CD57-positive cells, particularly with the formation of rosettes around large cells, would also favor lymphocyte predominance. On the other hand, the identification of monoclonal immunoglobulin heavy and/or light chain gene rearrangements would strongly favor T-cell/histiocyte-rich B-cell lymphoma. Some hematopathologists have reported T-cell/histiocyte-rich B-cell lymphoma to occur following a diagnosis of lymphocyte predominance, but I would consider these cases as recurrences of lymphocyte predominance even though such recurrences have been associated with clinical disease progression and other aggressive behavior.

BURKITT LYMPHOMA[322–327]

Burkitt lymphoma is a distinctive high-grade malignant lymphoma composed of monomorphic neoplastic lymphoid cells of intermediate size showing consistent

Table 36. St. Jude Modification of Ann Arbor Staging System for Burkitt Lymphoma[328]

Stage	
I	Single anatomic area or single extranodal site, excluding intrathoracic, abdominal, or paraspinal lesion
II	Single extranodal site with regional lymph node involvement
	Primary gastrointestinal tract tumor, completely resected
	Two or more anatomical areas or extranodal sites on same side of diaphragm
III	Two or more anatomical areas or extranodal sites on both sides of diaphragm
	All primary intrathoracic tumors
	All extensive primary abdominal disease
	All primary paraspinal or epidural tumors
IV	Central nervous system or bone marrow involvement

translocation of the c-myc gene. Outside the setting of immunosuppression, there are two main clinical forms. In equatorial Africa and Papua New Guinea, endemic Burkitt lymphoma is seen. In this form, the peak of incidence is in children over the age of 2, with a 2:1 M:F ratio, and a universal association with EBV. The disease most often presents with jaw involvement, often with coexisting orbital involvement, although most patients also have subdiaphragmatic disease as well. In Western countries, a sporadic form is seen. In this form, both children and adults are affected, again with a 2:1 M:F ratio and with a 20% association with EBV. An abdominal presentation is most frequently seen, most often with a mass in the ileocecal region and regional mesenteric lymph nodes. Unusual sites such as bilateral breasts (occurring in pubertal girls or lactating women), ovaries, kidneys, or the pancreas are not uncommonly also involved. Bone marrow involvement is common in the sporadic form, and some patients may present with a leukemic form of the disease, formerly known as the L3 subtype of acute lymphoblastic leukemia. The central nervous system may be involved in up to 20% of cases, more frequent in endemic than sporadic cases. A form transitional between endemic and sporadic Burkitt lymphoma occurs in North Africa, South Africa, equatorial South America, and parts of Asia. A staging system that takes into account the unique features of Burkitt lymphoma has been developed (Table 36).[328] Burkitt lymphoma associated with immunodeficiency is further discussed in Chapter 9.

Involved lymph nodes usually have a fleshy appearance on cut section, often with areas of hemorrhage and/or necrosis. At low magnification, diffuse effacement of nodal architecture typically is seen, although some cases of focal involvement may show preferential involvement of the follicles (Figures 187 and 188). A starry-sky appearance is almost always seen. This is due to the presence of scattered tingible-body macrophages with abundant phagocytosed debris (representing remnants of apoptotic tumor cells) in a background of a monomorphic population of atypical lymphoid cells, with an extremely high mitotic rate. The proliferating cells are medium sized, with nuclei approximately the size of normal histiocytes. The cytoplasm is generally moderate in amount, basophilic, and

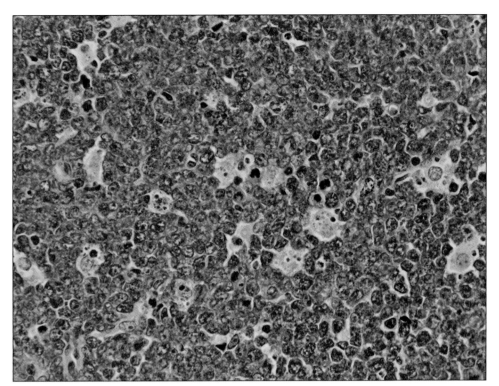

Figure 187. Classical Burkitt lymphoma. A starry-sky appearance is seen, with regularly spaced tingible-body macrophages and a uniform population of lymphoid cells.

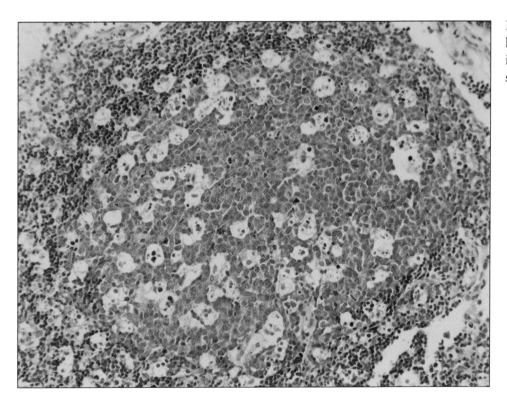

Figure 188. Classical Burkitt lymphoma. Preferential involvement of a follicle is seen in this focus.

tends to *square off* with adjacent cells. Multiple lipid vacuoles are often discernible in imprint preparations. Small lymphocytes, plasma cells, or granulocytes are typically not seen, unless there are secondary changes, such as necrosis.

At least two cytologic variants have been recognized. In classical Burkitt lymphoma, the neoplastic nuclei are round and uniform in size, with a somewhat

Figure 189. Classical Burkitt lymphoma. The cells have medium-sized nuclei, with generally several nucleoli, and small rim of cytoplasm. Note the high mitotic rate.

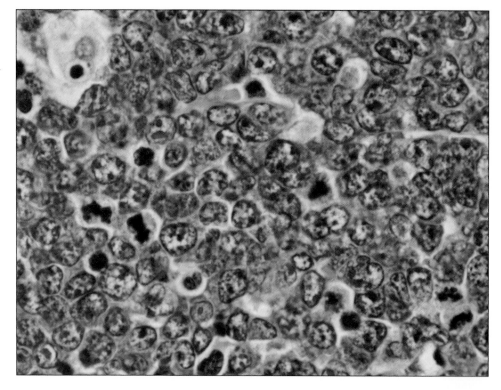

Figure 190. Burkitt-like lymphoma. The presence of prominent nucleoli distinguishes this case from classical Burkitt lymphoma. This case had a c-myc translocation.

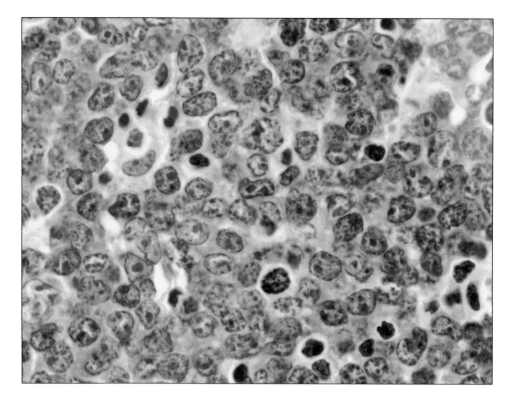

vesicular chromatin pattern and typically several randomly disposed medium-sized nucleoli (Figure 189), while in atypical Burkitt lymphoma, the neoplastic nucleoli are more variable in size and shape and tend to have fewer, but more prominent, nuclei (Figure 190). Classical cytology is said to be more common in endemic cases and those cases occurring in children, while atypical cytology is

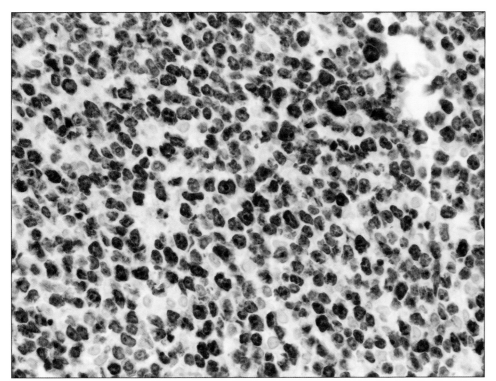

Figure 191. Burkitt lymphoma, Ki-67 stain. All or virtually all the lymphoid cells are positive. Any significant degree of negative staining would not be compatible with Burkitt lymphoma.

said to be more common in sporadic cases, particularly those cases occurring in adults. However, I believe that the two cytologic appearances are overlapping and more a function of fixation than real. The important message is that whether one uses the terminology classical or atypical to modify a diagnosis of Burkitt lymphoma, the use of the term Burkitt is really what is of importance, implying a high-grade neoplasm as defined above. The term *Burkitt-like* derives from the Working Formulation. It probably represents a wider group of neoplasms than Burkitt lymphoma as used here, including some cases of aggressive diffuse large B-cell lymphoma and some cases of blastic transformation of follicular lymphoma; therefore, it should no longer be used.

Burkitt lymphoma has a relatively homogeneous immunophenotype. There is consistent expression of CD45 and pan-B-cell markers, including CD20, CD79a, CD19, CD22, and PAX-5, as well as the B-cell transcription factors BOB.1 and OCT-2. The cells express surface IgM with light chain restriction, although the latter is usually not demonstrable in paraffin sections. There is also consistent expression of the germinal center cell markers CD10 and bcl-6. Although it has been stated that bcl-2 is consistently negative, recent studies have shown positivity in up to 33% of cases. There may be aberrant coexpression of CD43, seen in up to 50% of cases. The Ki-67 index is consistently close to 100%, and T-cell stains reveal very few infiltrating T-cells (Figure 191). Despite the blastic appearance of the cells, terminal deoxyribonucleotidyl transferase, CD117, and CD34 are consistently negative.

The genetic hallmark of Burkitt lymphoma is a relatively simple karyotype containing a c-myc translocation. This is most often a t(8;14)(q24;q32) involving the immunoglobulin heavy chain locus (85% of cases), but may alternatively be a t(2;8) involving the kappa–light chain gene (10% of cases) or a t(8;22) involving the lambda–light chain gene (5% of cases), with the unifying features being the deregulation of the c-myc gene. Because the breakpoints occur at different loci at the molecular level, the translocations are not readily detected by routine PCR studies. FISH studies using *break-apart* probes are often the most optimal technique for detecting the translocation; in addition, these studies usually can be performed on paraffin-embedded tissue. Similar to other B-cell lymphomas, Burkitt lymphoma also shows clonal rearrangements of the immunoglobulin heavy and/or light chain genes.

Prognostic factors include bulk of disease, presence of residual disease after surgical excision, presence of involvement of the blood, bone marrow and the central nervous system, and high lactate dehydrogenase levels. There is a staging system for Burkitt lymphoma in children that takes into account many of the unique features of this neoplasm. When aggressive chemotherapy is given, often with intrathecal chemotherapy, recent survival rates have exceeded those of diffuse large B-cell lymphoma, particularly in children.

The differential diagnosis of Burkitt lymphoma is limited, but it is important to establish a correct diagnosis. The distinction from diffuse large B-cell lymphoma is the most difficult and may be impossible in some cases; however, it is important to attempt as Burkitt lymphoma is often treated more aggressively, including central nervous system chemoprophylaxis, than diffuse large B-cell lymphoma. One should consider Burkitt lymphoma in any diffuse intermediate- to large-cell lymphoma with a monomorphic appearance and a very high mitotic rate. The next step would be to perform immunostains to confirm B-lineage and furthermore to assess CD10, bcl-6, and Ki-67. CD10 and bcl-6 should be positive, and the Ki-67 index should be close to 100%. Other supportive results would be a negative bcl-2 (although it may still be positive in 33% of cases of Burkitt lymphoma) and aberrant coexpression of CD43 (seen in 50% of cases of Burkitt lymphoma). If Burkitt lymphoma is still being considered after the immunostudies, then FISH studies for the presence of a c-myc translocation are indicated. FISH studies for c-myc are probably not warranted unless Burkitt lymphoma is being strongly considered, as about 10% of cases of diffuse large B-cell lymphomas have a c-myc translocation, usually in the context of a complex karyotype containing many other abnormalities. Multiparameter studies, including karyotyping and mRNA microarrays, have validated this approach, although these studies have shown that potential misdiagnosis may still occur in a small minority of cases.

Lymphoblastic lymphoma may have a superficial similarity to Burkitt lymphoma, with a monomorphic population of blastic-appearing cells. However, the cells of lymphoblastic lymphoma have a finer chromatin pattern, less prominent nucleoli, generally a lower mitotic rate, and less abundant cytoplasm that does not square off against adjacent cells. In difficult cases, immunophenotyping is of great utility, as lymphoblastic lymphoma is mostly of T-lineage and shows consistent expression of terminal deoxynucleotidyl transferase. The blastic variant of mantle cell lymphoma may also resemble Burkitt lymphoma. Again, the cells have a finer chromatin pattern, less prominent nucleoli, generally a lower mitotic rate, and less abundant cytoplasm. Although both mantle cell lymphoma and

Burkitt lymphoma are of B-lineage, the blastic variant of mantle cell lymphoma is cyclin D1 positive, often CD5 positive, and is negative for CD10. Lymph node involvement by acute myeloid leukemia may also simulate Burkitt lymphoma. With acute leukemia, there is often more variability in the neoplastic cells as well as more variability in the cell population, with scattered eosinophils sometimes present. Acute myeloid leukemia usually expresses CD117, CD34, and/or myeloperoxidase, markers consistently negative in Burkitt lymphoma.

Finally, a blastic transformation of follicular lymphoma may be difficult to distinguish from Burkitt lymphoma. The neoplastic cells may have a very close morphologic appearance, and, in addition, both express the germinal center markers CD10 and bcl-6. Patients with a blastic transformation of follicular lymphoma are generally older than the typical Burkitt patient and often have a history of previous follicular lymphoma. In fact, a bone marrow biopsy may reveal the underlying follicular lymphoma. While blastic transformation of follicular lymphoma often contains a c-myc translocation, it almost always also has a t(14;18) characteristic of the underlying follicular lymphoma.

PRECURSOR B-LYMPHOBLASTIC LYMPHOMA/LEUKEMIA[329]

Precursor B-lymphoblastic lymphoma/leukemia is a high-grade neoplasm of immature B-lymphocytes. About 80% of cases occur in young childhood. Although the distinction is artifactual, cases with greater than 25% marrow involvement at presentation are generally regarded as leukemia, while cases presenting with a mass lesion and less than 25% marrow involvement at presentation are generally regarded as lymphoma. The disease presents as lymphoma in about 10% of cases. Patients with a lymphoma presentation are somewhat older, with a median age of about 20 years. Extranodal sites, including skin, bone, and soft tissue, are most frequently the presenting site. About 10% of cases present in lymph nodes, although regional lymph nodes are commonly involved in patients presenting with extranodal disease. Patients with precursor B-lymphoblastic leukemia/lymphoma are treated with multidrug chemotherapy, with a greater than 50% survival rate.

Involved lymph nodes often show infiltration of the lymph node capsule with extension of the proliferation into the perinodal fat. The proliferation is centered in the paracortical region, often with sparing of the follicles, and a focal or diffuse starry-sky appearance may be seen. Cytologically, the involved areas show a monotonous infiltrate of small- to medium-sized cells with a fine chromatin pattern, inconspicuous nucleoli, and scant cytoplasm (Figure 192). The nuclear outlines may be round, irregular, or highly convoluted.

Immunophenotyping studies demonstrate an immature B-cell lineage. Most, but not all, cases express CD45, and there is uniform expression of terminal deoxyribonucleotidyl transferase. PAX-5 and CD19 are the mostly consistently expressed pan-B-cell markers, positive in virtually all cases, and BOB.1 and CD79a are also expressed in 90 and 80% of cases, respectively. In contrast, CD20

Figure 192. B-precursor lymphoma/leukemia. The cells are medium sized and show a little variation in size and shape. The chromatin pattern is somewhat fine. This morphology probably corresponds to and L2 appearance on smears.

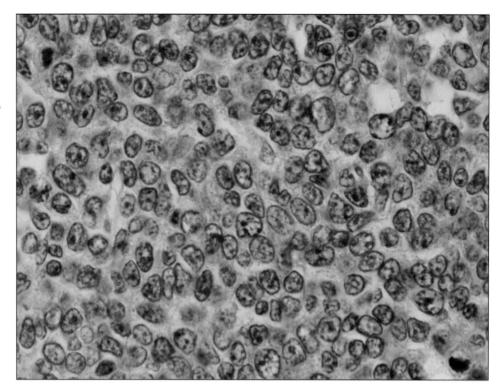

and OCT-2 are positive in only a minority of cases. CD10 is expressed in about one-half of cases, being negative in the most immature cases (early precursor stage). Surface immunoglobulin is usually (but not always) negative, but cytoplasmic mu may be expressed in the most mature stage (pre-B). There is also usually expression of CD43 and CD34, and there may be expression of the myeloid markers CD13 and CD33. The Ki-67 index is highly variable, but generally ranges from 50 to 90%. Molecular studies usually demonstrate clonal gene rearrangements of the immunoglobulin heavy and/or light chain genes. Cytogenetic studies show several types of cases of prognostic significance, including a hypodiploid group, a low hyperdiploid group, a high hyperdiploid group, a group with one of a set of characteristic translocations, and a pseudodiploid group. It is beyond the scope of this book to discuss the various findings and their clinical and biologic significance.

The differential diagnosis is that of the blastic neoplasm involving lymph nodes and includes precursor T-lymphoblastic lymphoma/leukemia, acute myeloid leukemia, the blastic variant of mantle cell lymphoma, Burkitt lymphoma, precursor plasmacytoid dendritic cell neoplasm, and diffuse large B-cell lymphoma (see Table 34). Precursor T-lymphoblastic lymphoma/leukemia has virtually identical morphologic features and also shares expression of terminal deoxynucleotidyl transferase and CD43. Clinically, precursor T-lymphoblastic lymphoma/leukemia often shows involvement of the mediastinum. Immunophenotyping studies demonstrate the presence of one or more pan-T-cell markers and the absence of pan-B-cell markers. Acute myeloid leukemia usually shows more prominent nuclei and more abundant cytoplasm. Although a subset of cases may express terminal deoxyribonucleotidyl transferase and cases of precursor B-cell leukemia/lymphoma may express CD11 and CD33, the latter consistently lack myeloperoxidase and lysozyme and expresses multiple pan-B-lineage antigens. The blastic variant of mantle cell lymphoma may show a close morphologic similarity to precursor B-lymphoblastic lymphoma/leukemia. For this reason, cyclin D1 stains are recommended (along with terminal deoxyribonucleotidyl transferase) in any case of a blastic hematolymphoid neoplasm involving the lymph node. Burkitt lymphoma usually has a more prominent starry-sky appearance and is composed of cells with more prominent nucleoli and more abundant cytoplasm. In contrast to the precursor B-lymphoblastic lymphoma/leukemia, Burkitt lymphoma has consistent expression of CD20, has a near 100% Ki-67 index, has consistent translocations involving c-myc, and lacks expression of terminal deoxynucleotidyl transferase. Large-cell lymphoma has larger nuclei with a more vesicular chromatin pattern and more prominent nuclei, consistent expression of CD20, and also lacks expression of terminal deoxynucleotidyl transferase. Precursor plasmacytoid dendritic cell neoplasm may express terminal deoxyribonucleotidyl transferase, but lacks B-lineage markers and expresses CD123 and CD56.

PRECURSOR T-LYMPHOBLASTIC LYMPHOMA/LEUKEMIA[330-334]

Precursor T-lymphoblastic lymphoma/leukemia is a high-grade neoplasm of immature T-lymphocytes. Although the distinction is artifactual, cases with greater than 25% marrow involvement at presentation are generally regarded as leukemia, while cases presenting with a mass lesion and less than 25% marrow involvement at presentation are generally regarded as lymphoma. Precursor lymphoblastic lymphoma/leukemia presents at all ages, although the peak of incidence is in young adults and children. There is a male predominance. Most patients present with a mediastinal mass, often with an accompanying pleural effusion. A majority of patients also have involvement of peripheral blood, bone marrow, and lymph nodes at presentation. Common sites of lymph node involvement include the neck and axillary regions. Other less common areas of infiltration include the central nervous system, liver, and testis. Patients are generally treated with intensive combination chemotherapy, with autologous stem cell transplantation in first remission.

Involved lymph nodes show either preferential involvement of the paracortex or, more commonly, diffuse effacement, often with extension of the proliferation outside the capsule (Figure 193). Involvement of the capsule often manifests as a single-file pattern of infiltration, simulating lobular carcinoma of the breast (Figure 194). A starry-sky pattern may be seen, but this is more often a focal finding than diffusely seen throughout the neoplasm such as observed in Burkitt lymphoma. Cytologically, the cells are small to intermediate in size (Figures 195 and 196). The nuclei are round to oval and have a fine chromatin pattern with small nucleoli. The nuclear outlines may vary from smooth to convoluted. Mitoses are usually easily seen, but are not as numerous as in Burkitt lymphoma. Cytoplasm is typically scant. Precursor T-lymphoblastic lymphoma/leukemia associated with a t(8;13) may

Figure 193. Precursor
T-lymphoblastic lymphoma/
leukemia. A diffuse
proliferation of
monomorphic blastic cells is
seen. Although there are
scattered tingible-body
macrophages, a
well-developed starry-sky
pattern is not seen. Note the
numerous degenerating cells
with pyknotic nuclei.

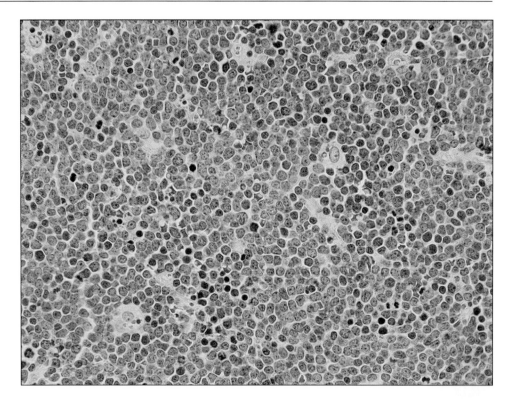

Figure 194. T-precursor
lymphoma/leukemia. There is
often a tendency toward
sclerosis with a single-cell
pattern of infiltration,
particularly in the lymph
node capsule and adjacent
soft tissue.

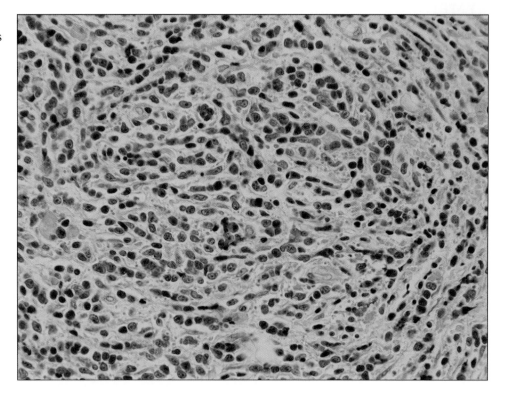

show scattered eosinophils and a biphasic pattern, with areas resembling lympho-blastic lymphoma along with other areas more resembling acute blastic leukemia.

Immunophenotyping studies usually show an immature thymocyte phenotype, at varying stages of maturation. The neoplastic cells consistently express CD45, the immature marker terminal deoxyribonucleotidyl transferase (Figure 197), and

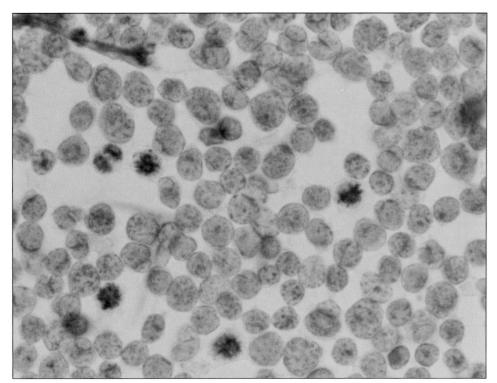

Figure 195. Precursor T-lymphoblastic lymphoma/ leukemia. This scrape preparation shows the fine blastic chromatin pattern. Note the numerous mitotic figures.

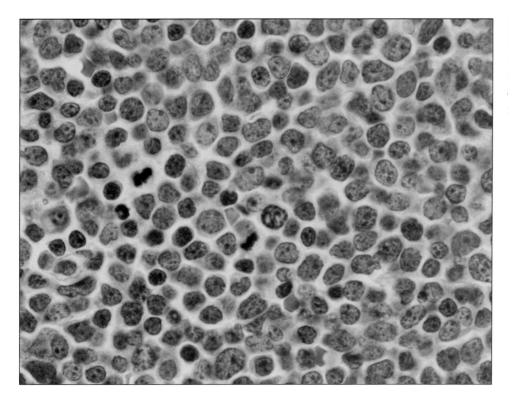

Figure 196. T-precursor lymphoma/leukemia. The uniform cells are small to medium sized, with a fine chromatin pattern and small nucleoli.

CD99. At the earliest stage of maturation, CD7 and cytoplasmic CD3 (detectable in paraffin sections) are expressed, soon followed by CD2 and CD5. At the intermediate stage, there is expression of CD1a and coexpression of CD4 and CD8. At the most mature stage, there is loss of CD1a, membrane CD3 expression, and the cells become either CD4 or CD8 positive but no longer show coexpression of these latter

Figure 197. T-precursor lymphoma/leukemia, terminal deoxyribonucleotidyl transferase stain. There is strong nuclear positivity.

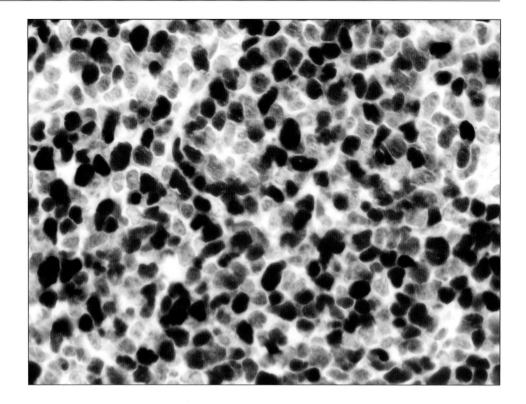

two markers. Occasional cases may be CD79a positive, and a subset of cases are positive for CD10, but other B-lineage markers are consistently negative. Some cases may express some myeloid antigens, such as CD13, CD33, and/or CD117. The Ki-67 index may be quite variable, but is usually greater than 50%.

Precursor T-lymphoblastic lymphoma/leukemia usually shows rearrangement of the gamma and beta T-cell receptor genes. In addition, about one-third of cases have translocations involving the alpha/delta, beta, or gamma chain genes. Gene expression microarray studies have confirmed the different stages of thymic maturation among these neoplasms.

Adverse prognostic clinical factors include older age; advanced stage; high International Prognostic Index; the presence of bone marrow, blood, and central nervous system involvement; B symptoms; and serum lactate dehydrogenase. Most pathologic factors are not of prognostic significance, although there may be a correlation between early phenotype and expression of pan-T-cell antigens and good outcome. Specifically, the presence of specific translocations does not seem to correlate with clinical outcome.

The differential diagnosis of precursor T-lymphoblastic lymphoma/leukemia includes precursor B-lymphoblastic lymphoma/leukemia, acute myeloid leukemia, the blastic variant of mantle cell lymphoma, Burkitt lymphoma, diffuse large B-cell lymphoma, precursor plasmacytoid dendritic cell neoplasm, and peripheral T-cell lymphoma (see Table 34).[335] Precursor B-lymphoblastic lymphoma/leukemia has an identical morphologic appearance and also shows consistent expression of terminal deoxyribonucleotidyl transferase. However, it more often occurs in children, almost always presents as acute leukemia, rarely presents as a mediastinal mass, and more often involves skin and bone. Immunostains are definitive, showing consistent expression of the B-lineage markers CD19, PAX-5, and cytoplasmic CD79a and an absence of pan-T-cell markers. Acute myeloid leukemia usually shows more prominent nucleoli and more abundant cytoplasm. Although a subset of cases may express terminal deoxyribonucleotidyl transferase, immunostains show frequent expression of myeloperoxidase and/or lysozyme as well as the absence of multiple pan-T-cell markers. The blastic variant of mantle cell lymphoma expresses multiple B-lineage markers along with cyclin D1, along with the absence of terminal deoxyribonucleotidyl transferase. Burkitt lymphoma and diffuse large B-cell lymphoma similarly express multiple B-lineage markers and are negative for terminal deoxyribonucleotidyl transferase. Peripheral T-cell lymphoma is composed of T-cells with a more mature chromatin pattern, greater pleomorphism from cell to cell, and a wider range of reactive cells. Immunohistochemically, it shares the expression of pan-T-cell markers with precursor T-lymphoblastic lymphoma/leukemia, but lacks terminal deoxyribonucleotidyl transferase, CD1a, and CD99 expression. Precursor plasmacytoid dendritic cell neoplasm may express terminal deoxyribonucleotidyl transferase, but expresses CD123 and CD56.

MATURE T-CELL AND NK-CELL NEOPLASMS[213,336–338]

The WHO Classification of mature T-cell and NK-cell neoplasms is given in Table 25. Collectively, they comprise less than 10% of all cases of malignant lymphomas. In general, they are a heterogeneous group of neoplasms. Classification is based on a constellation of clinical, histologic, phenotypic, genotypic, and viral findings. Only a few types have a predilection for lymph nodes, even with recurrences. However, those few comprise the majority of cases. The T-cell lymphomas that predominantly present in lymph nodes include peripheral T-cell lymphoma, unspecified; angioimmunoblastic T-cell lymphoma; and anaplastic large-cell lymphoma. In addition, lymph nodes are commonly involved in patients with adult T-cell leukemia/lymphoma and mycosis fungoides/Sezary syndrome. In the other types, lymph node involvement is rare and generally only occurs as a late manifestation of disease long after a definitive diagnosis is established.

ANGIOIMMUNOBLASTIC T-CELL LYMPHOMA[339–344]

Angioimmunoblastic T-cell lymphoma is a specific type of peripheral T-cell lymphoma probably arising from intrafollicular T-helper cells. It comprises about 15% of all cases of T/NK-cell lymphoma. It almost exclusively affects adults, particularly the elderly, and has a slight male predilection. Patients usually present with systemic symptoms along with generalized lymphadenopathy, hepatosplenomegaly, and skin rash. Patients often have a polyclonal hypergammaglobulinemia, associated with hemolytic anemia or circulating immune complexes, and the bone marrow is often involved at presentation. Some hematopathologists, including myself, believe that there may be a preneoplastic state (angioimmunoblastic

Figure 198.
Angioimmunoblastic
lymphadenopathy–like T-cell
lymphoma. Intense
hypervascularity is seen.

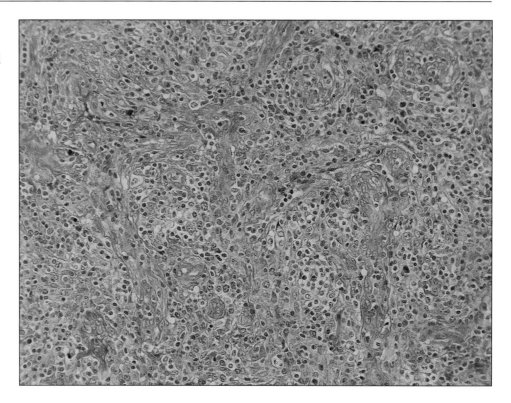

lymphadenopathy), often characterized by oligoclonal proliferations of T-cells. Greater than normal numbers of EBV-infected B-cells and, to a lesser extent, T-cells are present, but probably represent a consequence of the relative immuno-deficiency that is a part of the disease process rather than of etiologic significance. Patients with angioimmunoblastic-like T-cell lymphoma are generally treated with multidrug chemotherapy if they are healthy enough to withstand the therapy. Alternatively, some patients may be treated with prednisone.

Involved lymph nodes are usually only moderately enlarged. At low magnification, partial to diffuse effacement is typical, often with some extension outside the capsule. At medium magnification, regressed follicles are usually seen, although occasionally reactive germinal centers may be present or even a prominent finding throughout the lymph node. The paracortical region is dominant, although highly vascular and often somewhat cell poor, and subcapsular sinuses are often patent (Figure 198). At high magnification, one sees a mixed cell population, including varying numbers of small round lymphocytes, eosinophils, histiocytes, plasma cells, immunoblasts, and a population of small- to medium-sized lymphocytes, often with clear cytoplasm and usually clustered around small blood vessels (Figure 199). The histiocytes may or may not be epithelioid and are sometimes quite prominent. Focal areas may contain an interstitial eosinophilic substance; these areas usually represent the residuum of follicles. The blood vessels consist mostly of high endothelial venules and small veins.

Immunohistochemical studies show a predominance of T-cells of CD4-positive helper phenotype. The T-cells usually do not show loss of pan-T-cell antigens, or at most, loss of one antigen, most frequently CD7. However, the T-cells frequently show aberrant expression of CD10 and bcl-6, along with CXCL13. CD10 and bcl-6

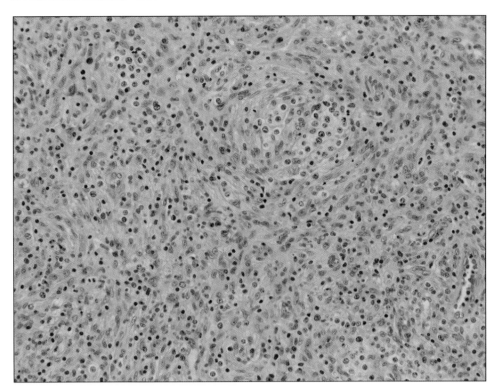

Figure 199.
Angioimmunoblastic-like
T-cell lymphoma. A cell-poor
appearance is seen at low
magnification. Note small
clusters of larger cells with
clear cytoplasm, particularly
adjacent to blood vessels.

are expressed on normal T-helper cells of the germinal center, while CXCL13 is a chemokine highly upregulated in germinal center T-helper cells, consistent with an origin of angioimmunoblastic T-cell lymphoma from T-helper cells. B-lineage stains identify hyperplastic or regressed germinal centers, the residua of follicles, as well as varying numbers of B-immunoblasts. CD21, CD23, and/or CD35 stains demonstrate follicular dendritic cells in these follicles as well as extended networks infiltrating around and between the high endothelial venules, suggesting a follicular origin for these areas as well. The Ki-67 index is variable but usually not high.

Gene rearrangement studies show clonal rearrangements of the T-cell receptor genes in about 75% of cases; conversely, about 25% of cases may lack T-cell receptor gene rearrangements. Clonal rearrangements of the immunoglobulin heavy and/or light chain genes are detectable in about 25% of cases. These latter rearrangements are thought to derive from oligoclonal or clonal populations of B-immunoblasts. In situ hybridization studies have shown that many of the B-immunoblasts are often EBV positive (although usually EBV-LMP negative), which may be driving the proliferation in the setting of relative immunosuppression. A variety of cytogenetic abnormalities have been identified, mostly gains of chromosomes, and the presence of multiple chromosomal abnormalities may be associated with poor prognosis.

The differential diagnosis is wide and consists of reactive proliferations, Hodgkin lymphoma, and other non-Hodgkin lymphomas, including other types of peripheral T-cell lymphomas. Reactive paracortical hyperplasia may show intense hypervascularity, while angioimmunoblastic-like T-cell lymphoma may show numerous immunoblasts, and, moreover, many of the immunoblasts may be EBV positive by in situ hybridization studies. Usually, reactive paracortical hyperplasia also shows varying degrees of reactive follicular hyperplasia, but this may also be a feature of some cases of angioimmunoblastic-like T-cell lymphoma. The presence of significant numbers of CD10- and/or bcl-6–positive T-cells or the demonstration of large meshworks of follicular dendritic cells around vessels supports a diagnosis of lymphoma. One must keep in mind that clonal T-cell gene rearrangements may be found in some cases of reactive paracortical hyperplasia. In borderline cases, I would err on the side of benign; if the diagnosis is lymphoma, then rebiopsy of another site or at a later period in time should clarify the situation. Some cases of possible angioimmunoblastic-like T-cell lymphoma lack a clear-cut population of small to intermediate T-cells with clear cell features, but otherwise have typical features. I obtain gene rearrangement studies in these cases. If there are clonal T-cell gene rearrangements, then a diagnosis of angioimmunoblastic-like T-cell lymphoma is appropriate. However, if gene rearrangements are not identified, I diagnose such cases as angioimmunoblastic lymphadenopathy without diagnosing lymphoma, with a note that these cases usually progress to overt angioimmunoblastic-like T-cell lymphoma, therefore requiring close clinical follow-up.

Some cases of angioimmunoblastic-like T-cell lymphoma may contain Reed-Sternberg–like cells, usually associated with EBV positivity. The key to the diagnosis is to view these cells in their background – which includes small- to intermediate-sized T-cells with clear cytoplasm, as well as other immunoblasts. A more difficult differential diagnostic consideration is angioimmunoblastic-like T-cell lymphoma complicated by diffuse large B-cell lymphoma. This presumably occurs when there is a clonal proliferation of EBV-positive immunoblasts, complicated by a transformation event. I do not diagnose transformation to diffuse large B-cell lymphoma unless there are patternless sheets of large B-cells. Finally, other peripheral T-cell lymphomas should be distinguished from angioimmunoblastic-like T-cell lymphoma. Many cases of peripheral T-cell lymphoma, not otherwise specified, have a paracortical localization with hypervascularity, although they usually have a more polymorphic and pleomorphic neoplastic population. Positivity for CD10 and/or bcl-6 and the presence of meshworks of follicular dendritic cells around high endothelial venules would strongly favor angioimmunoblastic-like T-cell lymphoma.

PERIPHERAL T-CELL LYMPHOMA, UNSPECIFIED[340,345–349]

Peripheral T-cell lymphoma, unspecified, is a category in the WHO Classification that probably represents a mixed bag of entities awaiting further elucidation. Essentially, it represents cases of mature T-cell lymphoma that lack clinicopathologic features characteristic of other known categories of mature T-cell lymphoma. These lymphomas comprise about 4% of all non-Hodgkin lymphomas and about one-half of all mature T-cell lymphomas in Western countries. They have a wide age range, but occur mainly in older adults. There is no sex predominance. Patients tend to present with lymph node enlargement and are generally

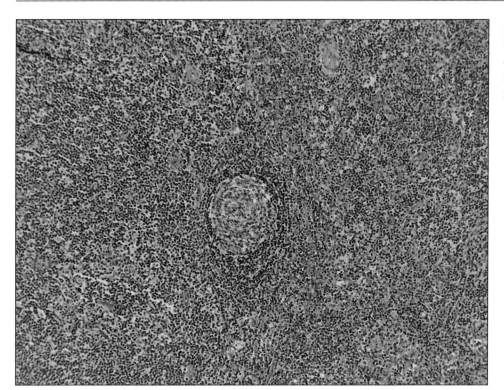

Figure 200. Peripheral T-cell lymphoma, T-zone variant. A *T-zone* pattern of involvement is seen, with residual germinal centers.

in high stage and with frequent B symptoms and a low performance index. Involvement of extranodal sites is frequent, with bone marrow, skin, liver, and spleen particularly common sites. Treatment usually consists of the same multi-drug chemotherapy regimens that are used for diffuse large B-cell lymphoma, although patients with peripheral T-cell lymphoma have a worse prognosis than similarly matched patients with diffuse large B-cell lymphoma. Autologous bone marrow transplantation has also been employed as a treatment, with preliminary results comparable to that seen in diffuse large B-cell lymphoma. Adverse prognostic factors include stage and International Prognostic Index. Histologic factors do not appear to correlate with clinical outcome.

Involved lymph nodes are usually moderately to markedly enlarged and show a fish-flesh appearance on cut section. At low magnification, diffuse effacement of architecture is usually seen although some cases show preferential involvement of the paracortical region with sparing of the follicles (so-called T-zone pattern) (Figure 200). Rare cases may show preferential involvement of follicles (Figure 201). Vascularity is generally increased, although not usually to the extent seen in angioimmunoblastic-like T-cell lymphoma. At high magnification, a polymorphic and pleomorphic population of cells is most often seen. Typically, there is a mixture of cell types, including small, round lymphocytes, eosinophils, plasma cells, histiocytes, which may be epithelioid, and a population of neoplastic T-cells (Figure 202). The neoplastic cells within individual cases usually vary from small to large, with varying degrees of hyperchromatism and nuclear irregularities. However, in some cases, the neoplastic cells are relatively monomorphic. Cytoplasm varies in amount, from scanty to abundant, and may be pale or clear in some cases (Figure 203). The mitotic rate is variable, but typically high.

Figure 201. Peripheral T-cell lymphoma, unspecified. Occasionally, there is preferential involvement of the follicles.

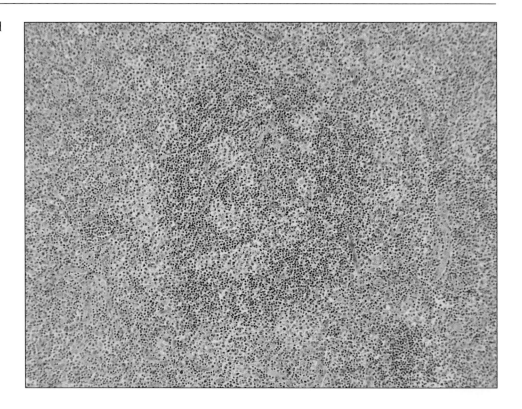

Figure 202. Peripheral T-cell lymphoma, unspecified. A mixed population of neoplastic cells is seen. There are scattered eosinophils, plasma cells, and histiocytes in the background.

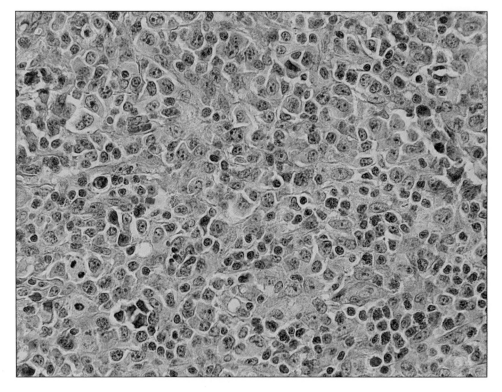

There are two histologic variants that are recognized in the 2001 WHO Classification. The T-zone variant has an interfollicular growth pattern with normal or hyperplastic follicles (Figure 200). The infiltrate is polymorphic, containing a mixture of reactive cells. Cytologically, the neoplastic cells are relatively monomorphic and are usually small to medium in size. They

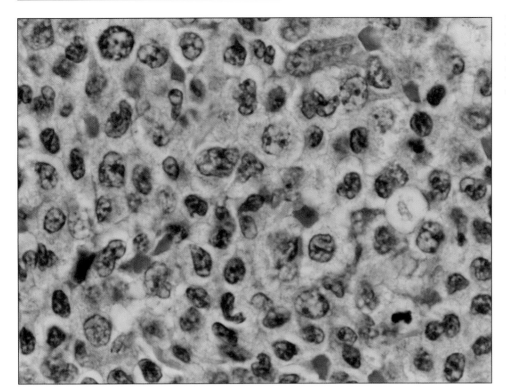

Figure 203. Peripheral T-cell lymphoma, unspecified. This case has a predominance of large cells with pale to clear cytoplasm.

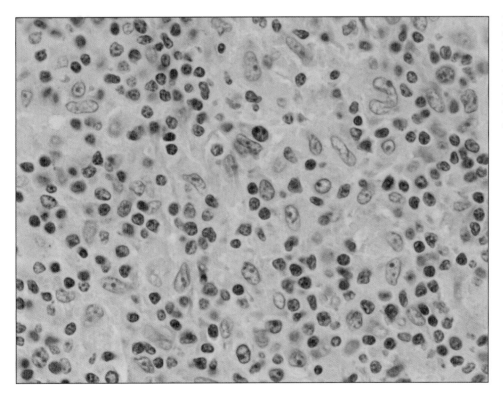

Figure 204. Peripheral T-cell lymphoma, lymphoepithelioid (Lennert) variant. There are numerous histiocytes, and atypical lymphoid cells are difficult to clearly identify.

generally lack significant pleomorphism, although the presence of Reed-Sternberg–like cells has been described. In the lymphoepithelioid cell variant (Lennert lymphoma), there are numerous epithelioid histiocytes, present singly and organized into small aggregates (Figure 204). The neoplastic cells may be difficult to identify, obscured by the massive histiocytic infiltrate, but

Figure 205. Peripheral T-cell lymphoma, unspecified, CD3 stain. The CD3 stain labels the atypical cells. A predominantly cytoplasmic pattern of reactivity is seen even though CD3 usually marks the membrane of normal T-cells.

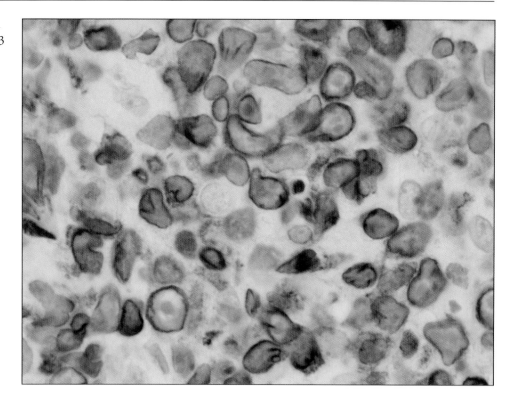

usually are small with subtle nuclear irregularities and only scattered large atypical cells.

By definition, this lymphoma shows a mature T-cell phenotype (Figure 205). There is often loss of one or more pan-T-cell markers, most often CD7 followed by CD5, and loss of the usual bcl-2 expression of a normal phenotype may also be seen. Most cases are CD4 positive, but CD8-positive or double-positive or double-negative phenotypes may be seen (Figures 206 and 207). CD1a and terminal deoxyribonucleotidyl transferase, markers of immature thymocytes, are consistently negative. CD30 may be variably positive on the large cells, and CD15 occasionally shows cytoplasmic positivity, usually with a granular pattern of staining. Usually, there is no expression of B-cell lineage markers, although some well-documented cases have shown aberrant expression of CD20 without other B-cell markers. Some cases may express CD56, and cases that preferentially involve follicles are usually bcl-6 and CD10 positive. The Ki-67 index is variable, but usually high. Gene rearrangement studies usually demonstrate clonal rearrangement of the gamma and beta T-cell receptor genes. Complex karyotypes are frequent and, with the exception of a trisomy 3 in the lymphoepithelioid variant, do not seem to be consistent from case to case. EBV in situ hybridization studies often identify scattered positive cells, but these appear to be bystander cells, mainly of B-cell lineage.

The differential diagnosis is wide and includes granulomatous inflammation, reactive paracortical hyperplasia, Hodgkin lymphoma, B-cell lymphoma, and other types of T-cell lymphoma. Granulomatous inflammation may be confused with the lymphoepithelioid variant of peripheral T-cell lymphoma. Generally, the epithelioid histiocytes in granulomatous inflammation are organized at least focally into

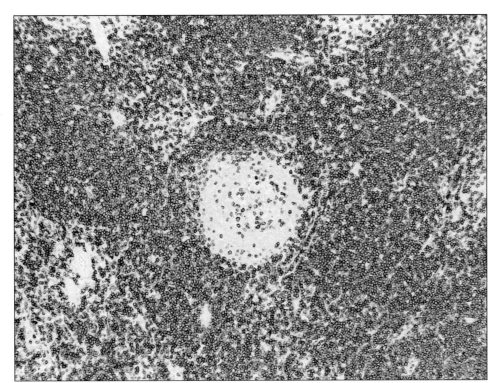

Figure 206. Peripheral T-cell lymphoma, T-zone variant (same case as Figures 200 and 207), CD3. The neoplastic cells are positive for CD3.

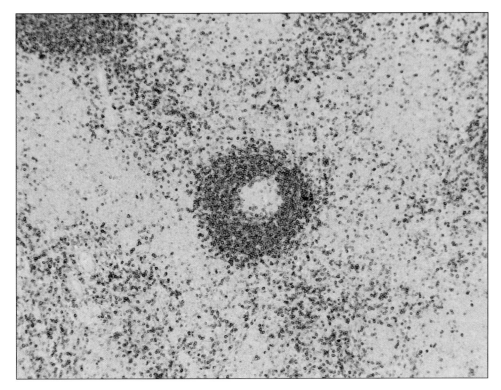

Figure 207. Peripheral T-cell lymphoma, T-zone variant, bcl-2 (same case as Figures 200 and 206). The T-cells are aberrantly negative for bcl-2, consistent with a neoplastic T-cell process.

well-formed granulomas with giant cells and may show focal areas of necrosis in the granulomas. The epithelioid histiocytes in the lymphoepithelioid variant of peripheral T-cell lymphoma typically form small aggregates, but not well-formed granulomas, and giant cells are not seen. In addition, necrosis, if it occurs, is regional and not restricted to the epithelioid cell aggregates. Peripheral T-cell lymphomas showing an interfollicular/paracortical pattern may be easily confused with reactive paracortical hyperplasia. These cases often share the polymorphic infiltrate seen in hyperplasia and may lack significant cytologic atypia. Cases of reactive paracortical hyperplasia usually have large number of admixed large B-immunoblasts and are usually associated with florid reactive follicular hyperplasia. Sometimes, T-cell gene rearrangement studies are necessary to help in the distinction, with the caveat that rare cases of reactive paracortical hyperplasia may have detectable oligoclonal or even seemingly monoclonal T-cell gene rearrangements.

Classical Hodgkin lymphoma may share a similar polymorphic background with peripheral T-cell lymphoma. The mere presence of cells resembling diagnostic Reed-Sternberg cells is not sufficient to establish a diagnosis of Hodgkin lymphoma. There is usually a higher mitotic rate and a greater range of cytologic atypia in peripheral T-cell lymphoma, including atypical small, medium, and large cells. The large cells in peripheral T-cell lymphoma may be CD30 positive, but they are also positive for CD45 and T-cell antigens. In contrast, Hodgkin cells usually express PAX-5 and CD15 in a majority of cases.

Most cases of diffuse large B-cell lymphoma show a relatively monomorphic population of cells, while this is seen in only a minority of cases of peripheral T-cell lymphoma. That having been said, immunphenotyping is the only truly reliable way to ensure the correct lineage. While CD20 may be negative in some cases of diffuse large B-cell lymphoma and CD20 may be aberrantly expressed in rare cases of T-cell lymphoma, a battery of studies can nearly always sort this out. Diffuse follicular center cell lymphoma and T-cell/histiocyte-rich B-cell lymphoma are harder to distinguish morphologically from peripheral T-cell lymphoma. In diffuse follicular center cell lymphoma, many cells, including atypical small and large cells, should type as B-cell. In T-cell/histiocyte-rich B-cell lymphomas, the B-cells represent, by definition, the distinct minority of the cellular population. Some cases of peripheral T-cell lymphoma may have scattered immunoblasts, but they are not usually as regularly dispersed throughout the infiltrate as in T-cell/histiocyte-rich B-cell lymphoma. Furthermore, both small and large cells should show significant degrees of cytologic atypia in peripheral T-cell lymphoma. However, one does occasionally need B- and/or T-cell receptor gene rearrangements to resolve the diagnostic dilemma.

Finally, peripheral T-cell lymphoma, unspecified, should be distinguished from angioimmunoblastic-like T-cell lymphoma and anaplastic large-cell lymphoma. There may be intense hypervascularity and a range of cytologic atypia in both neoplasms. In addition, angioimmunoblastic-like T-cell lymphoma may also have large numbers of epithelioid histiocytes. Angioimmunoblastic-like T-cell lymphoma occurs in a characteristic clinical setting and has a cell-poor appearance at low magnification. If there are large aggregates of follicular dendritic cells or widespread expression of bcl-6 and/or CD10, then a diagnosis of angioimmunoblastic-like T-cell lymphoma is appropriate. In anaplastic large-cell lymphoma, the CD30 expression is usually uniformly strongly positive in the entire neoplastic cell population, which often shows at least a focal sinusoidal pattern of involvement. While peripheral T-cell lymphoma, unspecified, may have positivity for CD30, it is

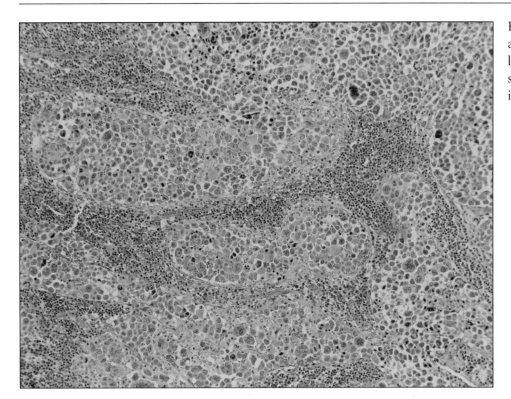

Figure 208. ALK-negative anaplastic large-cell lymphoma. An exquisite sinusoidal pattern of involvement is seen.

usually restricted to a subset of cells – typically the largest, most atypical ones. ALK positivity would exclude peripheral T-cell lymphoma, unspecified, by definition. Confusion of peripheral T-cell lymphoma with ALK-negative anaplastic large-cell lymphoma probably does not have clinical significance, at least at this point in time.

ANAPLASTIC LARGE-CELL LYMPHOMA, ALK-NEGATIVE TYPE[350–354]

Anaplastic large-cell lymphoma, ALK-negative type, is a non-Hodgkin lymphoma of T or *null* phenotype, composed of anaplastic-appearing cells, with uniform or near-uniform expression of CD30, and the absence of ALK protein expression/ALK translocation. As defined here, it is probably closely related to peripheral T-cell lymphoma, unspecified. It occurs mainly, but not exclusively, in older adults, without a striking sex predilection. Patients generally present in lymph nodes, although extranodal sites are not uncommonly involved. Most patients are in clinical stage III or IV and often have B symptoms. These patients are generally treated in the same manner as those with other peripheral T-cell lymphomas, with a similar overall poor outcome. Prognostic factors are those found for peripheral T-cell lymphoma, unspecified, such as stage, performance status, and the International Prognostic Index.

Involved lymph nodes may be normal in size or enlarged. At low magnification, there may be a distinctly sinusoidal pattern of growth with retention of the normal architecture, a mixed sinusoidal or paracortical pattern of involvement, or diffuse effacement of architecture (Figure 208). There may be capsular fibrosis, or,

Figure 209. ALK-negative anaplastic large-cell lymphoma. Large bizarre cells are seen.

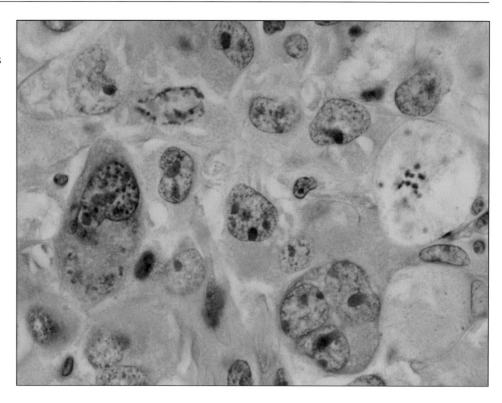

occasionally, even broad bands mimicking nodular sclerosis Hodgkin lymphoma. The hallmark at high magnification is the presence of bizarre anaplastic cells, which may be so odd as to suggest carcinoma or malignant melanoma (Figure 209). Nucleoli are single or multiple, and may be quite large, resembling Hodgkin cells. Cytoplasm is generally abundant and may show squaring off against adjacent cells. A relatively pure population of neoplastic cells may be seen, although in many cases there may be a significant admixture of other cells, which may include, histiocytes, plasma cells, eosinophils, and neutrophils.

The immunophenotypic hallmark of anaplastic large-cell lymphoma, ALK-negative type, is uniform or near-uniform expression of CD30, along with negativity for ALK protein (Figure 210). CD45 and CD43 are expressed in about two-thirds of cases. CD2 is expressed in about one-half of cases. Other T-cell markers, including CD3, CD5, and CD7 are expressed in up to 25% of cases. Cases that lack specific T-cell markers have been regarded by some to be of null phenotype, but probably still represent T-lineage neoplasms. Most cases express cytotoxic markers, including TIA-1, granzyme B, and/or perforin. CD4 is positive in most cases, and CD8 is usually negative. In addition to CD30, the activation marker CD25 (IL-2R) is also consistently expressed. There is no expression of B-lineage markers, including CD20 and PAX-5. CD15 may show positivity in about 10% of cases, usually cytoplasmic in distribution. Although there may be some positivity for CD68, the histiocytic marker CD163 is consistently negative. The Ki-67 index is variable, but usually high.

Both T- and null-cell anaplastic large-cell lymphomas, ALK-negative type, show clonal T-cell receptor gene rearrangements in greater than 90% of cases. Translocations involving the ALK gene are not found, consistent with the ALK

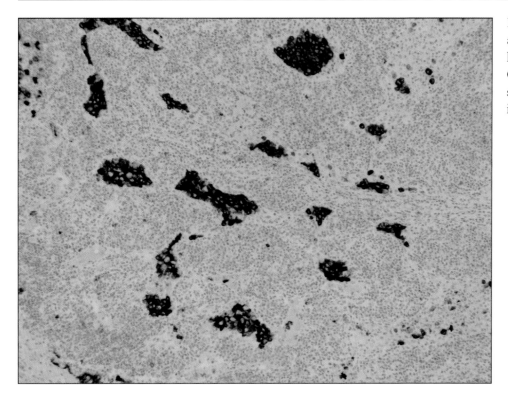

Figure 210. ALK-negative anaplastic large-cell lymphoma, CD30 stain. This CD30 stain highlights the sinusoidal pattern of involvement.

protein negativity. In fact, no consistent cytogenetic abnormalities have been reported. EBV is consistently negative outside the setting of immunosuppression.

The differential diagnosis includes reactive paracortical proliferations; metastatic carcinoma and malignant melanoma; Hodgkin lymphoma; malignant histiocytosis; true histiocytic lymphoma; peripheral T-cell lymphoma, unspecified; cutaneous anaplastic large-cell lymphoma; transformation of other malignant lymphomas; and ALK-positive anaplastic large-cell lymphoma. I have seen cases of acute infectious mononucleosis mistaken for anaplastic large-cell lymphoma, when there are areas of sheets of CD30-positive cells. The clinical setting may suggest the diagnosis, as may other areas showing features more typical of mononucleosis. Studies for EBV may be useful, as anaplastic large-cell lymphoma is EBV negative outside of the setting of immunosuppression. Cases of anaplastic large-cell lymphoma with a predominantly sinusoidal localization may simulate metastatic carcinoma and malignant melanoma. Immunostains for keratin, S-100 protein, CD30, and other markers should usually sort this out, although rare cases of anaplastic large-cell lymphoma may show a punctate cytoplasmic positivity for keratin. When Hodgkin lymphoma forms sheets, it may simulate anaplastic large-cell lymphoma, and anaplastic large-cell lymphoma may have areas of fibrosis and an inflammatory background that may simulate Hodgkin lymphoma. Although both neoplasms share consistent CD30 positivity, Hodgkin lymphoma is usually CD45 and CD43 negative, negative for cytotoxic markers, and CD15 and PAX-5 positive, while anaplastic large-cell lymphoma is usually CD45 and CD43 positive, positive for one or more cytotoxic markers, and CD15 and PAX-5 negative. B-cell lymphomas may show anaplastic cytologic features and/or consistent expression of CD30. These cases should not be diagnosed as anaplastic large-cell lymphoma, since they behave similar to other cases of diffuse large B-cell lymphoma. They can be distinguished by expression of B-lineage markers, including CD20, PAX-5, CD79a, and/or B-cell–specific transcription factors. Most cases diagnosed as malignant histiocytosis in the old literature have been found to be cases of anaplastic large-cell lymphoma upon modern phenotypic analysis. Rare cases of true histiocytic sarcoma may be distinguished by their positivity for CD163, negativity for CD30- or T-lineage–specific markers, and the absence of clonal rearrangements of the T-cell receptor genes.

It may be difficult to distinguish some cases of peripheral T-cell lymphoma, unspecified, from ALK-negative anaplastic large-cell lymphoma, as there may be a gradient of cases of peripheral T-cell lymphoma with increasing pleomorphism and CD30 expression. To date, fortunately, there are no clinical or even biologic reasons to distinguish the two neoplasms, and it may well be that ALK-negative anaplastic large-cell lymphoma should be considered a histologic variant of peripheral T-cell lymphoma, unspecified. Cutaneous anaplastic large-cell lymphoma may have a close histologic resemblance to anaplastic large-cell lymphoma, ALK-negative type; but by definition, the former presents in skin and is a much more indolent disease, which usually lacks lymph node involvement until late in its course. Peripheral T-cell lymphoma, including mycosis fungoides, may also show histologic transformation to neoplasms indistinguishable from ALK-negative anaplastic large-cell lymphoma, requiring clinical information and review of previous specimens to separate this *secondary* anaplastic large-cell lymphoma from primary cases. Finally, there are several clinical and histologic differences between ALK-positive and ALK-negative anaplastic large-cell lymphoma. Patients with the ALK-positive anaplastic lymphoma tend to be much younger and show a male predominance. Histologically, these cases are much less pleomorphic and have hallmark cells – cells with kidney-shaped nuclei, often with a paranuclear eosinophilic hof. Occasionally, the histologic findings may be overlapping; therefore, I recommend ALK stains in all cases before making a diagnosis of anaplastic large-cell lymphoma, ALK-negative type.

ANAPLASTIC LARGE-CELL LYMPHOMA, ALK-POSITIVE TYPE[311,352–360]

Anaplastic large-cell lymphoma, ALK-positive type, is defined as a T-cell/null-cell neoplasm that has expression of CD30 and ALK protein. In contrast to ALK-negative anaplastic large-cell lymphoma, this neoplasm appears to be a distinct clinicopathologic entity different from other types of peripheral T-cell lymphoma. It occurs most often in children or young adults, with a striking male predominance. Patients most often present with lymphadenopathy and are usually in high stage. Involvement of extranodal sites, including skin, bone, and soft tissue, and bone marrow is frequent. Patients with ALK-positive anaplastic large-cell lymphoma tend to have a relatively good prognosis after multidrug chemotherapy. In contrast to most other large-cell lymphomas, there is often a good response to chemotherapy even after first relapse.

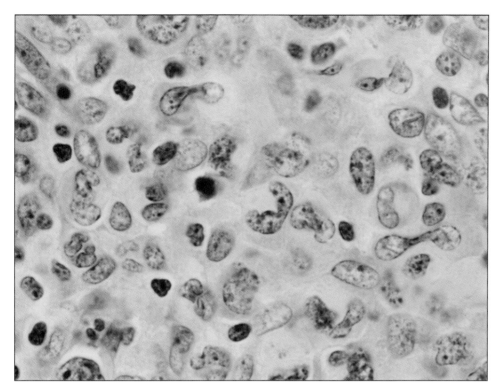

Figure 211. ALK-positive anaplastic large-cell lymphoma. Some of the characteristic cells of this neoplasm are seen, including *hallmark* cells, with reniform nuclei.

Histologically, a wide variety of patterns may be seen. The lymph node architecture may be intact, with only focal involvement, or there may be diffuse effacement. Focal involvement may be either sinusoidal, paracortical, or a combination of the two. The neoplastic element can show a range in cell size, from small to large. The most distinctive appearance is a large cell with a large reniform to horseshoe-shaped nucleus, called a hallmark cell (Figure 211). Similar smaller cells may also be present. Occasionally, the nucleus may be multinucleated and may even form a wreathlike structure (so-called doughnut cells) (Figure 212). The cytoplasm is typically abundant, eccentrically placed, often with a hof adjacent to the indented nucleus. Several histologic variants have been described. In the common variant, the neoplastic cells described above are the predominant element and may show a monomorphic or pleomorphic pattern. Occasionally, the neoplastic cells are found in an abundant lymphohistiocytic background, the lymphohistiocytic variant. The neoplastic element may be masked by the reactive cells, but can be often found in greater numbers around blood vessels. In the small-cell variant, small- to medium-sized cells predominate; occasionally, these cases show transformation to a more typical histologic appearance, signally a worsening of the clinical course (Figure 213). Other more rare patterns include a giant-cell variant, composed of numerous doughnut cells and other multinucleated neoplastic cells; a signet-ring variant; and a spindled variant, often containing a myxoid background.

By definition, all cases of ALK-positive anaplastic large-cell lymphoma express ALK protein. The pattern of expression varies from nuclear, cytoplasmic, to nuclear and cytoplasmic, depending upon the specific translocation causing the ALK overexpression (see Table 37) (Figures 214 and 215). In addition to the ALK expression, the neoplastic cells consistently express CD30, usually in a strong

Figure 212. ALK-positive anaplastic large-cell lymphoma. Several wreathlike cells are seen in this field.

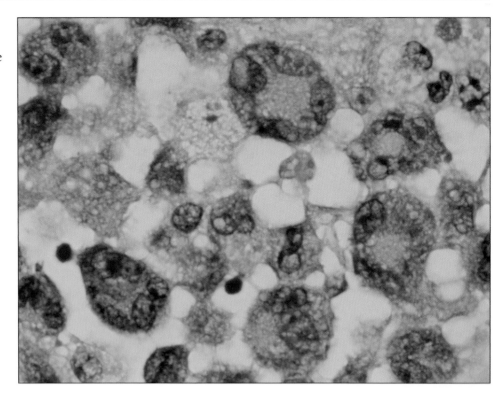

Figure 213. ALK-positive anaplastic large-cell lymphoma, small-cell variant. The predominant neoplastic cell type has small- to intermediate-sized nuclei that can be easily overlooked as histiocytic. Larger cells tend to cluster near blood vessels.

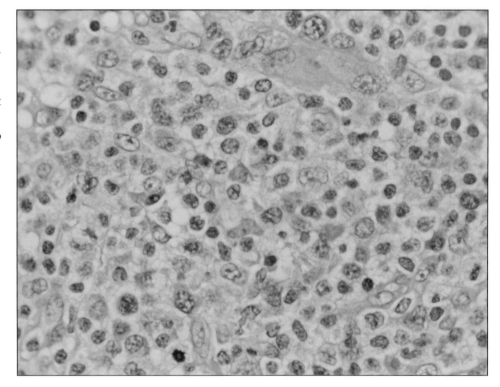

membrane and paranuclear pattern (Figure 216). Typically, the largest cells show the strongest staining. Epithelial membrane antigen is also expressed in a high proportion of cases. Otherwise, the phenotypic profile is similar to that seen in non–ALK-positive anaplastic large-cell lymphoma. CD45 and CD43 are positive in most cases. About two-thirds of cases express one or more specific

Table 37. ALK Fusion Partners[335]

Translocation	Genes	Incidence	Staining Pattern
t(2;5)(p23;q35)	ALK/NPM	75%	Cytoplasm, nucleus, and nucleolus
t(1;2)(q21;p23)	TPM3/ALK	15%	Cytoplasm and cell membrane
t(2;3)(p23;q21)	ALK/TFG	2%	Cytoplasm
Inv(2)(p23;q35)	ALK/ATIC	2%	Cytoplasm
t(2;17)(p23;q23)	ALK/CLTC	2%	Cytoplasm
t(X;2)(q11-12;p23)	MSN/ALK	1%	Cell membrane

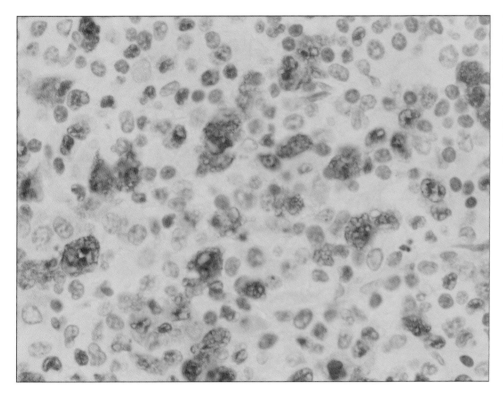

Figure 214. ALK-positive anaplastic large-cell lymphoma, lymphohistiocytic variant, ALK stain. The neoplastic cells show a nuclear pattern of staining for ALK. Note that both large and scattered small cells are positive.

T-cell markers, most often CD2. CD4 is positive much more often than CD8, although many cases express the cytotoxic cell–associated markers TIA-1, granzyme B, and/or perforin (Figure 217). There is no expression of B-lineage markers. The specific histiocytic marker CD163 is consistently negative, although the lysosomal marker CD68 may be positive in some cases.

Similar to ALK-negative anaplastic large-cell lymphoma, clonal T-cell receptor gene rearrangements may be detected in almost all cases. However, translocations associated with the ALK gene on chromosome 2 are consistently present that are not present in ALK-negative anaplastic large-cell lymphoma. In a majority of cases a t(2;5) involving the ALK and nucleophosmin genes is found, but a variety of other translocations have been reported in the remaining minority of cases (see Table 37). EBV and other viruses are consistently negative.

The differential diagnosis includes reactive lymphohistiocytic proliferations, diffuse large B-cell lymphoma with expression of ALK, Hodgkin lymphoma, and

Figure 215. ALK-positive anaplastic large-cell lymphoma, ALK stain. The cytoplasmic reactivity for ALK seen in this case is indicative of a variant translocation involving ALK – a translocation other than the t(2;5).

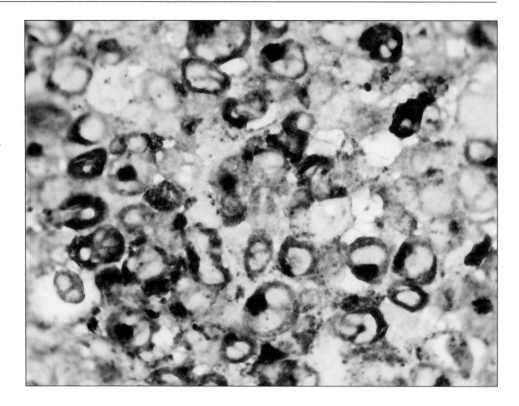

Figure 216. ALK-positive anaplastic large-cell lymphoma, CD30 stain. CD30 labels all or virtually all of the cells in a paranuclear and membrane distribution.

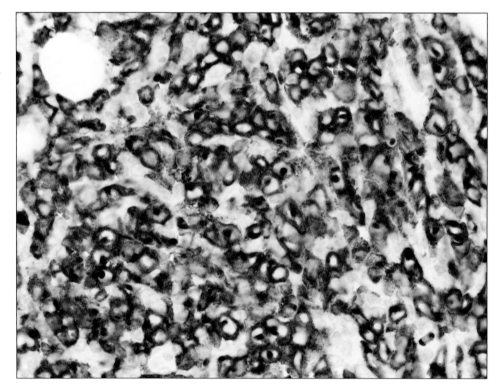

other peripheral T-cell lymphoma. Any lymphohistiocytic proliferation in a child or young adults should be stained for CD30 and/or ALK to rule out the lymphohistiocytic variant of ALK-positive anaplastic large-cell lymphoma. The CD30/ALK-positive cells tend to cluster around blood vessels. ALK positivity in lymphoid cells is not seen in reactive proliferations and is, at least at this point in time, diagnostic of

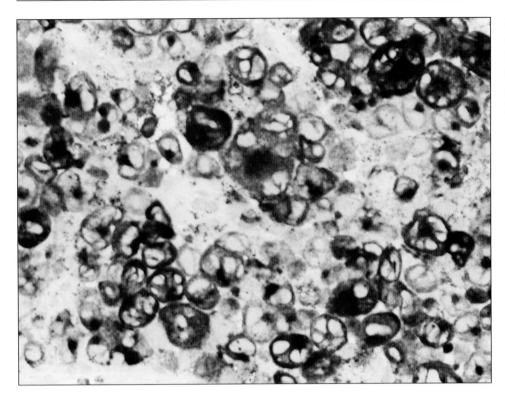

Figure 217. ALK-positive anaplastic large-cell lymphoma, granzyme B stain. Strong reactivity is typically seen in anaplastic large-cell lymphoma.

malignant lymphoma, although ALK expression has also been observed in myofibroblastic tumors and some cases of rhabdomyosarcoma. Diffuse large B-cell lymphoma with expression of ALK is the only other lymphoid neoplasm that has been reported to show ALK expression. These cases usually show plasmablastic cytologic features, have intracytoplasmic IgA expression with light chain restriction, and lack CD30 expression. The giant-cell variant of ALK-positive anaplastic large-cell lymphoma can mimic Hodgkin lymphoma, and some cases have broad fibrous bands, specifically mimicking the nodular Sclerosis subtype. However, ALK positivity and negativity for PAX-5 would exclude the latter diagnosis. ALK-positive anaplastic large-cell lymphoma may closely resemble ALK-negative anaplastic large-cell lymphoma. Some hematopathologists regard the presence of hallmark cells as a reliable marker of the ALK-positive cases. I recommend immunostaining for ALK in any case in which a diagnosis of anaplastic large-cell lymphoma is being considered, since the prognosis is much better for the ALK-positive cases.

MYCOSIS FUNGOIDES/SEZARY SYNDROME[361–366]

Mycosis fungoides and Sezary syndrome are very closely related cutaneous-based neoplasms of helper T-cells. Sezary syndrome is similar to mycosis fungoides, but includes erythroderma and blood involvement in addition to skin disease. Although regarded as primary lymphomas of the skin, involvement of lymph nodes occurs frequently in both. In Sezary syndrome, lymph node enlargement due to infiltrating by tumor cells usually occurs at presentation. In contrast, lymph node enlargement early in the course of mycosis fungoides is usually the result of

Figure 218. Mycosis fungoides with superimposed dermatopathic changes. Scattered atypical lymphoid cells are seen (LN-2).

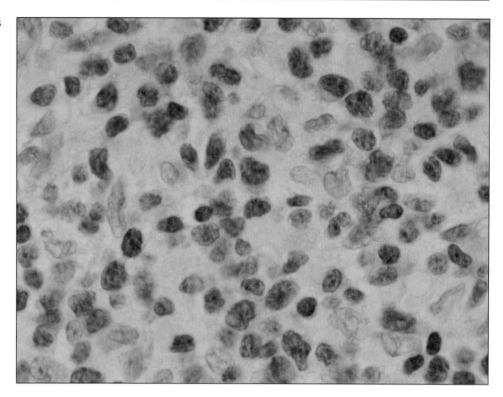

dermatopathic lymphadenitis, with involvement by tumor usually occurring after years of cutaneous disease. Clinical stage represents the single most important prognostic factor, with stage II representing clinical enlargement of lymph nodes and stage III representing lymph node involvement documented by histology.

Early involvement of the lymph node involved by Sezary syndrome or mycosis fungoides typically manifests as isolated single cells or small clusters, generally less than three to six cells, in the paracortex, invariably in a background of dermatopathic lymphadenitis (Figure 218). These cells have the typical cerebriform contours of the cells seen in the epidermis. Later, the clusters become larger, including aggregates of fifteen or more cells, until there is at first complete involvement of the paracortex, and then, ultimately, complete effacement of lymph node architecture (Figure 219). As the clusters get larger in size, there is usually an increase in the number of large cells. Just as tumor stage mycosis fungoides has a high incidence of large-cell transformation, large-cell transformation is frequently seen in lymph nodes showing diffuse effacement of architecture. Several grading systems have been proposed to assess lymph node involvement by mycosis fungoides (see Table 38).

Immunohistochemical studies show that, similar to the skin, mycosis fungoides in the lymph node has a CD4-positive/CD-8–negative phenotype, consistent with T-helper cells. There is often loss of one or more pan-T-cell markers, particularly CD7, but sometimes CD5, CD2, or even CD4. Large cells may express CD30, and large-cell transformation is frequently diffusely CD30 positive. Occasionally, cytotoxic markers such as TIA-1 or granzyme B may be positive in cases with transformation. There is consistent clonal rearrangement of the T-cell receptor genes. Chromosomal abnormalities may be present, particularly in transformed cases.

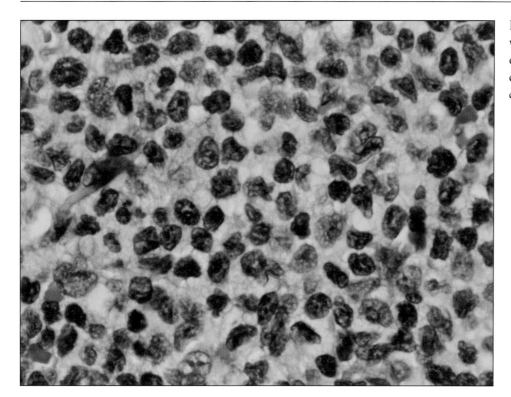

Figure 219. Mycosis fungoides with superimposed dermatopathic changes. Large clusters of atypical lymphoid cells are seen (LN-3).

Table 38. Grading of Lymph Node Involvement in Mycosis Fungoides[213]

I	LN-0–LN-2	Dermatopathic lymphadenopathy with no to scattered cerebriform lymphocytes
II	LN-3	Focal obliteration of architecture by clusters of cerebriform lymphocytes
III	LN-4	Complete replacement of architecture

Early lymph node involvement by mycosis fungoides or Sezary syndrome is extremely difficult to distinguish from dermatopathic lymphadenitis caused by other skin diseases, due to disruption of the skin barrier. Many lymphoid cells in dermatopathic lymphadenitis may have irregular nuclear contours, easily mimicking the cerebriform neoplastic cells seen in mycosis fungoides or Sezary syndrome. In addition, scattered reactive immunoblasts may be seen in dermatopathic lymphadenitis, mimicking the large cells that are part of the neoplastic process in mycosis fungoides or Sezary syndrome. Routine histologic assessment is usually not helpful in distinguishing benign from malignant unless there is some degree of architectural effacement or unless large-cell transformation, characterized by sheets of large cells, has occurred. Immunohistochemical studies are of limited utility in the differential diagnosis. Although CD7 is typically aberrantly absent in mycosis fungoides or Sezary syndrome, it may also be lost in cases of dermatopathic lymphadenitis due to a wide variety of reactive conditions. Although loss of other T-cell antigens is more specific, it is also much less frequent. For this reason, gene rearrangement studies have been recommended as the most effective way of distinguishing dermatopathic lymphadenitis due to reactive causes from that due to cutaneous T-cell lymphoma. Clonal T-cell receptor gene rearrangements can be identified in a subset of cases of Category I, usually those in LN-2, most of those cases of Category II, and in almost all cases of Category III. Some studies have found that the identification of clonal T-cell populations in Category I lymph nodes may adversely impact prognosis, so I recommend this study in all such patients.

Large-cell transformation of mycosis fungoides may be difficult to distinguish from other large-cell lymphomas. One may often also see small, cerebriform lymphocytes admixed with the large cells, suggesting the diagnosis; however, the key to the diagnosis in most cases is a good clinical history and the performance of immunohistochemical studies. Large-cell transformation is usually CD30 positive, but is always negative positive for ALK protein.

ADULT T-CELL LEUKEMIA/LYMPHOMA[337,367,368]

Adult T-cell leukemia/lymphoma is a peripheral T-cell lymphoma caused by the retrovirus HTLV-1. It occurs in regions of the world in which HTLV-1 is endemic, including parts of southwestern Japan, the Caribbean basin, and central Africa. It is rare in the United States. Because of the long latency time, it occurs most often in adults, with a male predominance. Four clinical variants have been recognized, including acute, lymphomatous, chronic, and smoldering. Generalized lymphadenopathy is commonly seen at presentation in the acute and lymphomatous variants. Lymph node involvement in the chronic variant is much less common and is essentially not seen in the smoldering variant. In the acute variant, the most common variant, the lymphadenopathy is associated with peripheral blood involvement and a skin rash, along with hypercalcemia. In the lymphomatous variant, blood involvement is absent and hypercalcemia is less often seen. Both the acute and the lymphomatous variants are clinically aggressive, with death usually occurring within 1 year. Prognostic factors include age, performance status, serum calcium, and serum lactate dehydrogenase.

Involved lymph nodes may show diverse histologic appearances. In many cases, the histologic appearance is indistinguishable from peripheral T-cell lymphoma, unspecified. The presence of highly pleomorphic cells, often with polylobated nuclear outlines, prominent nucleoli, and abundant basophilic cytoplasm may suggest the diagnosis (Figure 220). The cells are sometimes quite large, but occasional cases may be composed of cells that are small to medium sized. In the Hodgkin-like variant, seen most often in early or indolent presentations, there may be scattered cells resembling Hodgkin cells, in a background of small- to medium-sized atypical cells.

The neoplastic cells are usually of mature T-helper phenotype, with expression of pan-T-cell markers and an absence of B-lineage markers. CD25 (the IL-2R) is consistently expressed, and CD30 may be positive. The atypical large cells in the Hodgkin-like variant are usually of B-lineage; they also express CD30, CD15, and EBV-LMP; and their presence probably reflects an underlying immunodeficiency in these patients. Clonal rearrangements of the T-cell receptor genes are consistently detected, and, moreover, clonally integrated HTLV-1 is found in all cases.

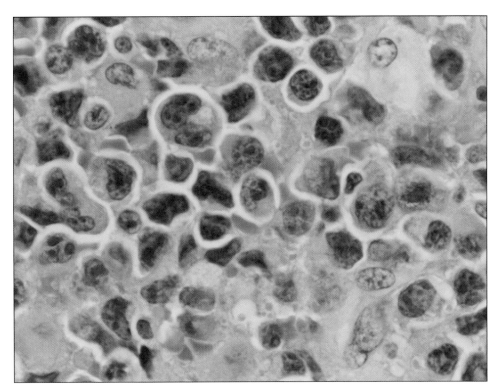

Figure 220. Adult T-cell leukemia/lymphoma. Highly pleomorphic cells are seen, but this appearance is not specific to this lymphoma type.

The primary differential diagnosis is with peripheral T-cell lymphoma, although cases of the Hodgkin-like variant can be confused with true Hodgkin lymphoma. A history of previous residence in an HTLV-1–endemic area should raise consideration of adult T-cell leukemia/lymphoma, and any case of peripheral T-cell lymphoma in which the patient has antibodies to HTLV-1 is adult T-cell leukemia/lymphoma until proven otherwise; and the demonstration of HTLV-1 genome in neoplastic tissue is diagnostic of the neoplasm. The presence of Hodgkin-like cells raises true Hodgkin lymphoma in the differential diagnosis. These cells share CD30, CD15, and EBV positivity with Hodgkin cells. In the Hodgkin-like variant, the large cells are found in a background of peripheral T-cell lymphoma, with small- and medium-sized cells showing varying degrees of cytologic atypia. A diagnosis of Hodgkin lymphoma should be made with great caution in anyone who has serologic evidence of HTLV-1, as many of these cases progress to overt adult T-cell leukemia/lymphoma, usually within a short period of time.

T-CELL PROLYMPHOCYTIC LEUKEMIA[369,370]

T-cell prolymphocytic leukemia is a rare leukemia of mature T-cells. Patients, usually adults, present with a leukemic picture, with a very high lymphocyte count (usually over 100×10^9 per liter), hepatosplenomegaly, and generalized lymphadenopathy. There is no association with viruses; in particular, HTLV-1 is negative by definition. The disease is usually aggressive with a median survival less than 1 year. The peripheral blood shows a predominance of prolymphocytes in most cases, although about 25% of cases show small lymphocytes and about

Figure 221. T-cell prolymphocytic leukemia. A relatively uniform population of cells small- to intermediate-sized nuclei and discernible nucleoli are seen.

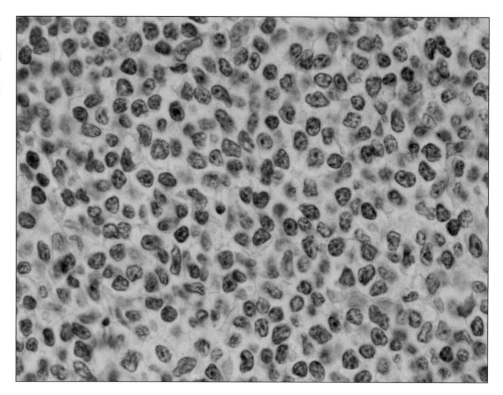

5% of cases show cerebriform cells. Involved lymph nodes show preferential paracortical localization, typically with preserved follicles. A monomorphous population of small atypical lymphoid cells is seen, often with infiltration of high endothelial venules (Figure 221). Immunophenotypic studies show a mature T-cell phenotype, usually without aberrant loss of pan-T-cell antigens. A CD4-positive/CD8-negative phenotype is seen in most cases, but about 25% are CD4 positive/CD8 positive, and 15% are CD4 negative/CD8 negative. Terminal deoxyribonucleotidyl transferase is negative. The T-cell receptor genes are clonally rearranged. There are a number of characteristic chromosomal abnormalities, including inversions or reciprocal translocations involving chromosomes at the sites of the T-cell receptor alpha/beta locus and the TCL1 and TCL1b genes. The differential diagnosis in lymph nodes is limited within the context of the entire disease picture, including the extensive leukemic population in the peripheral blood and bone marrow. Terminal deoxyribonucleotidyl transferase staining should provide clear distinction from T-precursor lymphoblastic neoplasm.

OTHER MATURE T- AND NK-CELL NEOPLASMS

Other mature T- and NK-cell neoplasms recognized by the WHO Classification include T-cell large granular lymphocytic leukemia, aggressive NK-cell leukemia, extranodal NK/T-cell lymphoma, nasal type, enteropathy-associated T-cell lymphoma, hepatosplenic T-cell lymphoma, subcutaneous panniculitis-like T-cell lymphoma, and blastic NK-cell lymphoma. Blastic NK-cell lymphoma is now considered to be a neoplasm of the precursor cells to plasmacytoid

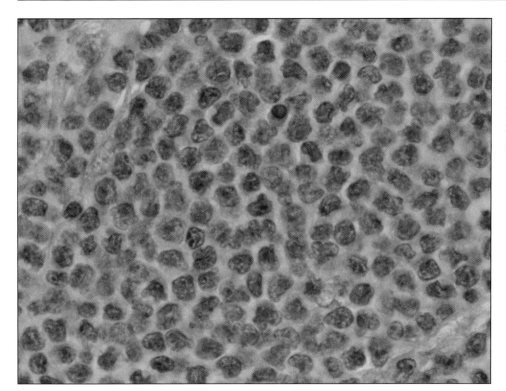

Figure 222. T-cell large granular lymphocytic leukemia. In paraffin sections, the cells are small to medium sized, with discernible nucleoli and irregular nuclear membranes. The cytoplasmic granules are not seen.

dendritic cells. It has been renamed precursor plasmacytoid dendritic cell neoplasm and is discussed in Chapter 10. Among the other neoplasms, involvement of lymph nodes is either rare, almost never the presenting site of disease, or clinically insignificant. Nonetheless, some of these neoplasms arise in differential diagnosis; therefore, a brief summary of each is given here.

T-Cell Large Granular Lymphocytic Leukemia[371]

T-cell large granular lymphocytic leukemia, also known as T-gamma lymphoproliferative disorder, is an indolent neoplasm primarily involving peripheral blood, bone marrow, liver, and spleen. It primarily occurs in adults, in whom lymphocytosis is seen along with neutropenia and splenomegaly. Blood and bone marrow smears show large granular lymphocytes, with abundant cytoplasm and azurophilic granules. Lymph node involvement is rare, and I have only seen one case, which had preferential involvement of the sinuses (Figures 222 and 223). A mature T-cell phenotype is seen, usually CD4 negative and CD8 positive. Markers of NK-cells, including CD57, are usually positive, and the cytotoxic marker TIA-1 is usually also positive. The neoplasm is clonal, with all cases showing rearrangement of the T-cell receptor beta and/or gamma chain genes.

Aggressive NK-Cell Leukemia[372,373]

Aggressive NK-cell leukemia is a rare neoplasm of NK-cells. Patients are usually in the second or third decade, without a striking sex predilection. Patients present with a leukemic picture, with involvement of peripheral blood and bone marrow

Figure 223. T-cell large granular lymphocytic leukemia. There was preferential involvement of the sinuses, including the subcapsular sinus shown here.

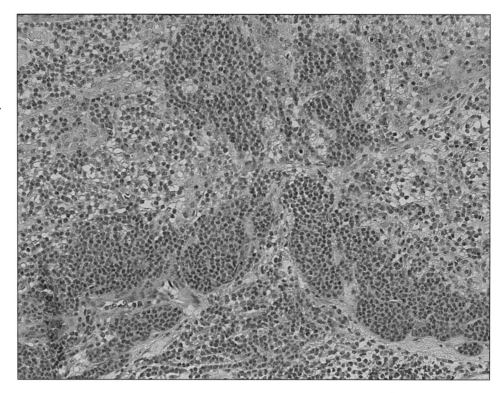

and hepatosplenomegaly. There is a strong association with Epstein–Barr, and some have speculated that this disease may represent a leukemic variant of extranodal NK/T-cell lymphoma, of nasal type. Lymph node involvement is rare. One usually sees effacement of the lymph node parenchyma by a monotonous population of atypical cells with round nuclei. There is a high mitotic rate, with frequent apoptosis. Immunophenotypic studies show expression of CD2, cytoplasmic CD3, CD56, and cytotoxic molecules. The antigen receptor genes are consistently in a germline configuration, even when EBV studies can demonstrate clonal episomal forms.

Extranodal NK/T-Cell Lymphoma, Nasal Type[374–376]

This is an uncommon but not rare neoplasm derived from activated NK-cells or less commonly cytotoxic T-lymphocytes. There is a strong association with EBV and a marked propensity to occur in the nasal region. It occurs more commonly in Asians and in South America, occurring primarily in adults, with a male predilection. Patients most often present with a nasal mass, often with extension to adjacent local structures, although a variety of extranodal organs may rarely be presenting sites of disease. The disease is aggressive, and the prognosis is poor, with the best outcomes seen in patients treated with aggressive regimens including multidrug chemotherapy combined with radiotherapy. Lymph node involvement is uncommon, but may be seen as a part of widespread disease. The histologic findings are similar to those seen elsewhere, with a polymorphous population of tumor cells, with angiocentricity and necrosis (Figures 224). Immunophenotypic studies usually show expression of CD2, cytoplasmic CD3, CD56,

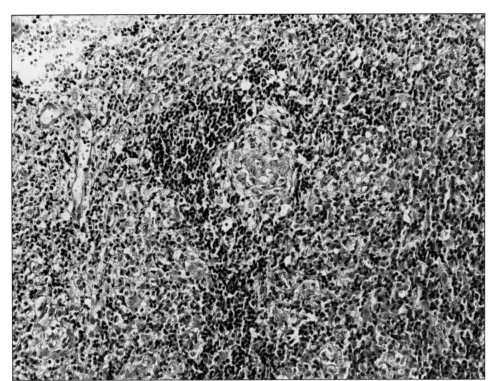

Figure 224. Extranodal NK/T-cell lymphoma, nasal type, involving lymph node. In this rare case showing lymph node involvement by nasal T/NK-lymphoma, a paracortical distribution is seen, compressing a residual germinal center.

and cytotoxic molecules, although a minority of cases may show surface CD3 and absence of CD56. Antigen receptor genes are in a germline configuration even when EBV studies can demonstrate clonal episomal forms.

Enteropathy-Associated T-Cell Lymphoma[373,377–379]

Enteropathy-associated T-cell lymphoma is a lymphoma derived from intra-mucosal T-cells. Patients usually present with abdominal pain, due to a mass or multiple masses, with or without accompanying perforation, in the jejunum, ileum, or less commonly in other sites. There is a strong association with celiac disease. Lymph node involvement is rare, even in lymph nodes draining sites of disease, with disease recurrence usually occurring in the gastrointestinal tract or other extranodal sites. The tumor may be monomorphic or pleomorphic (Figures 225 and 226). Immunophenotypic studies show expression of CD3, CD2, and CD7, as well as cytotoxic molecules. CD5, CD4, CD8, and CD56 are most often negative, although some cases composed of medium-sized cells may express CD8 and CD56 (Figure 226). CD30 is variably expressed. Molecular studies show consistent rearrangement of the T-cell receptor genes.

Hepatosplenic T-Cell Lymphoma[380–384]

Hepatosplenic T-cell lymphoma is an aggressive lymphoma that shows a re-markable tropism for sinusoidal involvement of spleen, liver, and bone marrow, and is usually derived from gamma-delta T-cells. It primarily affects patients in the second and third decades, with a predilection for females. Patients present

Figure 225.
Enteropathy-associated
T-cell lymphoma. The classic
cytologic appearance is seen,
with large lymphoid cells with
prominent nucleoli.

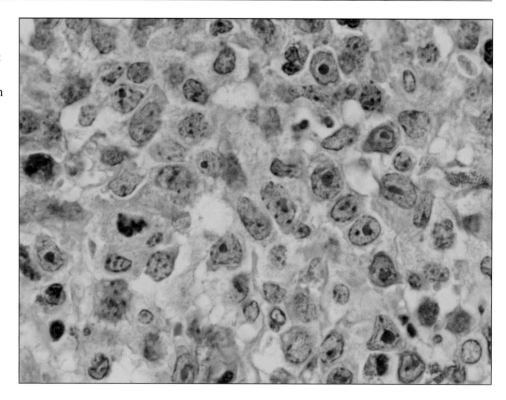

Figure 226.
Enteropathy-associated
T-cell lymphoma. Variant
small-cell cytology is seen.
These cases are usually
positive for CD8 and CD56.

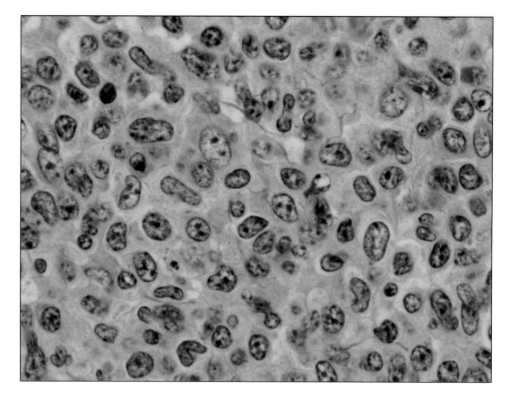

with hepatosplenomegaly, thrombocytopenia, and anemia. Lymph nodes are rarely involved. The median survival is usually about 1 year. One sees medium-sized lymphoid cells infiltrating the sinuses of the spleen, liver, and bone marrow, although the marrow infiltration may be quite subtle. The cells are CD3 positive, express TIA-1 (but not perforin), and usually have a gamma-delta

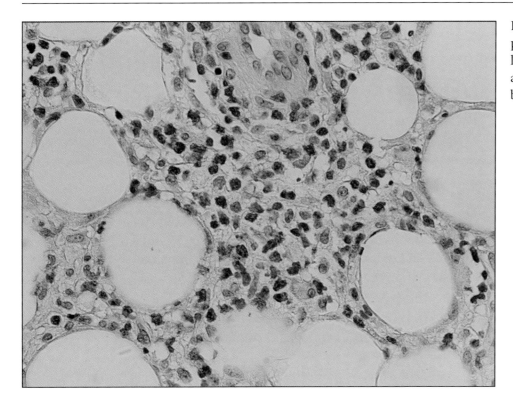

Figure 227. Subcutaneous panniculitic T-cell lymphoma. An infiltrate of atypical cells is present between lobules of fat.

phenotype, although a small subset of cases are alpha-beta type. They are usually negative for CD4, CD8, and CD56. Clonal rearrangements of the gamma T-cell receptor gene are found, and there is a characteristic isochromosome 7q.

Subcutaneous Panniculitis-Like T-Cell Lymphoma[381,385]

Subcutaneous panniculitis-like T-cell lymphoma is an aggressive T-cell lymphoma derived from cytotoxic T-cells with a remarkable tropism for the subcutaneous adipose tissue. It primarily affects young adults, with no age predilection. Patients present with multiple subcutaneous nodules, most commonly in the trunk and extremities, sometimes accompanied by a hemophagocytic syndrome. Histologically, one sees a polymorphous atypical lymphoid infiltrate involving subcutaneous adipose tissue, with substantial involvement of the overlying skin (Figure 227). There may be rimming of individual fat cells by the infiltrate, which also involves the septae. Lymph nodes may be involved late in the clinical course and may show diffuse effacement of architecture. Immunophenotypic studies show a mature T-cytotoxic phenotype, with expression of pan-T-cell antigens, CD8, and cytotoxic molecules. Most cases are of alpha-beta phenotype, but a subset are gamma-delta; these cases are negative for CD4 and CD8 and express CD56. There are no recurrent cytogenetic abnormalities described.

8 COMPOSITE LYMPHOMAS AND INTERFACE BETWEEN CLASSICAL HODGKIN AND NON-HODGKIN LYMPHOMA

Composite Classical Hodgkin and B-Cell Non-Hodgkin Lymphoma	216
Sequential Hodgkin Lymphoma and B-Cell Lymphoma	217
B-Cell Lymphoma with Features Intermediate Between Diffuse Large B-Cell Lymphoma and Classical Hodgkin Lymphoma (Gray-Zone Lymphoma)	217
Hodgkin Lymphoma and T-Cell Lymphoma	219

Classical Hodgkin lymphoma has been found to be a neoplasm of B-lymphocytes in virtually all cases; thus, it is not surprising that there may be some biological and clinical overlap between Hodgkin and non-Hodgkin lymphoma. This section will discuss composite classical Hodgkin and B-cell non-Hodgkin lymphoma, sequential classical Hodgkin and B-cell lymphoma, possible gray-zone lymphoma combining features of classical Hodgkin lymphoma and B-cell lymphoma, and the relationship between classical Hodgkin lymphoma and T-cell lymphoma.

COMPOSITE CLASSICAL HODGKIN AND B-CELL NON-HODGKIN LYMPHOMA[386]

Composite lymphoma is defined as the simultaneous occurrence of Hodgkin and non-Hodgkin lymphoma at the same anatomic site; it is a rare but well-described phenomenon. Since Hodgkin lymphoma is now known to be a lymphoma of B-cell derivation, it should not be surprising that almost all composite lymphomas represent the combination of Hodgkin lymphoma and a B-cell lymphoma. Diffuse large-cell lymphoma and follicular lymphoma represent the types of B-cell lymphoma usually involved, although all of the major B-cell lymphoma types have been described as part of a composite lymphoma. Composite Hodgkin lymphoma and chronic lymphocytic leukemia/small lymphocytic lymphoma have already been described in the section Chronic Lymphocytic Leukemia/Small Lymphocytic Lymphoma.

Patients with composite Hodgkin and non-Hodgkin lymphoma tend to be older adults. In most cases, there is a distinct separation of the Hodgkin lymphoma and the B-cell lymphoma. However, occasionally the two components are more closely intermingled. Nonetheless, typical histologic and immunohistochemical features should be seen for each component. Although difficult to study, the Hodgkin component has shown the same translocations as the non-Hodgkin component, consistent with evolution from the same clone. A subset of cases, particularly those cases in which Hodgkin lymphoma is composite with diffuse large B-cell lymphoma, are associated with EBV, present in both components.

Perhaps even more rarely identified, Hodgkin lymphoma and B-cell lymphoma may simultaneously occur at separate anatomic sites.

SEQUENTIAL HODGKIN LYMPHOMA AND B-CELL LYMPHOMA[387,388]

B-cell lymphoma may occur in patients who have been successfully treated for Hodgkin lymphoma, and conversely, Hodgkin lymphoma may even more rarely occur in patients who have been successfully treated for B-cell lymphoma. About 5% of patients develop B-cell lymphoma after successful treatment for Hodgkin lymphoma. Most patients present with abdominal disease and are usually of diffuse large B-cell or Burkitt type. Very limited data are available, but all of it is consistent with the lymphomas representing neoplasms derived from two completely distinct clones. Although it has been speculated that these cases occur due to the relative immunosuppression that patients treated for Hodgkin lymphoma have, only about 10% of these cases have been associated with EBV infection.

Hodgkin lymphoma occurring in patients treated for B-cell lymphoma is very rare, although it still represents the most common cancer in this setting, and occurring with a four-fold increase over expected. Follicular lymphoma and diffuse large B-cell lymphoma are the most common initial histologies, usually occurring in adults. The Hodgkin lymphoma follows after a median of about 5 years, presenting in lymph nodes. To date, there is no convincing evidence that the two neoplasms derive from the same clone of cells. There does not appear to be an association with EBV.

B-CELL LYMPHOMA WITH FEATURES INTERMEDIATE BETWEEN DIFFUSE LARGE B-CELL LYMPHOMA AND CLASSICAL HODGKIN LYMPHOMA (GRAY-ZONE LYMPHOMA)[389]

Gray-zone lymphoma is the term that has been applied to a hypothetical malignant lymphoma combining features of B-cell lymphoma and classical Hodgkin lymphoma and possibly representing a biologic transition between the two neoplasms. It has been particularly used in the context of mediastinal masses whose

Figure 228. Gray-zone lymphoma. Sheets of atypical cells are seen in this mediastinal biopsy. The cells were uniformly positive for CD30, CD15, and CD20.

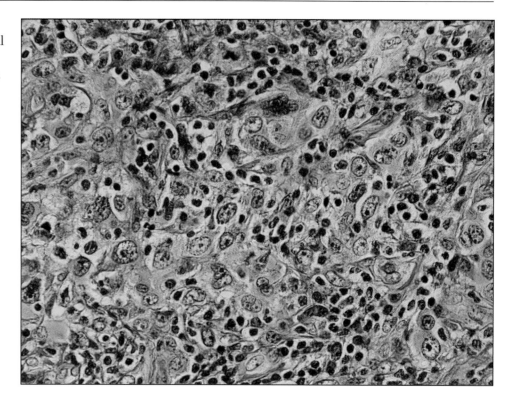

pathology shows confusing features or to the circumstance in which a biopsy taken within 1 year of a diagnosis of mediastinal Hodgkin lymphoma shows pathologic features more consistent with mediastinal large B-cell lymphoma, raising consideration that this latter lymphoma was present at the time of the initial biopsy (Figure 228). Biologically, there is some rationale for a true overlap between Hodgkin lymphoma and mediastinal B-cell lymphoma. Both neoplasms commonly occur in young women, with frequent involvement of the mediastinum. Immunophenotyping and other studies demonstrate an immunoglobulin-negative cell at a similar state of B-cell differentiation for both. Furthermore, there are some similar recurrent karyotypic abnormalities, including 2p15 (the site of the REL oncogene) and 9p24 (the site of the tyrosine kinase gene JAK2). Recent gene expression profiling studies have shown a closer relationship between mediastinal B-cell lymphoma with classical Hodgkin lymphoma than other types of diffuse large B-cell lymphoma.

Given the predilection for females of mediastinal large B-cell lymphoma, it may be surprising that most of the patients with gray-zone lymphomas are men. At low magnification, fibrous bands are either absent or focal, although a vague nodularity may still be seen, and there is often infiltration of fibrous tissue. At high magnification, sheets of large atypical cells are usually seen in a sparse reactive background. The typical phenotype overlaps that of Hodgkin cells and B-cells, with frequent expression of CD45, CD30, CD15, CD20, and CD79a. EBV is consistently negative. Clinically, treatment for the most aggressive component is recommended, typically doxorubicin-based chemotherapy with rituximab. The pattern of relapse in reported cases has been more typical of mediastinal B-cell lymphoma than Hodgkin lymphoma.

HODGKIN LYMPHOMA AND T-CELL LYMPHOMA[390]

Given the fact that virtually all or all cases of Hodgkin lymphoma are of B-cell lineage, one would not necessarily expect an association with T-cell lymphoma. The T-cell lymphoma most reported to be associated with Hodgkin lymphoma is mycosis fungoides. Most often, the Hodgkin lymphoma occurs following a long history of mycosis fungoides, although the opposite sequence has been reported as has simultaneous presentations. Studies purporting to show an association are hampered by the fact that Reed-Sternberg–like cells of both T- and B-cell lineage may be part of the pathologic findings in peripheral T-cell lymphoma.

9 IMMUNODEFICIENCY-ASSOCIATED LYMPHOPROLIFERATIVE DISORDERS

Primary Immunodeficiency Syndromes	220
HIV-Associated Malignant Lymphomas	224
Posttransplantation Lymphoproliferative Disorders	228
Immunosuppression Associated with Treatment of Other Diseases	231
Methotrexate-Associated Lymphoproliferative Disorders	231
Fludarabine-Associated Lymphoproliferative Disorders	231
Immunosuppression Associated with Aging	231

Immunodeficiency-associated lymphoproliferative disorders[391] occur in several main categories, including primary immunodeficiency syndromes, HIV infection, posttransplantation immunosuppression, immunosuppression associated with treatment of other diseases, and the immunosuppression associated with aging. The incidence and specific types of lymphoproliferative disorders depend on the specific category of immunosuppression, but some generalizations can be made. Most, but not all, of the lymphoproliferations represent B-cell disorders, although T-cell neoplasms and Hodgkin lymphoma may still occur. Although the specific etiologies may be multifactorial, many of the lymphoproliferations are associated with viruses such as EBV and HHV-8, sometimes with a preceding phase of polyclonal hyperplasia. Finally, some of the lymphoproliferations may respond to reduction in immunosuppression, implying a less than complete malignant phenotype.

PRIMARY IMMUNODEFICIENCY SYNDROMES[392-394]

The congenital immunodeficiencies most commonly associated with lymphoproliferative disorders include Wiskott-Aldrich syndrome, common variable immunodeficiency, ataxia telangiectasia, severe combined immunodeficiency, X-linked lymphoproliferative disorder, hyper-IgM syndrome, and autoimmune lymphoproliferative syndrome (ALPS). The common theme underlying these disorders is abnormal regulation of lymphoid proliferation due to specific but varying defects in the immunologic system.

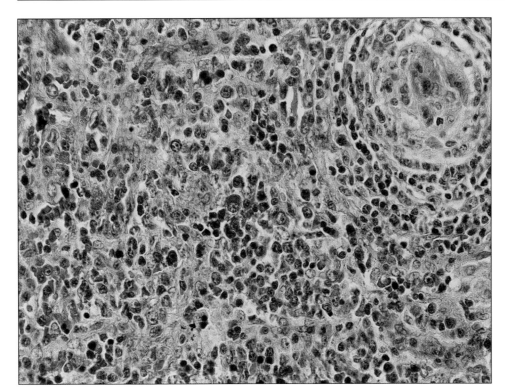

Figure 229. Wiskott-Aldrich syndrome. The paracortex shows lymphocyte depletion. Note the eosinophilic myelocyte and scattered plasma cells.

Wiskott-Aldrich syndrome is an X-linked recessive disorder that usually presents with bacterial infections and thrombocytopenia. Patients have defective antibody formation and T-cell dysfunction. Lymph nodes show depletion of small lymphocytes from the paracortical region, with a prominence of the stroma, atypical plasma cells, and extramedullary hematopoiesis (Figure 229). Occasionally, there are increased numbers of eosinophils, hemophagocytosis, and progressive depletion of follicles. Approximately 20% of patients develop malignant lymphoma, usually in childhood. Most cases represent diffuse large B-cell lymphoma, particularly of immunoblastic subtype, and usually occur in extranodal sites. The majority of cases are associated with EBV. About 5% of cases represent classical Hodgkin lymphoma. Monoclonal expansion of B-lymphocytes has also been described in lymph nodes, along with concomitant serum monoclonal peaks. Some lymphoproliferations may show spontaneous regression, even ones demonstrated to be monoclonal.

Common variable immunodeficiency is a heterogeneous group of disorders characterized by hypogammaglobulinemia, which generally, but not always, affects all antibody classes. The specific defect varies, but most involve abnormalities in T-cell signaling, particularly affecting B- and T-cell interactions, preventing proper B-cell activation. It usually first presents in teens or young adults who present with clinical manifestations of antibody deficiency – usually recurrent infections. Most biopsied lymph nodes show reactive or atypical lymphoid hyperplasia. Cases with atypical lymphoid hyperplasia may show histologic architectural effacement, although immunohistochemical studies may show retained immunoarchitecture, with florid hyperplasia of both the B- and T-cell compartments. Gene rearrangement studies generally show no evidence of clonal rearrangements, but clonal B- and T-cell populations may be detected in the absence of other indications of malignancy. Some cases may show chronic granulomatous inflammation. Malignant lymphoma occurs in about 5% of patients, mostly adult women. Most occur in extranodal sites and consist primarily of diffuse large B-cell lymphoma, with or without immunoblastic features; many are associated with EBV. Some cases may have histologic features consistent with classical Hodgkin lymphoma.

Ataxia telangiectasia is an autosomal recessive disorder due to mutations in the ATM gene on chromosome 11q22–23. Patients present in childhood with immunodeficiency, usually manifesting as recurrent sinopulmonary infections, and neurologic deficits, particularly cerebellar degeneration (giving rise to ataxia) and oculocutaneous telangiectasia. Many patients are deficient in IgA, and some have a deficiency of IgG as well. Patients are prone to develop precursor lymphoblastic neoplasms, usually of T-cell phenotype, T-cell prolymphocytic leukemia, classical Hodgkin lymphoma, as well as non-Hodgkin lymphoma, including diffuse aggressive B-cell lymphoma and peripheral T-cell lymphoma.

Severe combined immunodeficiency is a family of genetic defects manifesting as severe defects in B- and T-cell function. Infants, usually boys, present with recurrent severe infections. About 50% of patients have an X-linked recessive pattern of inheritance due to a mutation in the cytokine receptor gamma chain, while other cases have an autosomal recessive pattern, most often due to genetic defects leading to an absence of purine degradation enzymes. Lymph nodes from these patients are tiny and show an absence of lymphocytes, with only sinuses and a connective tissue framework. About 5% of patients develop malignant lymphoma, mostly non-Hodgkin lymphoma with a minority of cases of classical Hodgkin lymphoma.

X-linked lymphoproliferative disorder is due to a mutation of the SH2D1A gene, which codes for a protein called SAG that probably is a signal transduction molecule for activated T-cells. Affected patients appear well until their first exposure to EBV, leading to severe or fatal acute infectious mononucleosis. Involved lymph nodes show a marked immunoblastic hyperplasia, along with extensive areas of necrosis, followed by a plasmacytoid proliferation. Most patients who survive the initial infectious mononucleosis develop lymphoid depletion along with hypogammaglobulinemia. Malignant lymphoma, usually an EBV-associated high-grade B-cell lymphoma, ultimately develops in a majority of patients. There is a predilection for extranodal sites, particularly the ileocecal region, although lymph nodes are also commonly involved.

Hyper-IgM syndrome is a group of disorders characterized by normal or elevated serum IgM and low IgG and IgA. It most often has an X-linked pattern of inheritance, due to mutation of the gene for CD40L, or, less commonly, is autosomal recessive. Patients present in early childhood with recurrent bacterial infections or *P. carinii*. In this syndrome, the B-cell lymphocytes only express surface IgM and IgD, without switching to IgG or IgA. Lymph nodes show an absence of germinal centers, but otherwise show normal immunoarchitecture. There is a predilection for the development of non-Hodgkin lymphoma, mostly

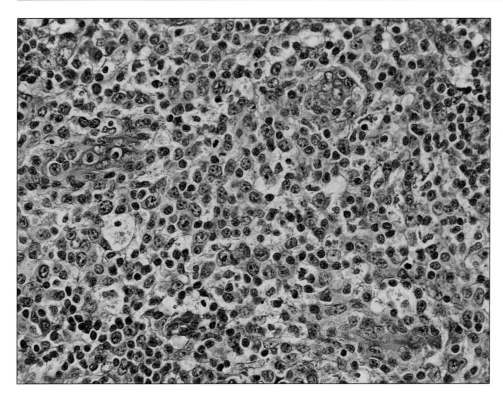

Figure 230. Autoimmune lymphoproliferative disease. The paracortical region shows an immunoblastic proliferation. The T-cells in this case were *double negative*, lacking CD4 and CD8 expression.

extranodal high-grade B-cell lymphomas, but also classical Hodgkin lymphoma. In addition, some patients develop a massive polyclonal IgM plasma cell proliferation, also usually extranodal.

ALPS is a disorder characterized by childhood onset generalized lymphadenopathy, hypergammaglobulinemia, lymphocytosis, splenomegaly, and autoimmune phenomena. It is most often due to mutations encoding the TNFRSF6 gene encoding CD95 (Fas/Apo-1), although the etiology is still obscure in some patients. The CD95 mutations lead to defective lymphocyte apoptosis; however, there is not a 1:1 correspondence between in vitro studies and clinical findings. The enlarged lymph nodes found in these patients show reactive changes. The most striking finding in most patients is a marked paracortical hyperplasia (Figure 230). Immunophenotyping studies show that the paracortical areas have large numbers of CD3-positive/CD4-negative/CD8-negative/CD45RO-negative cells (*double-negative cells*), along with an increase of CD45RA-positive cells. These cells also usually express the cytotoxic markers perforin and TIA-1, as well as CD57. In addition, there is usually florid follicular hyperplasia, often with focal transformation of germinal centers, and in some cases, follicular involution. A polyclonal plasmacytosis is also frequently seen. In about 40% of patients, there is a histiocytic proliferation resembling Rosai-Dorfman disease, including the characteristic nuclear features, evidence of emperipolesis, and S-100 protein expression. This proliferation may be focal, multifocal, or diffuse.

The paracortical proliferation may be so extensive as to simulate a diagnosis of malignant lymphoma, although the identification of the distinctive phenotype including double-negative cells should resolve the diagnostic problem.

Table 39. 2001 WHO Classification of HIV-Associated Lymphomas[213]

Lymphomas commonly occurring in immunocompetent patients
Burkitt lymphoma
Classical
With plasmacytoid differentiation
Atypical
Diffuse large B-cell lymphoma
Centroblastic
Immunoblastic
Extranodal marginal zone B-cell lymphoma of mucosa-associated lymphoid tissue type (rare)
Peripheral T-cell lymphoma (rare)
Classical Hodgkin lymphoma
Lymphomas occurring more specifically in HIV+ patients
Primary effusion lymphoma
Plasmablastic lymphoma
Lymphomas also occurring in other immunodeficiency states
Polymorphic B-cell lymphoma (PTLD-like)

Although an increased risk of lymphoma has not been demonstrated in these patients, cases of lymphoma have been reported in family members of one affected individual.

HIV-ASSOCIATED MALIGNANT LYMPHOMAS[313,395,396]

The benign lymph node changes that may be observed in HIV infection have already been discussed in the section HIV-Related Benign Lymphadenopathy. The incidence of malignant lymphoma is greatly increased in patients with HIV infection. The relative risk of an aggressive B-cell lymphoma is increased 100- to 500-fold, the risk of low-grade B-cell lymphoma (particularly marginal zone B-cell lymphoma) is increased about 15-fold, and the risk of T-cell lymphoma also is increased among patients with a diagnosis of AIDS. Lymphoma is seen in all population groups at risk for HIV, in all ages, and more commonly in men than women. In the current era of HAART, the incidence of malignant lymphoma has decreased but is still markedly elevated over non–HIV-infected populations. In the post–HAART era, there has been an increase in the age of affected patients from the late 30s to the early 40s, with a decreased incidence among homosexuals and whites and an increase among women, those of nonwhite ethnicity (particularly Latino/Hispanic), and those who acquired HIV by heterosexual contact. In addition, the median CD4 count at lymphoma diagnosis has increased, along with a decrease in Burkitt histology and an increase in diffuse large B-cell histology.

The 2001 WHO Classification of HIV-associated lymphomas is given in Table 39. About one-third of cases represent Burkitt lymphoma, which

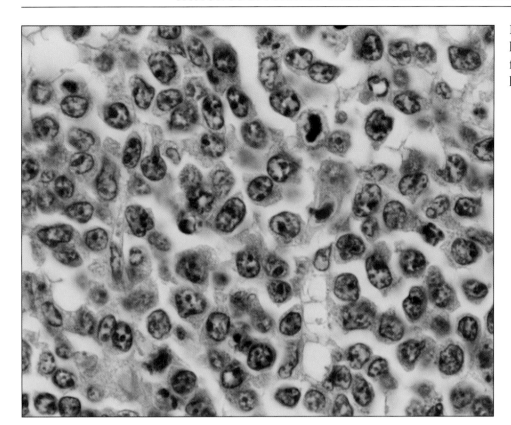

Figure 231. Burkitt-like lymphoma with plasmacytoid features. This patient had a history of AIDS.

more often presents extranodally or in bone marrow than in lymph nodes. Burkitt lymphoma typically occurs earlier in the natural history of HIV infection and is associated with a higher CD4 T-cell count than other lymphomas. It is usually preceded by reactive lymphadenopathy and presents in peripheral sites or bone marrow. About one-third of cases are associated with EBV infection, with a latency pattern 2 (EBNA-1 and latent membrane protein-1 expression), different from the latency pattern 1 seen in sporadic Burkitt lymphoma. The histologic appearance may resemble that seen in non–HIV-infected patients, but may also show a plasmacytoid appearance, with a more prominent, often centrally located nucleolus and more abundant amphophilic to basophilic cytoplasm (Figure 231). About two-thirds of these cases are associated with EBV.

About one-third of cases of HIV-associated lymphomas represent diffuse large B-cell lymphoma, which may present in nodal or extranodal sites. About 20% of cases are associated with EBV infection. Although the histologic appearance may resemble that seen in non–HIV-infected patients, about 20% of cases show an immunoblastic appearance, a percentage much higher than that seen in non–HIV-infected populations. This subtype usually is seen in extranodal sites, particularly the brain, and has a strong association with EBV infection. They particularly occur late in the course of HIV infection and are associated with low CD4 cell counts.

Classical Hodgkin lymphoma usually is of either mixed cellularity or lymphocyte depletion histology and may show areas of necrosis. There is usually a predominance of CD8-positive cells rather than the usual CD4 predominance.

225

Figure 232. Plasmablastic lymphoma associated with HIV infection. This case came from the oral cavity. The cells were negative for CD45 and CD20 and show striking plasmablastic features.

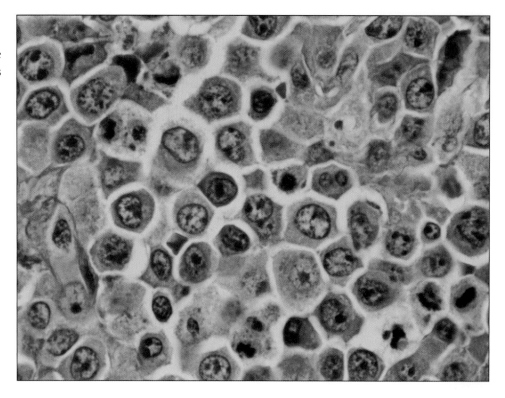

Almost all cases are associated with EBV infection. Cases of MALT lymphoma, other low-grade B-cell lymphomas, and peripheral T-cell lymphoma, including mycosis fungoides, have all been reported at an increased incidence in HIV-infected patients.

Plasmablastic lymphoma is a relatively recently described lymphoma that characteristically occurs in HIV-infected patients. It most frequently occurs near mucosal surfaces, particularly the oral cavity. Morphologically, the cells resemble those of immunoblastic lymphoma, but are distinguished by their immunophenotype (Figure 232). While immunoblasts are positive for both CD45 and CD20, plasmablasts are negative for CD45 and CD20 and, moreover, express cytoplasmic IgG and plasma cell markers such as CD138. These lymphomas have a strong association with EBV, but are negative for HHV-8.

Primary effusion lymphoma is a distinctive lymphoma that almost always occurs in effusions within body cavities. Most, but not all patients, have HIV infection. It is invariably associated with large amounts of HHV-8 within the tumor cells, which usually but not always also have EBV. Patients typically present with an effusion, although there may be extension to the adjacent soft tissue. Cytologically, the cells are immunoblastic, plasmablastic, or anaplastic. They almost always express CD45 and CD30, but usually lack expression of specific B- and T-cell markers. They lack immunoglobulin expression, but they may express the B-cell transcription factors BOB.1 or OCT-2, and they consistently have clonal rearrangements of the immunoglobulin heavy and/or light chain genes, consistent with a B-cell lineage. In addition, they usually express CD138 and CD38, are invariably positive for KSHV, and are usually also positive for EBV (although they consistently lack LMP-1 expression). I have

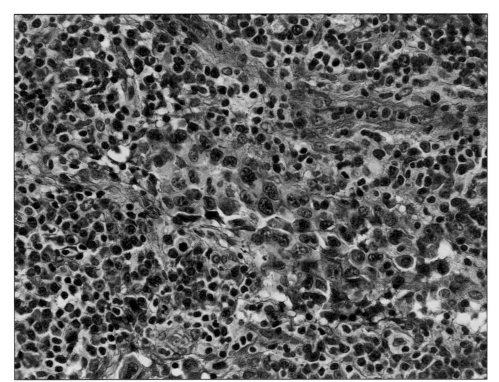

Figure 233. Diffuse large B-cell lymphoma, extracavitary pleural effusion lymphoma presenting in a lymph node. This case was strongly positive for KSHV (see next figure) and showed expression of BOB.1 and OCT-2, but was negative for CD45, CD20, and CD79a. The cells were largely confined to sinusoids. The nuclei are markedly atypical.

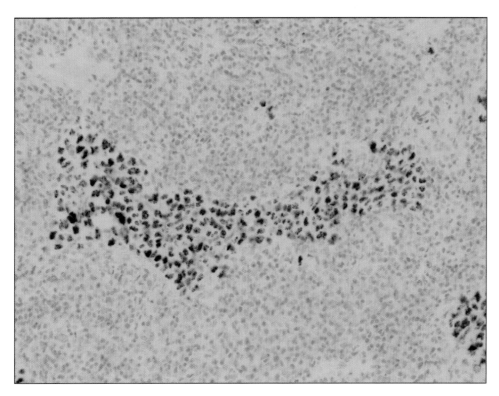

Figure 234. Diffuse large B-cell lymphoma, extracavitary pleural effusion lymphoma presenting in a lymph node, KSHV stain. There was positivity in all or virtually all the neoplastic cells.

only seen one case presenting in a lymph node, in which a sinusoidal distribution was seen (Figures 233 and 234). The CD45-positive, CD30-positive, and B- and T-antigen–negative phenotype may closely mimic null-cell anaplastic large-cell lymphoma; however, these cases will stain strongly for HHV-8 viral antigens.

Finally, HIV-associated lymphomas may rarely show a polymorphic appearance similar to what is more commonly observed in the posttransplant setting. Patients may present in extranodal sites or with enlarged lymph nodes. One sees a mixture of small lymphocytes, lymphoplasmacytic forms, plasma cells, and plasmacytoid immunoblasts. These lymphomas are usually EBV associated. Gene rearrangement studies usually show clonal rearrangements of the immunoglobulin heavy and/or light chain genes, although some cases may show an oligoclonal or polyclonal pattern or only small clonal populations within a polyclonal background.

POSTTRANSPLANTATION LYMPHOPROLIFERATIVE DISORDERS[397-400]

Posttransplantation lymphoproliferative disorders may occur after both solid-organ or allogenic bone marrow transplantation. The risk of disease depends on a number of factors, including the type of transplant, immunosuppressive regimen, age, and Epstein–Barr seropositivity prior to transplant. There is about a less than 1% incidence in kidney recipients, a 1–2% incidence in liver or allogenic bone marrow recipients, a 2–5% incidence in heart recipients, and a 5–8% incidence in lung or multiple-organ recipients. Much of these differences are probably due to the type of immunosuppressive regimen, as the stronger the regimen, the greater the incidence of posttransplantation lymphoproliferative disorder. Thus, patients with treatment with anti–T-cell antibodies have a much higher incidence than patients who do not receive such therapy. Young patients are much more likely to develop posttransplantation lymphoproliferative disorders, probably due to the fact that seronegative recipients are much more likely to be affected. About 80% of cases of posttransplantation lymphoproliferative disorders are associated with EBV infection, in which a type 1 latency pattern is most often seen. Most cases occurring in solid-organ recipients are of host origin, while most cases occurring in bone marrow recipients are donor in origin. Clinically, patients may present either early or late after transplantation. When they present within the first year of transplantation, patients tend to have widespread disease, with systemic symptoms and enlargement of the tonsils and cervical lymph nodes and often have rapid progression of disease. Patients presenting later than 1 year after transplant tend to have fewer constitutional symptoms and often present with extranodal disease with visceral nodal involvement. The allograft is the site of the lymphoma in about 20% of cases. The treatment varies based on the clinical circumstances but may include reduction in the degree of immunosuppression, rituximab, surgical resection, localized radiotherapy, low- to high-dose chemotherapy, or experimental therapies such as adoptive T-cell therapy.

Histologically, a wide variety of patterns may be seen. The 2001 WHO Classification of posttransplant lymphoproliferative disorders is given in Table 40. The early lesions include reactive plasmacytic hyperplasia and an infectious mononucleosis–like proliferation. Both of these lesions tend to occur in EBV-seronegative individuals and occur primarily in lymph nodes or tonsils. Reactive

Table 40. 2001 WHO Classification of Posttransplant Lymphoproliferative Disease (PTLD)[213]

Early lesions

    Reactive plasmacytic hyperplasia

    Infectious mononucleosis–like

Polymorphic PTLD

Monomorphic PTLD

    B-cell neoplasms

        Diffuse large B-cell lymphoma (immunoblastic, centroblastic, anaplastic)

        Burkitt/Burkitt-like lymphoma

        Plasma cell myeloma

        Plasmacytoma-like lesions

    T-cell neoplasms

        Peripheral T-cell lymphoma, not otherwise specified

        Other types

Hodgkin lymphoma/Hodgkin lymphoma–like PTLD

plasmacytic hyperplasia consists of a proliferation of small lymphocytes, polyclonal plasma cells, and infrequent immunoblasts that do not efface the underlying architecture. Scattered EBV-positive cells are always present. Infectious mononucleosis–like lesions resemble infectious mononucleosis in immunocompetent individuals, but may be difficult to distinguish from polymorphic lesions. Many EBV-infected cells are seen by in situ hybridization studies. Immunohistochemical studies show polyclonal populations, although small clonal B-cell populations may be demonstrated in some cases by PCR or EBV clonality studies.

Polymorphic posttransplant lymphoproliferative disorder has a histologic resemblance to infectious mononucleosis–like lesions, but shows complete architectural effacement. One sees a mixture of small lymphocytes, plasmacytoid lymphocytes, and plasmacytoid immunoblasts, including possibly atypical forms (Figure 235). Focal areas of necrosis may be present. Both immunophenotyping and molecular studies demonstrate B-cell clones, which may be multiple, and a subset may have bcl-6 mutations. Monomorphic posttransplant lymphoproliferative disorder shows the histologic appearance of specific lymphoma types. These include diffuse aggressive B-cell lymphomas, such as diffuse large B-cell lymphoma and Burkitt/Burkitt-like lymphoma, and peripheral T-cell lymphoma. Most cases are diagnosed as diffuse large B-cell lymphoma, often of immunoblastic subtype. Mutations of the bcl-6 gene are seen in almost all cases, and mutations of the RAS or P53 genes are also common. About 15% of cases represent peripheral T-cell lymphoma, including the entire range of subtypes. These cases tend to occur later in the posttransplant period, are less likely to be associated with EBV, and are less likely to respond to a decrease in

Figure 235.
Posttransplantation
lymphoproliferative disorder,
polymorphous variant.
A range of cells is seen, from
cells resembling plasma cells
through immunoblasts.

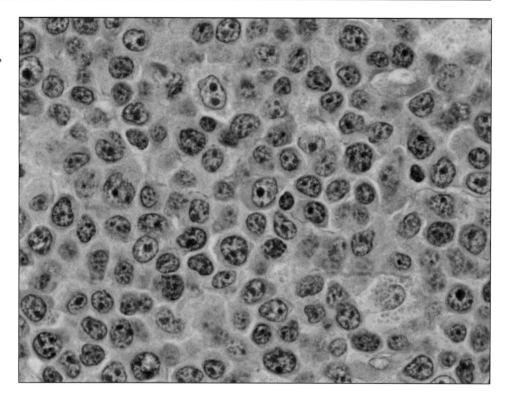

immunosuppression. About 1% of cases represent classical Hodgkin lymphoma. These cases have similar characteristics to de novo Hodgkin lymphoma, although almost all cases are EBV associated.

Plasmacytic hyperplasia may be difficult to distinguish from nonspecific reactive hyperplasia. One should not diagnose plasmacytic hyperplasia if EBV-positive cells are not identified by in situ hybridization. Infectious mononucleosis–like lesions may be difficult to distinguish from polymorphic lesions. In some cases, the distinction may be impossible (and fortunately not critical), but, at least theoretically, polymorphic lesions should show complete effacement, while infectious mononucleosis–like lesions should have at least some retention of architecture. Clonality studies may be of help; the demonstration of a large clonal population would strongly favor a polymorphic lesion. Hodgkin lymphoma in the posttransplant setting needs to be distinguished from Hodgkin-like posttransplant lymphoproliferative disorder. This rare lesion morphologically simulates classical Hodgkin lymphoma of mixed cellularity or lymphocyte depletion subtype, but can be distinguished on the basis of immunohistochemical and molecular studies. Immunohistochemicals show the large atypical cells of the Hodgkin-like lesions to consistently express CD45 and multiple B-lineage markers, show variable expression of CD30, and consistently lack CD15. In addition, the demonstration of a significant clonal B-cell population as well as the presence of EBV in both the large Hodgkin cells as well as a substantial subset of smaller lymphocytes would support a diagnosis of a Hodgkin-like lesion. The differentiation is important to make as these lesions should be treated similarly as other posttransplantation lymphoproliferative disorders and as classical Hodgkin lymphoma.

IMMUNOSUPPRESSION ASSOCIATED WITH TREATMENT OF OTHER DISEASES[401–403]

Methotrexate-Associated Lymphoproliferative Disorders

A small proportion of patients treated with methotrexate for autoimmune disease develop a lymphoproliferative disorder. About 80% of patients have a history of rheumatoid arthritis, while about 5% each have dermatomyositis or psoriasis. It is still not clear what the increased risk is, or even that there truly is an increased risk. Most patients present with nodal disease, although extranodal masses are almost as frequent. About 50% of cases are associated with EBV. The important clinical feature of these lesions is their propensity to show at least partial regression upon withdrawal of the methotrexate, particularly seen in the EBV-positive cases. Histologically, most cases show histologic features of a diffuse large-cell lymphoma. A subset of cases may have histologic features consistent with Hodgkin lymphoma, while others have Hodgkin-like or polymorphic features. The Hodgkin-like cases morphologically resemble Hodgkin lymphoma, but the large atypical cells express CD45 and multiple B-lineage antigens and lack CD15. Cases showing Hodgkin-like features typically regress following withdrawal of methotrexate therapy. Other cases may show features more suggestive of polymorphous posttransplant lymphoproliferative disorders with lymphoplasmacytic features (Figure 236).

Fludarabine-Associated Lymphoproliferative Disorders[404]

Fludarabine is a drug commonly used to treat chronic lymphocytic leukemia/small lymphocytic lymphoma and other low-grade B-cell lymphomas. Rarely, patients treated with fludarabine for low-grade lymphoma (often in combination with other therapies) may develop transformation to EBV-positive lymphoproliferative disorders. Some of the cases show Hodgkin-like lymphoma, with or without foci of large-cell transformation, while other cases show a polymorphic appearance similar to that seen in the posttransplantation setting. Most are clonally distinct from the original lymphoma. Some of these lymphoproliferations have regressed upon withdrawal of therapy.

IMMUNOSUPPRESSION ASSOCIATED WITH AGING[405,406]

EBV-associated B-cell lymphoproliferative disorders have been reported in the elderly (senile EBV-positive lymphoproliferations), suggesting that this disease may be related to the decline in immunologic competence that occurs during the normal aging process. There is a median age of about 71 years, with an equal incidence in men and women. There is no evidence for an overt immunodeficiency other than aging. The disease presents in lymph nodes in a majority of

Figure 236.
Methotrexate-associated
lymphoproliferation.
A polymorphous appearance
is seen.

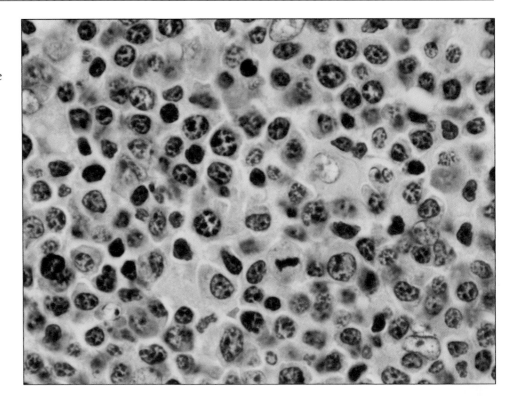

Figure 237. Senile
EBV-associated
lymphoproliferative disorder.
A polymorphous infiltrate
is seen. Note the
Reed-Sternberg–like
cell at the center.

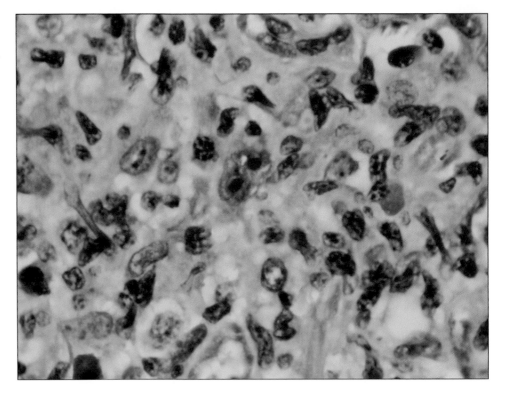

cases, although about 40% present in a variety of extranodal sites, including
Waldeyer ring and stomach. About 60% of cases show the histologic appearance
of diffuse large B-cell lymphoma, but about 40% show a polymorphic subtype,
with varying numbers of Hodgkin-like cells (Figure 237). Patients with the
Hodgkin-like subtype have a significantly better prognosis than the large-cell

subtype. EBV is consistently identified in all of the tumor cells, regardless of the histologic findings.

The differential diagnosis includes other spontaneous non-Hodgkin lymphomas and Hodgkin lymphoma. The identification of EBV in the tumor cells is definitional to this entity and would rule out spontaneous non-Hodgkin lymphoma. The differential diagnosis of the Hodgkin-like subtype with true classical Hodgkin lymphoma is much more problematic as both neoplasms may be EBV associated. Histologically, one often sees a range of atypia, with a greater number of large atypical cells than usually encountered in classical Hodgkin lymphoma. Immunohistochemical studies may also be helpful, as the large atypical cells in the Hodgkin-like subtype express multiple B-lineage antigens, including consistent expression of CD20 and CD79a, and is usually CD45 positive and CD15 positive, in contrast to the CD45-negative/CD15-positive phenotype seen in true Hodgkin cells.

10 HISTIOCYTIC AND DENDRITIC CELL NEOPLASMS

Histiocytic Sarcoma	234
Langerhans Cell Histiocytosis	237
Langerhans Cell Sarcoma	241
Interdigitating Dendritic Cell Sarcoma	241
Follicular Dendritic Cell Sarcoma	244
Fibroblastic Reticulum Cell Neoplasm	247
Precursor Plasmacytoid Dendritic Cell Neoplasm	248

Histiocytic and dendritic cell neoplasms[407] are uncommon diseases. Histiocytes are mobile but generally noncirculating cells derived from and are the tissue-based equivalent of monocytes. They express the specific marker CD163 and the lysosomal marker CD68. Dendritic cells are a family of antigen-presenting cells, including the myeloid-derived Langerhans cells and interdigitating dendritic cells, the fixed and probably non–hematopoietic-derived follicular dendritic cells of follicles, and the probably lymphoid-derived plasmacytoid dendritic cells, which upon stimulation with IL-3 become another subset of interdigitating dendritic cells.

HISTIOCYTIC SARCOMA[408–415]

Histiocytic sarcoma is a malignant neoplasm of post–bone marrow histiocytes. It is extremely rare, less than 1000-fold as frequent as malignant lymphoma. It occurs most commonly in adults, although it has been reported in all ages. A subset of cases may be associated with mediastinal germ cell tumors, usually malignant teratoma with or without a yolk sac component. Lymph nodes are the most common site of presentation, although any other site may be affected, particularly skin, liver, spleen, bone, and intestinal tract. Patients generally present at stage III or IV. Occasionally, patients show a systemic pattern of spread, reminiscent of the old term malignant histiocytosis. It is an aggressive neoplasm, generally with a poorer response to therapy than non-Hodgkin lymphoma, and most patients die of progressive disease. Nonetheless, some patients may respond to chemotherapy and have a more indolent course.

Diffuse effacement of lymph node architecture is usually seen, although some cases show a sinusoidal or paracortical distribution of disease (Figure 238).

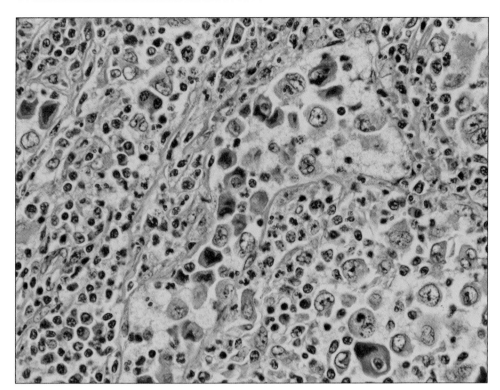

Figure 238. Histiocytic sarcoma. Most areas of the case showed diffuse effacement of nodal architecture, but a sinusoidal appearance was seen at the edges of the lesion.

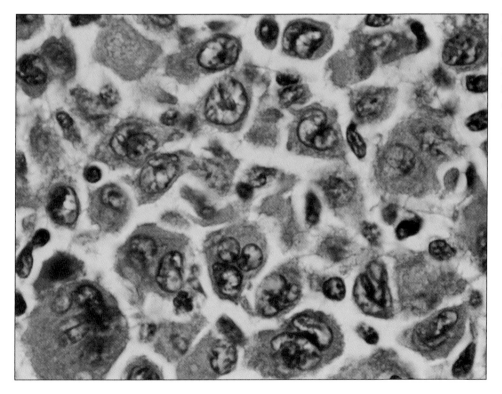

Figure 239. Histiocytic sarcoma. The cells in this case are large, with multilobated or multinucleated, and have abundant eosinophilic cytoplasm.

The neoplastic cells are generally large, with large nuclei with round to oval outlines, often eccentrically placed (Figure 239). Occasionally, the nuclear outlines may be irregular or multilobated, and truly multinucleated cells may be present. Nuclear atypia varies from mild to severe. The chromatin pattern

Figure 240. Histiocytic sarcoma, CD163. CD163 is a relatively sensitive and specific marker for nonneoplastic and neoplastic histiocytes.

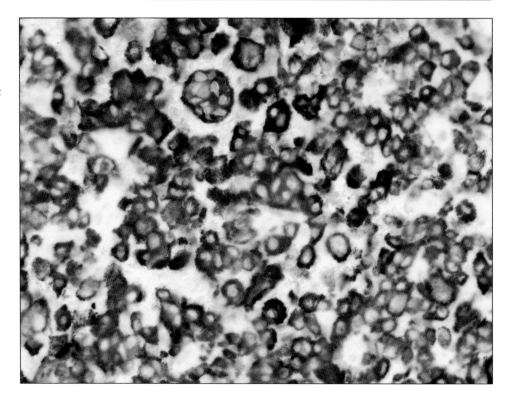

generally resembles that of large-cell lymphoma – usually vesicular, with nucleoli ranging from indistinct to large. Cytoplasm is moderate to abundant and sometimes eosinophilic. There may be some cells with foamy cytoplasm. Cytophagocytosis, usually hemophagocytosis may be present, but is not essential for the diagnosis. Scattered small lymphocytes, plasma cells, benign histiocytes, and eosinophils may be present.

Immunohistochemical studies show expression of the histiocytic marker CD163 along with lysozyme and the lysosomal-associated marker CD68 (Figure 240). In addition, the histiocytic markers CD11c and CD14 are also positive, although these markers are best detected in frozen sections or flow cytometry. CD45, HLA-DR, CD43, and CD4 (a marker of histiocytes in addition to T-helper cells) are usually positive, although, by definition, there is no expression of specific T- and B-cell markers. S-100 protein may be positive, but the expression is usually weak and focal. Langerin may occasionally be focally positive. CD30 and other markers of dendritic cells such as CD1a, CD21, CD23, CD35, and CD123 are negative. The Ki-67 index is highly variable. Rarely, there may be clonal immunoglobulin or T-cell receptor gene rearrangements. No recurrent cytogenetic abnormalities have been consistently reported.

The differential diagnosis includes reactive histiocytic proliferations, dendritic cell proliferations, non-Hodgkin lymphoma, and metastatic neoplasms such as malignant melanoma. Both reactive histiocytic proliferations and histiocytic sarcoma may have hemophagocytosis, multinucleated cells, and cells with foamy cytoplasm. The distinction with reactive histiocytic proliferations rests on cytologic features. Histiocytic sarcoma features cells with cytologically malignant

Table 41. Histiocytic and Dendritic Cell Tumors: Immunohistochemical Features

	CD45	S-100	CD1a	Langerin	CD21/CD23/CD35
Histiocytic sarcoma	+	−/+	−	−/+	−
Langerhans cell histiocytosis/sarcoma	+/−	+	+	+	−
Interdigitating dendritic cell sarcoma	+/−	+	−	−	−
Follicular dendritic cell sarcoma	−/+	−/+	−	−	+
Fibroblastic reticular cell sarcoma	−	−	−	−	−

nuclei distinct from the bland nuclei found in most reactive histiocytic proliferations or the distinctive round nuclei with a fine chromatin pattern seen in Rosai-Dorfman disease. Dendritic cell sarcomas, particularly interdigitating dendritic cell sarcoma, may also be confused with histiocytic sarcoma, as there is overlap of the histologic features in some cases (Table 41). Histiocytic sarcoma tends to have a greater degree of pleomorphism, while interdigitating dendritic cell tumor tends to have a greater degree of cell spindling. Both neoplasms may have S-100 protein–positive cells, but the positivity tends to be stronger and more diffuse in interdigitating cell tumor. Anaplastic large-cell lymphoma is the non-Hodgkin lymphoma most frequently confused with histiocytic sarcoma, given its propensity for involvement of the sinusoids and its frequent cytologic pleomorphism. In fact, many cases previously regarded as malignant histiocytosis have been found to actually represent anaplastic large-cell lymphoma. The distinction with non-Hodgkin lymphoma rests on immunophenotyping studies, optimally, combined with gene rearrangement studies. The presence of CD30 expression, the demonstration of specific T- or B-cell antigens (excluding the nonlineage specific CD43 and CD3), and the demonstration of clonal immunoglobulin and/or T-cell receptor gene rearrangements generally excludes histiocytic sarcoma. Both T- and B-cell lymphomas may have large numbers of reactive histiocytes (e.g., T-cell/histiocytic-rich B-cell lymphoma), so it is important to evaluate staining on the cytologically atypical cells. Finally, although both histiocytic sarcoma and metastatic malignant melanoma may show S-100 protein and CD68 expression, histiocytic sarcoma lacks expression of more specific melanoma markers such as HMB-45, Melan-A, or tyrosinase, while malignant melanoma lacks expression of the specific histiocytic marker CD163.

LANGERHANS CELL HISTIOCYTOSIS[416–428]

Langerhans cell histiocytosis, formerly known as histiocytosis X, is a neoplastic proliferation of Langerhans cells. Langerhans cells are defined as dendritic cells that express S-100 protein and CD1a and possess Birbeck granules on ultrastructural examination. They primarily reside in the basal layer of the epidermis and drain via lymphatics to regional lymph nodes. Langerhans cells histiocytosis

Figure 241. Langerhans cell histiocytosis. A sinusoidal pattern of involvement is seen.

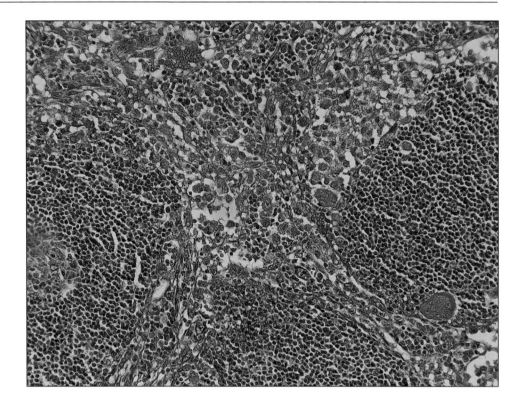

occurs as three main clinical syndromes, including unifocal disease (formerly, solitary eosinophilic granuloma), multifocal unisystem disease (formerly, Hand-Schüller-Christian disease), or multifocal, multisystem disease (formerly, Letterer-Siwe disease). Lymph node involvement occurs in several settings. First, it may be the only site of disease, occurring either isolated or involving multiple nodes, most often occurring in the cervical, inguinal, or axillary regions. Patients with isolated lymph node involvement typically lack systemic symptoms and present with lymphadenopathy. Second, it may be a part of multifocal multi-system disease, occurring in approximately 10% of children at presentation. These patients typically present with systemic symptoms, with frequent skin and bone disease. Third, lymph node involvement may occur as a focal process draining overlying skin or bone disease. Finally, it may occur as a focal process in association with another neoplasm, such as non-Hodgkin or Hodgkin lymphoma.

Several patterns of lymph node involvement may be seen. In the most common pattern, an exclusive or partial sinusoidal pattern of infiltration is seen (Figure 241). Less commonly, seen particularly in patients with multifocal, multisystem disease, there is partial to complete effacement of architecture. The capsule may be infiltrated, and clusters of Langerhans cells may be found in adjacent lymphatics. Rarely, one may see cohesive aggregates of Langerhans cells in the paracortical region resembling epithelioid granulomas, with more typical histology found at other sites. This pattern of involvement has been observed in abdominal lymph nodes, in which other sites of disease show more typical findings. At high magnification, one sees varying proportions of Langer-hans cells, multinucleate giant cells, eosinophils, neutrophils histiocytes, and small lymphocytes (Figure 242). Relatively pure populations of Langerhans

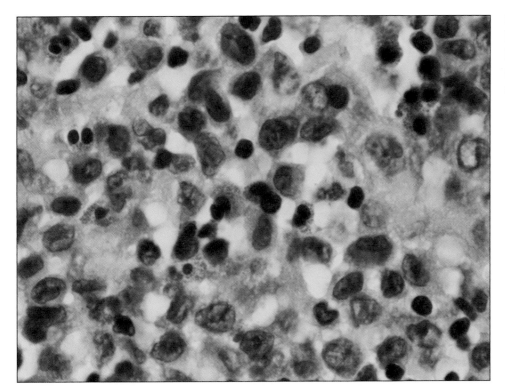

Figure 242. Langerhans cell histiocytosis. A mixture of Langerhans cells, eosinophils, and histiocytes is seen in this case.

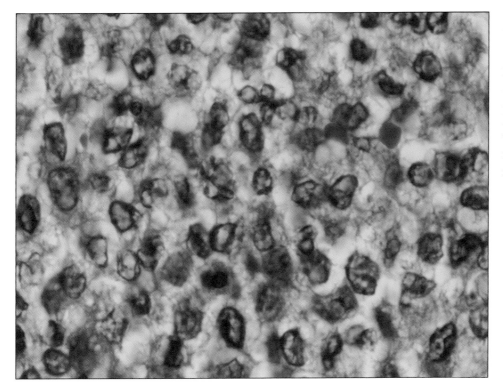

Figure 243. Langerhans cell histiocytosis. The nuclei have a histiocytic appearance, with prominent grooves. A relatively pure population is seen, as is typical of Langerhans cell histiocytosis when it occurs as a multisystem disease in infants.

may be seen, particularly in cases of partial or diffuse effacement occurring in infants and children (Figure 243). There may be areas of tumor necrosis, and one may observe hemophagocytosis in occasional Langerhans cells in these cases. Eosinophils and neutrophils are more common in early lesions, while foamy macrophages and plasma cells are more common in older lesions, often associated with areas of fibrosis. Eosinophils may occasionally be quite numerous, with the formation of eosinophilic microabscesses. The multinucleate giant cells may be of either histiocyte or Langerhans cell origin and may show phagocytosis. The histiocytes may be typical or epithelioid; the latter may also be of histiocyte or Langerhans cell origin. The Langerhans cells usually closely resemble nonneoplastic Langerhans cells. However, there may be some degree of cytologic atypia, but short of frank anaplasia. Many nuclei show a characteristic fine chromatin pattern with thin nuclear membranes, often with dented, folded, or grooved nuclei. Nucleoli are generally inconspicuous. Cytoplasm is usually moderately abundant and pale to intensely eosinophilic. Ultrastructural studies will reveal the presence of cytoplasmic Birbeck granules specific to Langerhans cells – membranous bodies with an osmiophilic core and a double outer sheath, often shaped like a tennis racket or a zipper. In addition, Langerhans cells have numerous lysosomes, small vesicles, and multivesicular bodies, but lack cell junctions.

The lesional cells of Langerhans cell histiocytosis have the phenotypic characteristics of Langerhans cells, with minor changes (Table 41). Thus, they express CD1a, S-100 protein, Langerin, HLA-DR, and peanut agglutinin lectin. In contrast to normal Langerhans cells, they express placental alkaline phosphatase. The Ki-67 index is usually low, but may be 25–50% in lesions occurring in infants. They are consistently negative for specific B- and T-lineage markers, CD30, CD34, and the follicular dendritic markers CD21, CD23, and CD35. They have been reported to be variably positive for CD45, CD68, CD163, CD4, and lysozyme, but most of the expression of histiocytic markers probably represents staining of nonneoplastic histiocytes, in my opinion. The lesions of Langerhans cell histiocytosis (with the exception of pulmonary Langerhans cell histiocytosis) represent clonal proliferations, as determined by X-linked androgen receptor gene studies. Clonal rearrangements of the antigen receptor genes are not found. Cytogenetic and other studies have shown abnormalities involving chromosomes 1p and 7. There is no association with viruses.

Prognostic factors include age, pattern of disease, and organ dysfunction. Cytologic features within the spectrum of Langerhans cell histiocytosis do not correlate with outcome.

The differential diagnosis includes dermatopathic lymphadenitis, Langerhans cell sarcoma, other dendritic proliferations, and occasionally Rosai-Dorfman disease. Dermatopathic lymphadenitis is the lesion most frequently mistaken for Langerhans cell histiocytosis. Although dermatopathic lymphadenitis may contain numerous Langerhans cells, the low-magnification appearance is distinctly different. While Langerhans cell histiocyte either shows a preferential sinusoidal pattern or partial or diffuse architectural effacement, dermatopathic lymphadenitis always shows a paracortical distribution with maintenance of the normal architecture and does not involve the sinuses. The distinction of Langerhans cell histiocytosis vs. Langerhans cell sarcoma rests on the cytologic features. While the proliferating cells of both have the phenotype of Langerhans cells, the presence of clearly cytologically malignant cells would warrant a diagnosis of Langerhans cell sarcoma. Several dendritic proliferations share S-100 protein expression with Langerhans cell histiocytosis, but all, with the exception of the indeterminate cell tumor, are negative for CD1a. The indeterminate cell tumor is a rare neoplasm that has been only reported in skin. It features cells that express CD1a and S-100 protein, but lack Birbeck granules on ultrastructural examination. Since large numbers of cases have not been reported, it is not clear whether it really represents a true clinicopathologic disorder or a case of Langerhans cell histiocytosis that lacks Birbeck granules, whether due to biology, sampling considerations, or other factors. I personally do not require electron microscopy to confirm a diagnosis of Langerhans cell histiocytosis when the histologic features are otherwise typical for the neoplasm. The sinusoidal architecture of Rosai-Dorfman disease may show a superficial resemblance to Langerhans cell histiocytosis (and shares S-100 protein expression), but the distinctive round nuclei with moderate nucleoli are very different from the bent, indented, and grooved nuclei of Langerhans cell histiocytosis.

LANGERHANS CELL SARCOMA[428–430]

Langerhans cell sarcoma is an extremely rare neoplasm composed of neoplastic Langerhans cells with anaplastic nuclei. It usually presents de novo but has been described as a transformation from typical Langerhans cell histiocytosis. There is a wide age range affected, including adults, and there may be a female predominance. Patients are generally in high stage when diagnosed, and an aggressive course is usually seen.

Histologically, most cases show diffuse effacement of architecture. By definition, a significant proportion of the proliferating cells show anaplastic cytologic features, although other cells may have nuclei more typical of Langerhans cells (Figure 244). There are usually few admixed reactive cells, but some cases have scattered eosinophils, histiocytes, giant cells, or neutrophils. The mitotic rate is consistently high. By definition, Birbeck granules are present by electron microscopy, and the cells have a phenotype typical of Langerhans cell histiocytosis, with expression of CD1a, Langerin, and S-100 protein (Figure 245 and Table 41). In keeping with the high mitotic rate, the Ki-67 index is usually greater than 50%.

The differential diagnosis includes Langerhans cell histiocytosis as well as large-cell lymphoma and other dendritic neoplasms. The presence of a significant population of cytologically malignant cells rules out Langerhans cell histiocytosis, while the CD1a/Langerin S-100–positive phenotype, particularly with the demonstration of Birbeck granules on ultrastructural examination, would rule out other malignant lymphoma or other dendritic neoplasms.

INTERDIGITATING DENDRITIC CELL SARCOMA[428,431–433]

Interdigitating dendritic cell sarcoma is a neoplasm differentiating toward normal myeloid interdigitating dendritic cells. Myeloid interdigitating dendritic

Figure 244. Langerhans cell sarcoma. Although the cells have nuclei reminiscent of Langerhans cells, striking cytologic atypia is present. Note the atypical mitotic figure. The neoplastic cells stained for CD1 and S-100 protein, consistent with Langerhans cells differentiation.

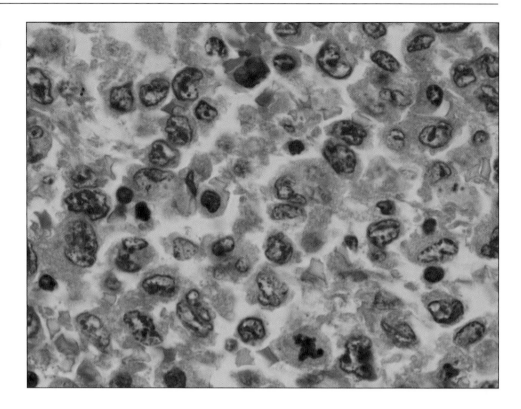

Figure 245. Langerhans cell sarcoma, CD1a stain. Despite the striking cytologic atypia, the cells stained for CD1a, consistent with Langerhans cells.

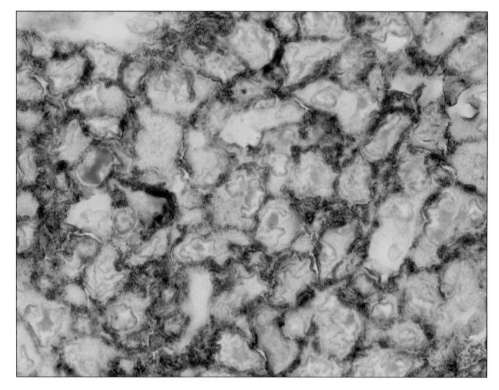

cells are CD1a-negative, S-100 protein–positive, antigen-processing dendritic cells of the paracortical region that are probably derived from Langerhans cells. Interdigitating dendritic cell sarcoma is a very rare neoplasm, even rarer than follicular dendritic cell sarcoma. Most reported cases have occurred in older adults, with no clear sex predilection, who usually present with solitary

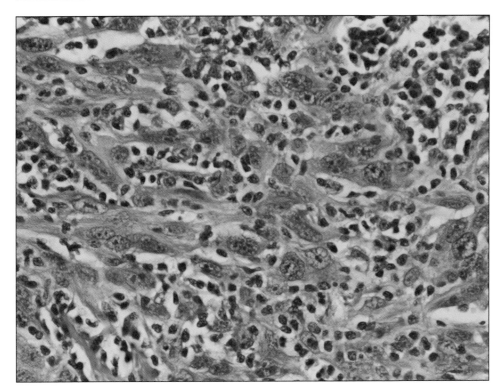

Figure 246. Interdigitating dendritic cell sarcoma. The neoplastic cells are predominantly spindled in this case, although some plumper cells are also present. Note the reactive lymphoplasmacytic background.

lymphadenopathy. The clinical course has been variable, but it is usually a more aggressive neoplasm than a follicular dendritic cell sarcoma, with more frequent metastases to visceral organs.

The neoplasm either shows a paracortical distribution with retained follicles or diffuse architectural effacement. The histologic appearance is somewhat variable ranging from a spindle-cell tumor closely resembling a follicular dendritic cell sarcoma to a more round-cell neoplasm mimicking a histiocytic sarcoma or a malignant lymphoma (Figure 246). The cytologic features may be bland, but more often some degree of cytologic atypia is usually present (Figure 247). The mitotic rate is usually low. Similar to follicular dendritic cell sarcoma, there are usually scattered admixed lymphocytes and plasma cells. Ultrastructural studies show complex interdigitating cell processes, without well-formed desmosomes or Birbeck granules.

The immunophenotype is somewhat nonspecific, more significant for what is negative rather than what is expressed (Table 41). S-100 protein is the most consistent positive stain and is usually strong and diffuse throughout the tumor. CD45, CD68, and lysozyme may show variable positivity. The tumor is negative for the follicular dendritic cell markers CD21, CD23, and CD35; the Langerhans cell markers CD1a and Langerin; the histiocytic marker CD163; the myeloid markers myeloperoxidase and CD34; specific B- and T-cell antigens; CD30; epithelial membrane antigen; and keratin. The Ki-67 index is variable but usually between 10 and 20%. The reactive lymphocytes usually type as T-cells. There are no detectable clonal antigen receptor gene rearrangements.

The differential diagnosis includes metastatic malignant melanoma, follicular dendritic cell sarcoma, fibroblastic reticulum cell sarcoma, and histiocytic

Figure 247. Interdigitating dendritic cell sarcoma. Plump, spindled cells are seen, with a moderate degree of cytologic atypia. The cells expressed S-100 protein, but were negative for CD21 and CD35.

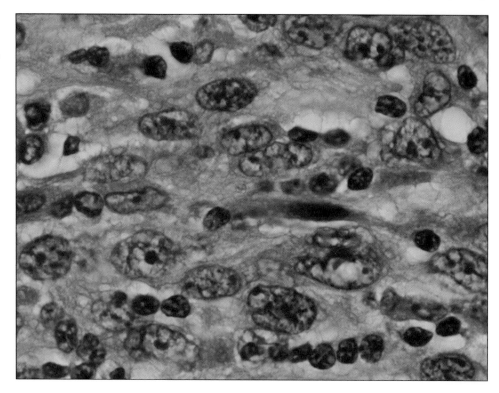

sarcoma (Table 41). Metastatic malignant melanoma shares consistent S-100 protein expression with interdigitating dendritic cell sarcoma, but usually also expresses one or more specific melanocytic markers, such as HMB-45, Melan-A, and/or tyrosinase. Fibroblastic reticulum cell sarcoma is consistently S-100 negative (by definition). Histiocytic sarcoma may show focal S-100 protein positivity, but is usually not strongly and diffusely S-100 protein positive and usually strongly expresses histiocytic markers such as CD163.

FOLLICULAR DENDRITIC CELL SARCOMA[39,428,431,434–440]

Follicular dendritic cell sarcoma is a neoplasm of follicular dendritic cells. As noted in the introduction, normal follicular dendritic cells are possibly a specialized form of myofibroblasts and may derive from bone marrow stromal cell progenitors. They represent the fixed antigen-presenting dendritic cells of follicles. It is an uncommon but not extremely rare tumor that occurs in all ages and without a sex predilection. A small subset of cases may occur in association with Castleman disease, particularly larger lesions, and some cases may be associated with schizophrenia. Patients typically present with a slow-growing mass, without any systemic symptoms. Treatment consists of surgical excision, with or without adjuvant therapy or local radiotherapy. Local recurrences occur in about 50% of patients, with distant metastases eventually occurring in about 25% of patients.

There is effacement of architecture by a spindle-cell tumor (Figure 248). The spindle cells may form fascicles or a storiform pattern with whorls (Figure 249).

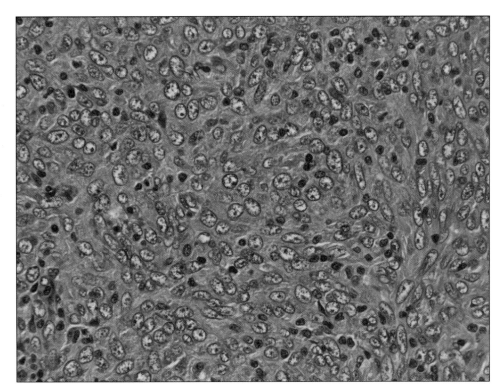

Figure 248. Follicular dendritic cell sarcoma. The cells are formed into whorls, mimicking a meningioma. This case was positive for CD21 and CD35.

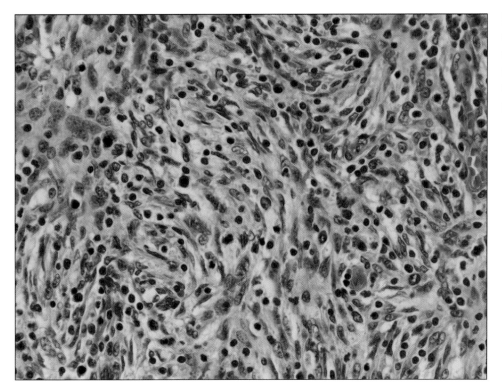

Figure 249. Follicular dendritic cell sarcoma. The cells are spindled, and contain an abundant admixture of reactive lymphocytes and plasma cells.

One characteristic feature that is usually present is an admixture of lymphocytes, which may be evenly interspersed or segregated into lymphoid aggregates. The spindle-cell nuclei are usually bland, but there may be varying degrees of atypia and mitotic activity, and these latter features are associated with more aggressive behavior (Figure 250). Occasional multinucleated spindle cells may be seen.

Figure 250. Follicular dendritic cell sarcoma. Note the cytologic atypia and the mitoses, including the atypical forms.

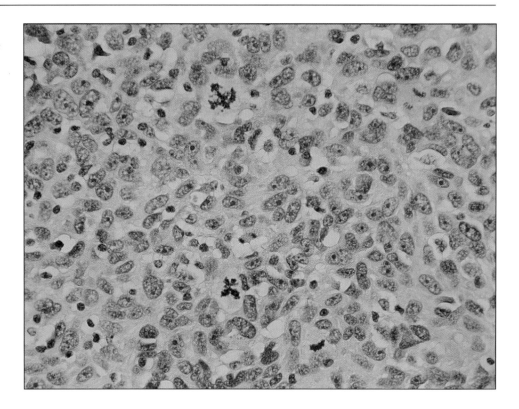

Ultrastructural studies show complex interdigitating processes with scattered mature desmosomes.

Follicular dendritic cell sarcoma has an immunophenotype identical to that of normal follicular dendritic cells (Table 41). Characteristically, there is expression of the follicular dendritic cell markers CD21, CD23, CD35, and clusterin, although not all four markers are positive in every case. In addition, vimentin, fascin, desmoplakin, and HLA-DR are positive, and S-100 protein, CD68, and epithelial membrane protein are variably positive. CD45 and CD20 are occasionally positive, while other B-lineage markers, T-lineage markers, CD30, CD1a, CD63, lysozyme, and myeloperoxidase are consistently negative. The Ki-67 index is variable, but usually around 10–20%. The reactive lymphocytes may be either predominantly B-cells or T-cells. There are no detectable clonal antigen receptor gene rearrangements.

The differential diagnosis is limited and includes other dendritic cell proliferations as well as metastatic malignant melanoma, carcinoma or sarcoma, and a fibroblastic reticulum cell tumor (Table 41). The expression of the follicular dendritic cell markers CD21, CD23, CD35, and/or clusterin in a spindle-cell tumor is specific for follicular dendritic cell tumor. Metastatic melanoma may show spindle-cell features, and while both neoplasms may share S-100 protein positivity, only melanoma may be positive for Melan-A, HMB-45, tyrosinase, or other specific melanocytic markers. Spindle-cell carcinoma will be keratin positive. The major distinction from fibroblastic reticulum cell tumor is the lack of expression of the follicular dendritic cell markers in the latter neoplasm.

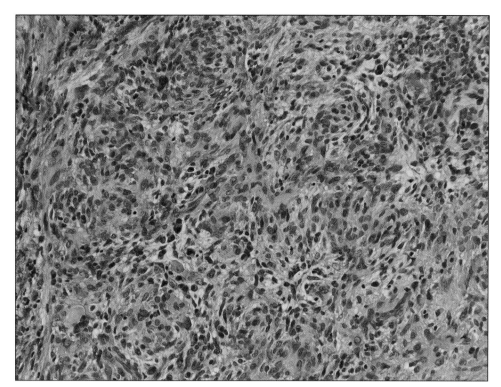

Figure 251. Fibroblastic reticulum cell tumor. A spindle-cell appearance is seen in this lymph node–based neoplasm. These neoplastic cells were negative for CD21, CD23, CD35, and S-100 protein.

FIBROBLASTIC RETICULUM CELL NEOPLASM[440]

While not strictly a neoplasm of dendritic cells, fibroblastic reticulum cell neoplasm is included here because of its morphologic similarities to follicular dendritic and interdigitating cell tumors. Fibroblastic reticulum cell neoplasm is defined as a tumor derived from fibroblastic reticular cells. Fibroblastic reticular cells normally reside in the parafollicular region and probably play a support role, being intimately associated with the nodal collagen framework. They are best seen in lymphocyte-depleted lymph nodes and probably represent a variant of myofibroblasts, with which they share close ultrastructural and immunohistochemical similarities. They express vimentin, smooth muscle actin, and desmin, and at least a subset may express some low–molecular weight keratins.

Only rare fibroblastic reticulum cell neoplasms have been reported. These cases have been reported primarily in teenagers or young adults, who have presented with solitary lymphadenopathy. Histologically, a spindle-cell proliferation is seen, usually in a paracortical distribution, often forming whorls (Figure 251). At high magnification, the cells are indistinguishable from those of follicular dendritic cell neoplasm (Figure 252). Nuclear pseudoinclusions have been described in one case. The diagnosis is established by immunohistochemical studies. The spindle cells are positive for the myofibroblastic markers, smooth muscle actin, and/or desmin and may also weakly express CD68. However, they are negative for the follicular dendritic cell markers CD21, CD23, and CD35; S-100 protein; CD1a; and the histiocytic marker CD163 (Table 41).

Figure 252. Fibroblastic reticulum cell tumor. The spindled cells are relatively bland in appearance.

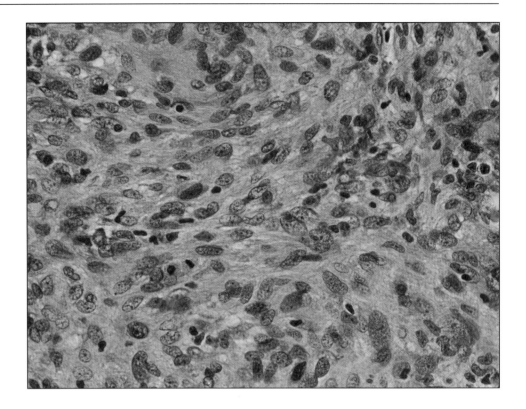

PRECURSOR PLASMACYTOID DENDRITIC CELL NEOPLASM[372,441–445]

Precursor plasmacytoid dendritic cell neoplasm, formerly blastic NK-cell lymphoma or hematodermic neoplasm, probably represents a neoplasm of precursor plasmacytoid dendritic cells. Plasmacytoid dendritic cells (formerly, plasmacytoid monocytes) are pre–dendritic cells of the lymph node paracortex that are a major source of alpha-interferon upon viral infection or CD154 stimulation. They consistently express CD123 (the IL-3 receptor), CD68, and CD4, and a subset express CD56. Precursor plasmacytoid dendritic cell neoplasms are uncommon but not extremely rare. Most patients are elderly, but a wide age range is seen. There is no known sex predilection. Most patients present with skin lesions, with or without lymphadenopathy, with lymph nodes representing the second most common presenting site. Most patients present in stage III or IV. There is a poor response to lymphoma therapy, but some response to regimens employed for acute leukemia is seen. There are no known etiologic factors.

Diffuse effacement of architecture is usually seen. At high magnification, a monomorphous blastic neoplasm is seen, with few admixed reactive cells (Figure 253). The cells are intermediate in size, with a fine chromatin pattern and small nucleoli, closely mimicking lymphoblastic lymphoma. The mitotic rate is high.

The immunophenotype is distinctive, with expression of the plasmacytoid dendritic marker CD123, along with CD4, CD56, and CD68. There is also positivity for CD45, CD43, HLA-DR, CD62L, and CXCR3; and there is frequent expression of terminal deoxyribonucleotidyl transferase and/or CD34. Other

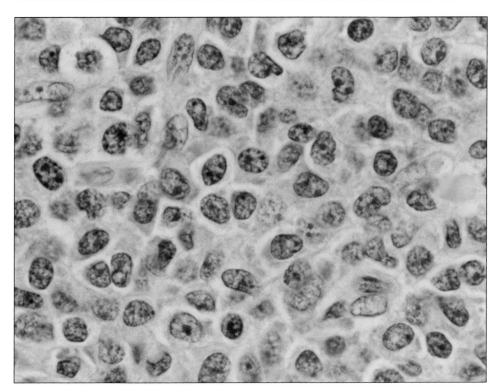

Figure 253. Precursor plasmacytoid dendritic cell neoplasm. A blastic neoplasm is seen. The differential diagnosis would include acute myeloid leukemia, lymphoblastic neoplasms, and a blastic variant of mantle cell lymphoma.

NK-cell markers or specific T- and B-cell markers are negative. The Ki-67 index is usually high. The antigen receptor genes are germline, and there is no association with EBV. There are no known recurring cytogenetic abnormalities.

The differential diagnosis includes blastic neoplasms such as B-, T-, or NK-precursor lymphoblastic neoplasms and acute myeloid leukemia (Table 34). Although CD4, CD56, or CD68 may be expressed in these other neoplasms, CD123 expression is relatively specific for precursor plasmacytoid dendritic cell neoplasm.

Extramedullary Hematopoiesis	250
Myeloid Sarcoma	251
Mast Cell Neoplasia	253

While myeloid and mast cell proliferations and neoplasms are primarily diseases of the bone marrow, lymph nodes may be involved and may rarely be the initial site of presentation.

EXTRAMEDULLARY HEMATOPOIESIS[446]

Even though the fetal lymph node is not traditionally thought of as a site of normal hematopoiesis, extramedullary hematopoiesis is not an unusual finding in the lymph nodes of infants and may persist in tiny amounts in children. However, the finding of a significant degree of extramedullary hematopoiesis in a child or the presence of any extramedullary hematopoiesis in an adult should prompt additional hematologic studies to search for a cause. In children, the most common causes are hereditary disorders of red cells, although any disorder that causes compensatory marrow hyperplasia or compromise of the marrow environment (such as osteopetrosis) may lead to extramedullary hematopoiesis. In adults, the most common causes are chronic myeloproliferative disorders, although treatment with hematopoietic cytokines has also been associated with extramedullary hematopoiesis.

Involved lymph nodes are rarely causes of lymphadenopathy, and excised lymph nodes are usually normal to minimally enlarged. Extramedullary hematopoiesis is generally seen in the sinuses, with extension to the adjacent paracortex (Figure 254). The morphologic manifestation varies with the underlying disorder; it may be predominantly erythroid, myeloid, or megakaryocytic. If the underlying disorder is marked by dysplasia, then the proliferation in the lymph node may also show dysplastic changes. Immunohistochemical studies for hemoglobin A, myeloperoxidase, and CD61 may be useful for confirming erythroid, myeloid, and megakaryocytic differentiation, respectively. The most important disease in the differentiation is myeloid sarcoma, which may be excluded by the lack of a monomorphic proliferation of immature elements, including

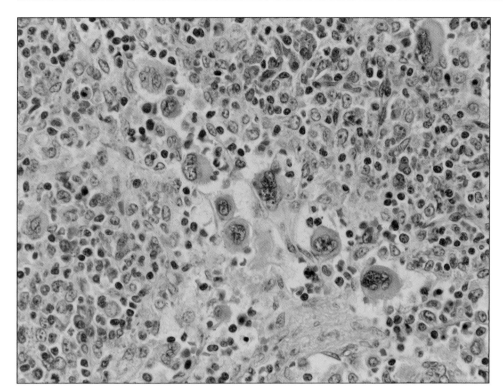

Figure 254. Extramedullary hematopoiesis. Numerous megakaryocytes are seen in sinuses and immature myeloid cells are seen in the adjacent paracortex.

blasts. Stains for immature cells, such as CD34 and CD117, may be helpful in making this distinction.

MYELOID SARCOMA[447,448]

Myeloid sarcoma, also known as extramedullary myeloid tumor, granulocytic sarcoma, or chloroma, is a tumor mass of immature myeloid cells occurring outside the bone marrow. It may occur in acute myeloid leukemia, chronic myeloid leukemia, other chronic myeloproliferative disorders, or in myelo-dysplastic syndromes. In acute myeloid leukemia, it may be the presenting and only site of disease, preceding the development of clinically obvious leukemia by days to months to years. It may also present concurrently with the leukemia and may also represent a site of relapse. In myeloproliferative and myelodysplastic disorders, it usually occurs at the time of blast transformation, and even when occurring alone may be considered as evidence of blast transformation. In general, patients are treated for their underlying leukemia, although localized radiotherapy may be used in isolated lesions occurring in patients in whom systemic disease is not yet evident.

Histologically, one may see diffuse effacement of architecture or selective involvement of the sinusoidal, paracortical, or the perinodal region (Figure 255). At high magnification, there is typically a monomorphic proliferation of cells with intermediate- to large-sized nuclei containing a fine to vesicular chromatin structure, a round or lobated nuclear outline, and small to prominent nucleoli (Figure 256). Cytoplasm may be scant or moderate in amount and may contain

Figure 255. Acute myeloid
leukemia, involving lymph
node. A paracortical
distribution is seen, isolating
a solitary germinal center.
A starry-sky appearance is
seen in the proliferating cells.

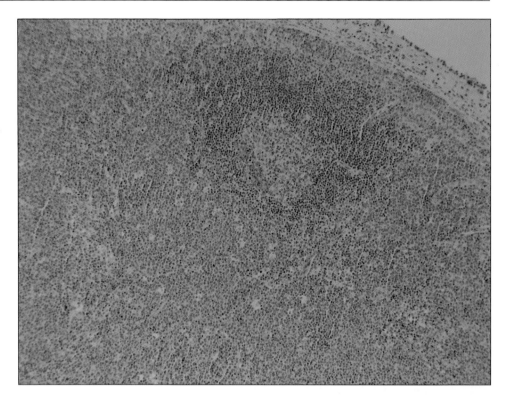

Figure 256. Acute myeloid
leukemia, involving lymph
node. The nucleoli are
somewhat prominent and the
chromatin is blastic. The
differential diagnosis would
include diffuse large-cell
lymphoma.

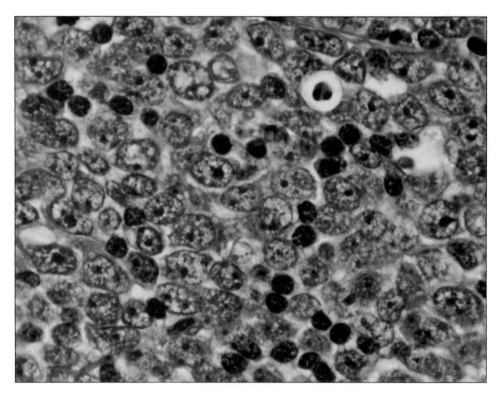

granules. In some cases there are scattered promyelocytes, and in other
cases there may even be scattered myelocytes or even mature neutrophils or
eosinophils. There is usually a high mitotic rate, and a starry-sky pattern may
be seen.

Immunophenotypic studies are important to establish the correct diagnosis. Myeloperoxidase is perhaps the most sensitive and specific myeloid stain, while lysozyme and CD68 are best in monocytic lesions. CD34, CD117, CD33, and CD13 may also be helpful to establish an immature myeloid phenotype, although the latter two markers are best used in flow cytometry and do not work well in paraffin sections. Similarly, CD14, CD116, and CD11c are useful flow cytometry markers for determining monoblastic differentiation. Cytochemical studies, such as myeloperoxidase or Sudan black B, may be performed on touch preparations. Myeloid sarcomas are particularly common in acute myeloid leukemia associated with the t(8;21) (acute myeloid leukemia with maturation) and inversion 16/t(16;16) (acute myelomonocytic leukemia with abnormal eosinophils).

The differential diagnosis includes blastic neoplasms such as precursor B- and T-lymphoblastic leukemia/lymphoma, blastic mantle cell lymphoma, Burkitt/Burkitt-like lymphoma, precursor plasmacytoid dendritic cell neoplasm, and diffuse large B-cell lymphoma. Of course, a history of acute myeloid leukemia, a chronic myeloproliferative disorder, or a myelodysplastic syndrome should certainly raise one's level of suspicion. Some features that are helpful in suggesting myeloid sarcoma would be an admixture of myelocytes or granulocytes, the presence of cytoplasmic granules (best seen in touch preparations), larger nuclei with larger nucleoli than typically seen in lymphoblastic neoplasms or blastic mantle cell lymphoma, and a finer chromatin pattern than typically seen in Burkitt/Burkitt-like lymphoma or diffuse large B-cell lymphoma. Inevitably, definitive diagnosis requires immunohistochemical studies. While some cases of myeloid sarcoma may express terminal deoxyribonucleotidyl transferase and virtually all cases of myeloid sarcoma express CD43, the expression of myeloperoxidase and/or lysozyme should provide a relatively specific diagnosis of myeloid sarcoma, while absence of other markers (see Table 34) should exclude other entities in the differential diagnosis. However, cases of stem cell leukemia/lymphoma syndrome with 8p11 (FGFR1) abnormalities may show a biphasic pattern, with some areas resembling acute myeloid leukemia but other areas more typical of precursor T-lymphoblast lymphoma/leukemia. It should also be kept in mind that acute myeloid leukemia with t(8;21) is often CD19 positive, and promyelocytic leukemia may be PAX-5 positive.

MAST CELL NEOPLASIA[449]

The WHO has divided mast cell neoplasia into several major categories (see Table 42). Lymph node involvement commonly occurs in systemic mastocytosis and its variants. There are specific major and minor criteria for the diagnosis of systemic mastocytosis (given in Table 43). It usually occurs in adults, with a slight female predilection. Patients may present with a myriad of symptoms, including symptoms due to direct tissue infiltration, as well as symptoms due to mediator effects. The bone marrow is usually involved, and there

Table 42. WHO Classification of Mastocytosis[213]

Cutaneous mastocytosis

Systemic mastocytosis

    Indolent systemic mastocytosis

    Systemic mastocytosis with associated clonal, hematologic non–mast cell lineage disease

    Aggressive systemic mastocytosis

    Mast cell leukemia

Mast cell sarcoma

Extracutaneous mastocytoma

Table 43. 2001 WHO Criteria for the Diagnosis of Systemic Mastocytosis[213]

Major criterion

    Multifocal, dense infiltrates of mast cells (fifteen or more mast cells in aggregates)

Minor criteria

    a. More than 25% of the mast cells in the infiltrate are spindle-shaped or have atypical morphology

    b. Detection of KIT point mutation at codon 816

    c. Mast cells that coexpress CD117 with CD2 and/or CD25

    d. Serum total tryptase persistently >20 ng/mL (unless there is an associated clonal myeloid disorder)

The diagnosis of SM may be made if one major and one minor criterion are present or if three minor criteria are fulfilled.

may also be a clonal hematologic non–mast cell lineage disorder. The skin, spleen, liver, and bone are also frequently involved. Peripheral lymphadenopathy occurs in about one-quarter of patients and central lymphadenopathy is present in about 20% of patients.

Involved lymph nodes range from showing very focal involvement to those showing diffuse architectural effacement. Any compartment of the lymph node may be primarily involved, including the paracortical region most often, followed by the follicles, the medullary cords, or, least commonly, the sinuses (Figure 257). Involvement of the sinuses may be particularly common in cases of mast cell leukemia. The mast cells are typically found in aggregates and small clusters or in sheets. Focal infiltrates usually show clusters of mast cells, often situated at the edge of the mantle zone of the follicles, closely simulating monocytoid B-cell hyperplasia, or in a perivascular location. The mast cells are round to oval or even spindled, with a moderate amount of clear to granular cytoplasm (Figure 258). The nuclei are round to oval or occasionally folded or lobated, with a relatively mature chromatin pattern and inconspicuous nucleoli. There is often an accompanying eosinophilic infiltrate, which may be abundant, forming eosinophilic microabscesses. There may also be an associated vascular proliferation,

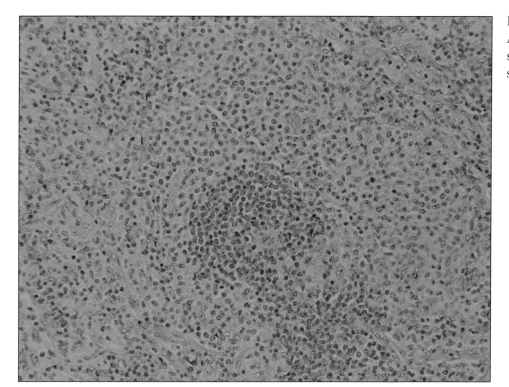

Figure 257. Mastocytosis. A paracortical distribution is seen, isolating a small follicle seen at center.

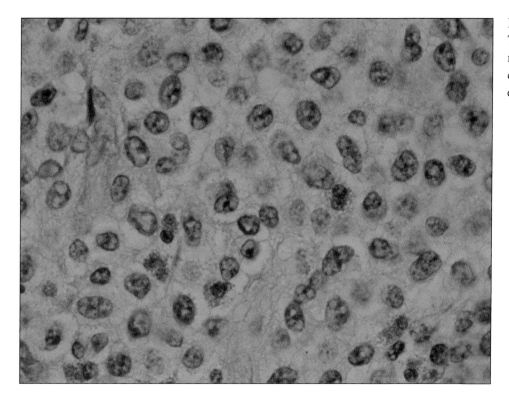

Figure 258. Mastocytosis. The cells are bland, with a moderate amount of pale cytoplasm. Note the scattered eosinophils.

reactive follicular hyperplasia, plasmacytosis, or collagen fibrosis. Some cases may also show extramedullary hematopoiesis.

Immunophenotypic studies show expression of CD45, CD68, CD33, CD117, and tryptase. Occasional cases may be CD2 and/or CD25 positive, aberrant findings that may be helpful in establishing a diagnosis, but mast cells lack other specific B- and T-cell markers or expression of the histiocytic marker CD163. Mast cell neoplasia shows consistent point mutations in the KIT gene, which encodes for CD117. A specific mutation involving codon 816 is present in most cases, although other mutations involving the KIT gene have also been reported.

The differential diagnosis of mast cell neoplasia in lymph nodes is wide and includes monocytoid B-cell hyperplasia, granulomatous inflammation, sinus histiocytosis, follicular hyperplasia and follicular lymphoma, a marginal zone B-cell lymphoma, peripheral T-cell lymphoma, and Langerhans histiocytosis. Tryptase is a relatively specific marker of mast cells and most helpful if a diagnosis of mast cell neoplasia is being considered. Monocytoid B-cell hyperplasia usually occurs in conjunction with hyperplasia in other compartments of the lymph node. It is usually associated with neutrophils, while mast cell infiltrates are usually associated with eosinophils. Its B-cell phenotype should provide easy distinction from mast cells. Mast cell infiltrates may show clusters similar to granulomas, but do not show giant cells and the often granular cytoplasm of mast cells is different from that of histiocytes, which also have more abundant cytoplasm. Mast cell neoplasia may be associated with eosinophilic micro-abscesses, which may simulate necrotizing granulomatous inflammation, but the identification of adjacent mast cell clusters should prompt the performance of a tryptase stain. Mast cell lesions associated with mast cell leukemia may show a prominent sinusoidal distribution. Knowledge of the clinical history and, in particular, examination of the peripheral blood smear should resolve that differential. Follicular hyperplasia and follicular lymphoma may be simulated by preferential follicular involvement by mast cell neoplasia, but there are usually foci of mast cells adjacent to the follicles as well that are usually easier to identify as mast cells. Marginal zone B-cell lymphoma often shows plasmacytoid differentiation and stains for B-cell markers. Peripheral T-cell lymphoma may have clear cells in a parafollicular distribution, but are usually composed of a more polymorphic population and stains for T-cell markers. Langerhans cell histiocytosis may share eosinophilic microabscesses with mast cell neoplasia, but the Langerhans cells have a characteristic nuclear appearance, with grooved nuclei, and stain for S-100 protein, CD1a, and Langerin.

REFERENCE LIST

1. Das D.K. (1999). Value and limitations of fine-needle aspiration cytology in diagnosis and classification of lymphomas: a review. *Diagn Cytopathol* **21**, 240–9.
2. Chu P.G., Chang K.L., Arber D.A., Weiss L.M. (1999). Practical applications of immunohistochemistry for hematolymphoid disorders: an updated review. *Ann Diagn Pathol* **3**, 104–33.
3. Bagg A. (2005). Molecular diagnosis in lymphoma. *Curr Hematol Rep* **4**, 313–23.
4. Staudt L. (2003). Molecular diagnosis of the hematologic cancers. *N Engl J Med* **348**, 1777–85.
5. Fan Y.S., Rizkalla K. (2003). Comprehensive cytogenetic analysis including multicolor spectral karyotyping and interphase fluorescence in situ hybridization in lymphoma diagnosis. A summary of 154 cases. *Cancer Genet Cytogenet* **143**, 73–9.
6. Baumgarth N., Roederer M. (2000). A practical approach to multicolor flow cytometry for immunophenotyping. *J Immunol Methods* **243**, 77–7.
7. Munoz-Fernandez R., Blanco F., Fresha C., Martin F., Kimatrai M., Abadia-Molina A., Garcia-Pacheco J., Olivares E. (2006). Follicular dendritic cells are related to bone marrow stromal cell progenitors and to myofibroblasts. *J Immunol* **177**, 280–9.
8. MacLennan I. (1994). Germinal centers. *Ann Rev Immunol* **12**, 117–39.
9. Butcher E.C. (1990). Cellular and molecular mechanisms that direct leukocyte traffic. *Am J Pathol* **136**, 3–12.
10. Moore S., Schneider J., Schaaf H. (2003). Diagnostic aspects of cervical lymphadenopathy in children in the developing world: a study of 1,877 surgical specimens. *Pediatr Surg Int* **19**, 240–4.
11. Dorfman R.F., Warnke R.A. (1974). Lymphadenopathy simulating the malignant lymphomas. *Hum Pathol* **5**, 519–50.
12. Segal G.H., Perkins S.L., Kjeldsberg C.R. (1995). Benign lymphadenopathies in children and adolescents. *Semin Diagn Pathol* **12**, 288–302.
13. Kojima M., Nakamura S., Itoh H., Yoshida K., Suchi T., Masawa N. (2001). Acute viral lymphadenitis mimicking low-grade peripheral T-cell lymphoma. A clinicopathological study of nine cases. *APMIS* **109**, 419–27.
14. Doggett R.S., Colby T.V., Dorfman R.F. (1983). Interfollicular Hodgkin's disease. *Am J Med* **78**, 22–8.
15. Lai R., Arber D.A., Chang K.L., Wilson C.S., Weiss L.M. (1998). Frequency of bcl-2 expression in non-Hodgkin's lymphoma. A study of 798 cases with comparison of marginal zone lymphoma and monocytoid B cell hyperplasia. *Mod Pathol* **11**, 864–9.
16. Nathwani B.N., Winberg C.D., Diamond L.W., Bearman R.M., Kim H. (1981). Morphologic criteria for the differentiation of follicular lymphoma from florid reactive follicular hyperplasia: a study of 80 cases. *Cancer* **48**, 1794–1806.
17. Osborne B.M., Butler J.J. (1991). Clinical implications of nodal reactive follicular hyperplasia in elderly patients with enlarged lymph nodes. *Mod Pathol* **4**, 24–30.

18. Segal G.H., Scott M., Jorgensen T., Braylan R.C. (1994). Standard polymerase chain reaction analysis does not detect t(14;18) in reactive lymphoid hyperplasia. *Arch Pathol Lab Med* **118**, 791–4.

19. Utz G.L., Swerdlow S.H. (1993). Distinction of follicular hyperplasia from follicular lymphoma in B5-fixed tissues: comparison of MT2 and bcl-2 antibodies. *Hum Pathol* **24**, 1155–8.

20. Wood B.L., Bacchi M.M., Bacchi C.E., Kidd P., Gown A.M. (1994). Immunocytochemical differentiation of reactive hyperplasia from follicular lymphoma using monoclonal antibodies to cell surface and proliferation-related markers. *Appl Immunohistochem* **2**, 48–53.

21. Kadin M.E., Vonderheid E.C., Weiss L.M. (1993). Absence of Epstein-Barr viral expression in lymphomatoid papulosis. *J Pathol* **170**, 145–8.

22. Hartsock R.J., Halling L.W., King F.M. (1970). Luetic lymphadenitis: a clinical and histologic study of 20 cases. *Am J Clin Pathol* **53**, 304–14.

23. Kojima M., Motoori T., Itoh H., Shimizu K., Iijima M., Tamaki Y., Murayama K., Ohno Y., Yoshida K., Masawa N., Nakamura S. (2005). Distribution of Epstein-Barr virus in systemic rheumatic disease (rheumatoid arthritis, systemic lupus erythematosus, dermatomyositis) with associated lymphadenopathy: a study of 49 cases. *Int J Surg Pathol* **13**, 273–8.

24. Kondratowicz G.M., Symmons D.P., Bacon P.A., Mageed R.A., Jones E.L. (1990). Rheumatoid lymphadenopathy: a morphological and immunohistochemical study. *J Clin Pathol* **43**, 106–13.

25. Weisenburger D.D., Nathwani B.N., Winberg C.D., Rappaport H. (1985). Multicentric angiofollicular lymph node hyperplasia: a clinicopathologic study of 16 cases. *Hum Pathol* **16**, 162–72.

26. Chen H., Thompson L., Aguilera N., Abbondanzo S. (2004). Kimura disease: a clinicopathologic study of 21 cases. *Am J Surg Pathol* **28**, 505–13.

27. Chan J.K.C., Hui P.K., Ng C.S., Yuen N.W.F., Kung I.T.M., Gwi E. (1989). Epithelioid hemangioma (angiolymphoid hyperplasia with eosinophilia) and Kimura's disease in Chinese. *Histopathology* **15**, 557–74.

28. Hui P.K., Chan J.K.C., Ng C.S., Kung I.T.M., Gwi E. (1989). Lymphadenopathy of Kimura's disease. *Am J Surg Pathol* **13**, 177–86.

29. Kuo T.T., Shih L.Y., Chan H.L. (1988). Kimura's disease. Involvement of regional lymph nodes and distinction from angiolymphoid hyperplasia with eosinophilia. *Am J Surg Pathol* **12**, 843–54.

30. Dorfman R.F., Remington J.S. (1973). Value of lymph node biopsy in the diagnosis of toxoplasmosis. *N Engl J Med* **289**, 878–81.

31. Stansfeld A.G. (1961). The histologic diagnosis of toxoplasmic lymphadenitis. *J Clin Pathol* **14**, 565–73.

32. Weiss L.M., Chen Y.Y., Berry G.J., Strickler J.G., Dorfman R.F., Warnke R.A. (1992). Infrequent detection of *Toxoplasma gondii* genome in toxoplasmic lymphadenitis: a polymerase chain reaction study. *Hum Pathol* **23**, 154–8.

33. Bowne W., Lewis J., Filippa D., Niesvizky R., Brooks A., Burt M., Brennan M. (1999). The management of unicentric and multicentric Castleman's disease: a report of 16 cases and a review of the literature. *Cancer* **85**, 706–17.

34. Casper C. (2005). The aetiology and management of Castleman's disease at 50 years: translating pathophysiology to patient care. *Br J Haematol* **129**, 3–17.

35. Nichols D., Diss T., Kellam P., Tulliez M., Du M.Q., Sicard D., Weiss R., Isaacson P., Boshoff C. (2000). HHV-8 is associated with a plasmablastic variant of Castleman's disease that is linked to HHV-8-positive plasmablastic lymphoma. *Blood* **95**, 1406–12.

36. Waterson A., Bower M. (2004). Fifty years of multicentric Castleman's disease. *Acta Oncol* **43**, 698–704.

37. Beck J.T., Hsu S.M., Wijdenes J., Bataille R., Klein B., Vesole D., Hayden K., Jagannath S., Barlogie B. (1994). Alleviation of systemic manifestations of Castleman's disease by monoclonal interleukin-6 antibody. *N Engl J Med* **330**, 602–5.

38. Bitter M.A., Komaiko W., Franklin W.A. (1985). Giant lymph node hyperplasia with osteoblastic bone lesions and the POEMS (Takatsuki's) syndrome. *Cancer* **56**, 188–94.

39. Chan J.K.C., Tsang W.Y.W., Ng C.S. (1994). Follicular dendritic cell tumor and vascular neoplasm complicating hyaline-vascular Castleman's disease. *Am J Surg Pathol* **18**, 517–25.

40. Danon A.D., Krishnan J., Frizzera G. (1993). Morpho-immunophenotypic diversity of Castleman's disease, hyaline-vascular type: with emphasis on a stroma-rich variant and a new pathogenetic hypothesis. *Virchows Arch A* **423**, 369–82.

41. Frizzera G., Massarelli G., Banks P.M., Rosai J. (1983). A systemic lymphoproliferative disorder with morphologic features of Castleman's disease: pathological findings in 15 patients. *Am J Surg Pathol* **7**, 211–31.

42. Frizzera G., Peterson B.A., Bayrd E.D., Goldman A. (1985). A systemic lymphoproliferative disorder with morphologic features of Castleman's disease: clinical findings and clinicopathologic correlations in 15 patients. *J Clin Oncol* **3**, 1202–16.

43. Frizzera G., Kaneko Y., Sakurai M. (1989). Angioimmunoblastic lymphadenopathy and related disorders: a retrospective look in search of definitions. *Leukemia* **3**, 1–5.

44. Gerald W., Kostianovsky M., Rosai J. (1990). Development of vascular neoplasia in Castleman's disease. *Am J Surg Pathol* **14**, 603–14.

45. Hanson C.A., Frizzera G., Patton D.F., Peterson B.A., McClain K.L., Gajl-Peczalska K.J., Hersey J.H. (1988). Clonal rearrangement for immunoglobulin and T-cell receptor genes in systemic Castleman's disease: association with Epstein-Barr virus. *Am J Pathol* **131**, 84–91.

46. Harris N.L., Bhan A.K. (1987). Plasmacytoid T cells in Castleman's disease: immunohistologic phenotype. *Am J Surg Pathol* **11**, 109–13.

47. Hsu S.M., Waldron J.A., Xie S.S., Barlogie B. (1993). Expression of interleukin-6 in Castleman's disease. *Hum Pathol* **24**, 833–9.

48. Keller A.R., Hochholzer L., Castleman B. (1972). Hyaline-vascular and plasma-cell types of giant lymph node hyperplasia of mediastinum and other locations. *Cancer* **29**, 670–83.

49. Radaszkiewicz T., Hannsmann M.L., Lennert K. (1989). Monoclonality and polyclonality of plasma cells in Castleman's disease of the plasma cell variant. *Histopathology* **14**, 11–24.

50. Soulier J., Grollet L., Oksenhendler E., Cacoub P., Cazals-Hatem D., Bbinet P., d'Agay M.-F., Clauvel J.-P., Raphael M., Degos L., Sigaux F. (1995). Kaposi's sarcoma-associated herpesvirus-like DNA sequences in multicentric Castleman's disease. *Blood* **86**, 1276–80.

51. Soulier J., Grollet L., Oksenhendler E., Miclea J.-M., Cacoub P., Baruchel A., Brice P., Clauvel J.-P., d'Agay M.-F., Raphael M., Sigaux F. (1995). Molecular analysis of clonality in Castleman's disease. *Blood* **86**, 1131–8.

52. Biberfeld P., Chayt K.J., Marselle L.M., Biberfeld G., Gallo R.C., Harper M.E. (1986). HTLV-III expression in infected lymph nodes and relevance to pathogenesis of lymphadenopathy. *Am J Pathol* **125**, 436–42.

53. Brynes R.K., Chan W.C., Spira T.J., Ewing E.P., Chandler F.W. (1983). Value of lymph node biopsy in unexplained lymphadenopathy in homosexual men. *JAMA* **250**, 1313–17.

54. Burns B.F., Wood G.S., Dorfman R.F. (1985). The varied histopathology of lymphadenopathy in the homosexual male. *Am J Surg Pathol* **9**, 287–97.

55. Chadburn A., Metroka C., Mouradian J. (1989). Progressive lymph node histology and its prognostic value in patients with acquired immunodeficiency syndrome and AIDS-related complex. *Hum Pathol* **20**, 579–87.

56. Ioachim H.L., Cronin W., Roy M., Maya M. (1990). Persistent lymphadenopathies in people at high risk for HIV infection. Clinicopathologic correlations and long-term follow-up in 79 cases. *Am J Clin Pathol* **93**, 208–18.

57. Pileri S., Rivano M.T., Raise E., Gualandi G., Gobbi M., Martuzzi M., Gritti F.M., Gerdes J., Stein H. (1986). The value of lymph node biopsy in patients with acquired immunodeficiency syndrome (AIDS) and the AIDS-related complex (ARC): a morphological and immunohistochemical study of 90 cases. *Histopathology* **10**, 1107–29.

58. Wood G.S., Garcia C.F., Dorfman R.F., Warnke R.A. (1985). The immunohistology of follicle lysis in lymph node biopsies from homosexual men. *Blood* **66**, 1092–7.

59. Burns B.F., Colby T.V., Dorfman R.F. (1984). Differential diagnostic features of nodular L&H Hodgkin's disease, including progressive transformation of germinal centers. *Am J Surg Pathol* **8**, 253–61.

60. Jones D. (2002). Dismantling the germinal center: comparing the processes of transformation, regression, and fragmentation of the lymphoid follicle. *Adv Anat Pathol* **9**, 129–38.

61. Chang C., Osipov V., Wheaton S., Tripp S., Perkins S. (2003). Follicular hyperplasia, follicular lysis, and progressive transformation of germinal centers. A sequential spectrum of morphologic evolution in lymphoid hyperplasia. *Am J Clin Pathol* **120**, 322–6.

62. Kojima M., Makamura S., Motoori T., Itoh H., Shimizu K., Yamane N., Ohno Y., Ban S., Yoshida K., Hoshi K., Oyama T., Shimano S., Sugihara S., Sakata N., Masawa N. (2003). Progressive transformation of germinal centers: a clinicopathological study of 42 Japanese patients. *Int J Surg Pathol* **11**, 101–7.

63. Hansmann M.L., Fellbaum C., Hui P.K., Moubayed P. (1990). Progressive transformation of germinal centers with and without association to Hodgkin's disease. *Am J Clin Pathol* **93**, 219–26.

64. Osborne B.M., Butler J.J. (1984). Clinical implications of progressive transformation of germinal centers. *Am J Surg Pathol* **8**, 725–33.

65. Osborne B.M., Butler J.J. (1987). Follicular lymphoma mimicking progressive transformation of germinal centers. *Am J Clin Pathol* **88**, 264–9.

66. Osborne B.M., Butler J.J., Gresik M.V. (1992). Progressive transformation of germinal centers: comparison of 23 pediatric patients to the adult population. *Mod Pathol* **5**, 135–40.

67. Poppema S., Kaiserling E., Lennert K. (1979). Nodular paragranuloma and progressively transformed germinal centers. Ultrastructural and immunohistologic findings. *Virchows Arch [Cell Pathol]* **31**, 211–25.

68. Nguyen P., Ferry J., Harris N.L. (1999). Progressive transformation of germinal centers and nodular lymphocyte predominance Hodgkin's disease: a comparative immunohistochemical study. *Am J Surg Pathol* **22**, 27–33.

69. Childs C.C., Parham D.M., Berard C.W. (1987). Infectious mononucleosis: the spectrum of morphologic changes simulating lymphoma in lymph nodes and tonsils. *Am J Clin Pathol* **53**, 304–14.

70. Gould E., Porto R., Albores-Saavedra J., Ibe M.J. (1988). Dermatopathic lymphadenitis. The spectrum and significance of its morphologic features. *Arch Pathol Lab Med* **112**, 1145–50.

71. Shin S.S., Berry G.J., Weiss L.M. (1991). Infectious mononucleosis: diagnosis by in situ hybridization in two cases with atypical features. *Am J Surg Pathol* **15**, 625–31.

72. Strickler J.G., Fedeli F., Horwitz C.A., Copenhaver C.A., Frizzera G. (1993). Infectious mononucleosis in lymphoid tissue. Histopathology, *in situ* hybridization, and differential diagnosis. *Arch Pathol Lab Med* **117**, 269–78.

73. Weiss L.M., Movahed L.A. (1989). In situ demonstration of Epstein-Barr viral genomes in viral-associated B cell lymphoproliferations. *Am J Pathol* **134**, 651–9.

74. Rushin J.M., Riordan G.P., Heaton R.B., Sharpe R.W., Cotelingam J.D., Jaffe E.S. (1990). Cytomegalovirus-infected cells express LeuM1 antigen. A potential source of diagnostic error. *Am J Pathol* **136**, 989–95.

75. Vago J.F., Titman W.E., Swerdlow S.H. (1989). CMV-associated lymphadenopathy in the "normal" host: a histopathologic and immunophenotypic description (abstract). *Lab Invest* **60**, 100A.

76. Younes M., Podesta A., Helie M., Buckley P. (1991). Infection of T but not B lymphocytes by cytomegalovirus in lymph nodes. An immunophenotypic study. *Am J Surg Pathol* **15**, 75–80.

77. Gaffey M.J., Ben-Ezra J., Weiss L.M. (1991). Herpes simplex lymphadenitis. *Am J Clin Pathol* **95**, 709–14.

78. Hartsock R.J. (1968). Postvaccinial lymphadenitis: hyperplasia of lymphoid tissue that simulates malignant lymphomas. *Cancer* **21**, 632–49.

79. Tamaru J.I., Mikata A., Horie H., Itoh K., Asai T., Hondo R., Mori S. (1990). Herpes simplex lymphadenitis. Report of two cases with review of the literature. *Am J Surg Pathol* **14**, 571–7.

80. Saltzstein S.L., Ackerman L.V. (1959). Lymphadenopathy induced by anticonvulsant drugs clinically and pathologically mimicking malignant lymphomas. *Cancer* **12**, 164–82.

81. Abbondanzo S.L., Irye N.S., Frizzera G. (1995). Dilantin-associated lymphadenopathy: spectrum of histopathologic patterns. *Am J Surg Pathol* **19**, 675–86.

82. Segal G.H., Cough J.D., Tubbs R.R. (1993). Autoimmune and iatrogenic causes of lymphadenopathy. *Semin Oncol* **20**, 611–26.

83. Burke J.S., Colby T.V. (1981). Dermatopathic lymphadenopathy. Comparison of cases associated and unassociated with mycosis fungoides. *Am J Surg Pathol* **5**, 343–52.

84. Weiss L.M., Beckstead J.H., Warnke R.A., Wood G.S. (1986). Leu 6 expressing lymph node cells are dendritic cells and closely related to interdigitating cells. *Hum Pathol* **17**, 179–84.

85. Black M.M., Speer F. (1958). Sinus histiocytosis of lymph node in cancer. *Surg Gynecol Obstet* **106**, 163–75.

86. Gould E., Perez J., Albores-Saavedra J., Legaspi A. (1989). Signet ring cell sinus histiocytosis: a previously unrecognized histologic condition mimicking metastatic adenocarcinoma in lymph nodes. *Am J Clin Pathol* **92**, 509–12.

87. Plank L., Hansmann M.L., Fischer R. (1993). The cytological spectrum of the monocytoid B-cell reaction: recognition of its large cell type. *Histopathology* **23**, 425–31.

88. Sheibani K., Fritz R.M., Winberg C.D., Burke J.S., Rappaport H. (1984). Mono-cytoid cells in reactive follicular hyperplasia with and without multifocal histio-cytic reactions: an immunohistochemical study of 21 cases including suspected cases of toxoplasmosis lymphadenitis. *Am J Clin Pathol* **81**, 453–8.

89. Sohn C.C., Sheibani K., Winberg C.D., Rappaport H. (1985). Monocytoid B lymphocytes: their relation to the patterns of the acquired immunodeficiency syndrome (AIDS) and AIDS-related lymphadenopathy. *Hum Pathol* **16**, 979–85.

90. Fleming J.L., Wiesner R.H., Shorter R.G. (1988). Whipple's disease: clinical, biochemical, and histopathologic features and assessment of treatment in 29 patients. *Mayo Clin Proc* **63**, 539–51.

91. Relman D.A., Schmidt T.M., McDermott R.P., Falkow S. (1992). Identification of the uncultured bacillus of Whipple's disease. *N Engl J Med* **327**, 293–301.

92. Sieracki J.C., Fine G. (1959). Whipple's disease – observations on systemic involvement: II. Gross and histologic observations. *Arch Pathol* **67**, 81–93.

93. Albores-Saavedra J., Vuitch F., Delgado R., Wiley E., Hagler H. (1994). Sinus histiocytosis of pelvic lymph nodes after hip replacement. A histiocytic prolifer-ation induced by cobalt-chromium and titanium. *Am J Surg Pathol* **18**, 83–90.

94. Ravel R. (1966). Histopathology of lymph nodes after lymphangiography. *Am J Clin Pathol* **46**, 335–40.

95. Truong L.D., Cartwright J., Goodman D., Woznicki D. (1988). Silicone lympha-denopathy associated with augmentation mammoplasty: morphologic features of nine cases. *Am J Surg Pathol* **12**, 484–91.

96. Warner N.E., Friedman N.B. (1956). Lipogranulomatous pseudosarcoid. *Ann Intern Med* **45**, 662–73.

97. Bonetti F., Chilosi M., Menestrina F., Scarpa A., Pelicci P.-G., Amorosi E., Fiore-Donati L., Knowles D.M. (1987). Immunohistological analysis of Rosai-Dorfman histiocytosis. A disease of S-100+CD1− histiocytes. *Virchows Arch* **411**, 129–35.

98. Eisen R.N., Buckley P.J., Rosai J. (1990). Immunophenotypic characterization of sinus histiocytosis with massive lymphadenopathy (Rosai-Dorfman disease). *Semin Diagn Pathol* **7**, 74–82.

99. Foucar E., Rosai J., Dorfman R.F. (1990). Sinus histiocytosis with massive lym-phadenopathy (Rosai-Dorfman disease). Review of the entity. *Semin Diagn Pathol* **7**, 19–73.

100. Komp D.M., Herson J., Starling K.A., Vietti T.J., Hvizdala E. (1981). A staging system for histiocytosis X: a Southwest Oncology Group Study. *Cancer* **147**, 798–800.

101. Naiem M., Gerdes J., Abdulaziz A., Stein H., Mason D.Y. (1983). Production of a monoclonal antibody reactive with human dendritic cells and its use in the immunohistological analysis of lymphoid tissue. *J Clin Pathol* **36**, 167–75.

102. Rosai J., Dorfman R.F. (1969). Sinus histiocytosis with massive lymphadenop-athy: a newly recognized benign clinicopathological entity. *Arch Pathol* **87**, 63–70.

103. Rosai J., Dorfman R.F. (1972). Sinus histiocytosis with massive lymphadenop-athy: a pseudolymphomatous benign disorder. Analysis of 34 cases. *Cancer* 1174–88.

104. Foucar E., Rosai J., Dorfman R.F. (1988). Sinus histiocytosis with massive lym-phadenopathy: current status and future directions. *Arch Dermatol* **124**, 1211–14.

105. Foucar E., Rosai J., Dorfman R.F. (1984). Sinus histiocytosis with massive lym-phadenopathy. An analysis of 14 deaths occurring in a patient registry. *Cancer* **54**, 1834–40.

106. Paulli M., Rosso R., Kindl S., et al (1992). Immunophenotypic characterization of the cell infiltrate in five cases of sinus histiocytosis with massive lymphadenopathy. *Hum Pathol* **6**, 647–54.

107. Janka G., Zur Stadt U. (2005). Familial and acquired hemophagocytic lymphohistiocytosis. *Hematology (Am Soc Hematol Educ Program)* 82–8.

108. Chen R.-L., Su I.-J., Lin K.-H., Lee S.-H., Lin D.-T., Chuu W.-M., Lin K.-S., Huang L.-M., Lee C.-Y. (1991). Fulminant childhood hemophagocytic syndrome mimicking histiocytic medullary reticulosis. An atypical form of Epstein-Barr virus infection. *Am J Clin Pathol* **96**, 171–6.

109. Favara B.E. (1992). Hemophagocytic lymphohistiocytosis: a hemophagocytic syndrome. *Semin Diagn Pathol* **9**, 63–74.

110. Kikuta H., Sakiyama T., Matsumoto S., Oh-Ishi T., Nakano T., Nagashima T., Oka T., Hironaka T., Hirai K. (1993). Fatal Epstein-Barr virus-associated hemophagocytic syndrome. *Blood* **82**, 3259–64.

111. Ladisch S., Holiman B., Poplack D.G., Blaese R.M. (1978). Immunodeficiency in familial erythrophagocytic lymphohistiocytosis. *Lancet* **1**, 581–3.

112. McKenna R.W., Risdall R.J., Brunning R.D. (1981). Virus associated hemophagocytic syndrome. *Hum Pathol* **12**, 395–8.

113. Risdall R.J., McKenna R.W., Nesbitt M.E., Krivit W., Balfour H.H., Simmons R.L., Brunning R.D. (1979). Virus associated hemophagocytic syndrome. A benign histiocytic proliferation distinct from malignant histiocytosis. *Cancer* **44**, 993–1002.

114. Falini B., Pileri S., DeSolas I., Martelli M.F., Mason D.Y., Delsol G., Gatter K.C., Fagioli M. (1990). Peripheral T-cell lymphoma associated with hemophagocytic syndrome. *Blood* **75**, 434–44.

115. Henter J., Arico M., Elinder G., Imashuku S., Janka G. (1998). Familial hemophagocytic lymphohistiocytosis. Primary hemophagocytic lymphohistiocytosis. *Hematol Oncol Clin North Am* **12**, 417–33.

116. Wong K., Chan J. (1991). Hemophagocytic disorders – a review. *Hematol Rev* **5**, 5–37.

117. Janka G., Schneider E. (2004). Modern management of children with haemophagocytic lymphohistiocytosis. *Br J Haematol* **124**, 4–14.

118. Cleary K.R., Osborne B.M., Butler J.J. (1982). Lymph node infarction foreshadowing malignant lymphoma. *Am J Surg Pathol* **6**, 435–42.

119. Norton A.J., Ramsey A.D., Isaacson P.G. (1988). Antigen preservation in infarcted lymphoid tissue: a novel approach to the infarcted lymph node using monoclonal antibodies effective in routinely processed tissues. *Am J Surg Pathol* **12**, 759–67.

120. Strickler J.G., Warnke R.A., Weiss L.M. (1987). Necrosis in lymph nodes. *Pathol Annu* **22** (*Pt* **2**), 253–82.

121. Chamulak G.A., Brynes R.K., Nathwani B.N. (1990). Kikuchi-Fujimoto disease mimicking malignant lymphoma. *Am J Surg Pathol* **14**, 514–23.

122. Dorfman R.F., Berry G.J. (1988). Kikuchi's histiocytic necrotizing lymphadenitis: an analysis of 108 cases with emphasis on differential diagnosis. *Semin Diagn Pathol* **5**, 329–45.

123. Facchetti F., Agostini C., Chilosi M., Mombello A., Grigolato P., van den Oord J. (1992). Suppurative granulomatous lymphadenitis. Immunohistochemical evidence for a B-cell-associated granuloma. *Am J Surg Pathol* **16**, 955–61.

124. Feller A.C., Lennert K., Stein H., Bruhn H.-D., Wuthe H.-H. (1983). Immunohistology and aetiology of histiocytic necrotizing lymphadenitis: report of three instructive cases. *Histopathology* **7**, 825–9.

125. Fujimoto Y., Kozima Y., Yamaguchi K. (1972). Cervical subacute necrotizing lymphadenitis. A new clinicopathologic entity. *Naika* **20**, 920–7.

126. Pileri S., Kikuchi M., Helbron D., Lennert K. (1982). Histiocytic necrotizing lymphadenitis without granulocytic infiltration. *Virchows Arch [Pathol Anat]* **395**, 257–71.

127. Medeiros L.J., Kaynor B., Harris N.L. (1989). Lupus lymphadenitis: report of a case with immunohistologic studies on frozen sections. *Hum Pathol* **20**, 295–9.

128. Petri M. (2005). Review of classification criteria for systemic lupus erythematosus. *Rheum Dis Clin North Am* **31**, 245–54.

129. Giesker D.W., Pastuszak W.T., Forouhar F.A., Krause P.J., Hine P. (1982). Lymph node biopsy for early diagnosis in Kawasaki disease. *Am J Surg Pathol* **6**, 493–501.

130. Goldsmith R.W., Gribetz D., Strauss L. (1976). Mucocutaneous lymph node syndrome (MLNS) in the continental United States. *Pediatrics* **57**, 431–5.

131. Braylan R.C., Long J.C., Jaffe E.S., Greco F.A., Orr S.L., Berard C.W. (1977). Malignant lymphoma obscured by concomitant extensive epithelioid granulomas: report of three cases with similar clinicopathologic features. *Cancer* **39**, 1146–55.

132. Hollingsworth H.C., Longo D.L., Jaffe E.S. (1993). Small noncleaved cell lymphoma associated with florid epithelioid granulomatous response: a clinicopathologic study of seven patients. *Am J Surg Pathol* **17**, 51–9.

133. Sacks E.L., Donaldson S.S., Gordon J., Dorfman R.F. (1978). Epithelioid granulomas associated with Hodgkin's disease: clinical correlations in 55 previously untreated patients. *Cancer* **41**, 562–7.

134. Chen K.T.K. (1992). Mycobacterial spindle cell pseudotumor of lymph nodes. *Am J Surg Pathol* **16**, 276–81.

135. Reid J.D., Wolinsky E. (1969). Histopathology of lymphadenitis caused by atypical mycobacteria. *Am Rev Respir Dis* **99**, 8–12.

136. Bagla N., Patel M., Patel R., Jarag M. (2005). Lepromatous lymphadenitis masquerading as lymphoma. *Lepr Rev* **76**, 87–90.

137. Alkan S., Morgan M.B., Sandin R.L., Moscinski L.C., Ross C.W. (1995). Dual role for *Afipia felis* and *Rochalimaea henselae* in cat-scratch disease (letter). *Lancet* **345**, 385.

138. Anderson B., Sims K., Regnery R., Robinson L., Schmidt M.J., Goral S., Hager C., Edwards K. (1994). Detection of *Rochalimaea henselae* DNA in specimens from cat scratch disease patients by PCR. *J Clin Microbiol* **32**, 942–8.

139. Korbi S., Toccanier M.F., Leyvraz G., Stalder J., Kapanci Y. (1986). Use of silver staining (Dieterle's stain) in the diagnosis of cat scratch disease. *Histopathology* **10**, 1015–21.

140. Naji A.F., Carbonell F., Barker H.J. (1962). Cat scratch disease: a report of three new cases, review of the literature, and classification of the pathologic changes in the lymph nodes during various stages of the disease. *Am J Clin Pathol* **38**, 513–21.

141. Wear D.J., Margileth A.M., Hadfield T.L., Fischer G.W., Schlagel C.J., King F.M. (1983). Cat-scratch disease: a bacterial infection. *Science* **221**, 1403–5.

142. Hadfield T.L., Lamy Y., Wear D.J. (1995). Demonstration of *Chlamydia trachomatis* in inguinal lymphadenitis of lymphogranuloma venereum: a light microscopy, electron microscopy and polymerase chain reaction study. *Mod Pathol* **8**, 924–9.

143. Schapers R.F.M., Reif R., Lennert K., Knapp W. (1981). Mesenteric lymphadenitis due to *Yersinia enterocolitica*. *Virchows Arch A [Pathol Anat Histol]* **390**, 127–38.

144. Davis R.E., Warnke R.A., Dorfman R.F. (1991). Inflammatory pseudotumor of lymph nodes. Additional observations and evidence for an inflammatory etiology. *Am J Surg Pathol* **15**, 744–56.

145. Perrone T., De Wolf-Peeters C., Frizzera G. (1988). Inflammatory pseudotumor of lymph nodes. A distinctive pattern of nodal reaction. *Am J Surg Pathol* **12**, 351–61.

146. Moran C.A., Suster S., Abbondanzo S.L. (1997). Inflammatory pseudotumor of lymph nodes: a study of 25 cases with emphasis on morphological heterogeneity. *Hum Pathol* **28**, 332–8.

147. Chan J.K.C., Warnke R.A., Dorfman R.F. (1991). Vascular transformation of sinuses in lymph nodes: a study of its morphologic spectrum and distinction from Kaposi's sarcoma. *Am J Surg Pathol* **15**, 732–43.

148. Cook P.D., Czerniak B., Chan J.K.C., MacKay B., Ordonez N.G., Ayala A.G., Rosai J. (1995). Nodular spindle cell vascular transformation of lymph nodes: a benign process occurring predominantly in retroperitoneal lymph nodes draining carcinomas that can simulate Kaposi's sarcoma or metastatic tumor. *Am J Surg Pathol* **19**, 1010–20.

149. Chan J.K.C., Lewin K.J., Lombard C.D., Teitelbaum S., Dorfman R.F. (1991). The histopathology of bacillary angiomatosis of lymph nodes. *Am J Surg Pathol* **14**, 430–7.

150. Relman D.A., Loutit J.S., Schmidt T.M., Falkow S., Tompkins L.S. (1990). The agent of bacillary angiomatosis. An approach to the identification of uncultured pathogens. *N Engl J Med* **323**, 1573–80.

151. Michaeli J., Niesvizky R., Siegel D., Ladanyi M., Lieberman P.H., Filippa D.A. (1995). Proteinaceous (angiocentric sclerosing) lymphadenopathy: a polyclonal systemic, nonamyloid deposition disorder. *Blood* **86**, 1159–62.

152. MacKenzie D.H. (1963). Amyloidosis presenting as lymphadenopathy. *Br Med J* **2**, 1449–50.

153. Ordi J., Grau J.M., Junque A., Nomdedeu B., Lalacin A., Cardesa A. (1993). Secondary (AA) amyloidosis associated with Castleman's disease. Report of two cases and review of the literature. *Am J Clin Pathol* **100**, 393–7.

154. Osborne B.M., Butler J.J., MacKay B. (1979). Proteinaceous lymphadenopathy with hypergammaglobulinaemia. *Am J Surg Pathol* **3**, 137–45.

155. Barnett R.N., Hull J.G., Vortel V., Schwarz J. (1969). Pneumocystis carinii in lymph nodes and spleen. *Arch Pathol Lab Med* **88**, 175–80.

156. Karp L.A., Czernobilsky B. (1969). Glandular inclusions in pelvic and abdominal paraaortic lymph nodes: a study of autopsy and surgical material in males and females. *Am J Clin Pathol* **52**, 212–18.

157. Holdsworth P.J., Hopkinson J.M., Leveson S.H. (1988). Benign axillary epithelial lymph node inclusions – a histological pitfall. *Histopathology* **13**, 226–8.

158. Cohn D.E., Folpe A.L., Gown A.M., Goff B.A. (1998). Mesothelial pelvic lymph node inclusions mimicking metastatic thyroid carcinoma. *Gynecol Oncol* **68**, 210–13.

159. Turner R.R., Ollila D.W., Krasne D.L., Giuliano A.E. (1997). Histopathologic validation of the sentinel lymph node hypothesis for breast carcinoma. *Ann Surg* **226**, 271–6.

160. Association of Directors of Anatomic and Surgical Pathology. (2001). ADASP recommendations for processing and reporting lymph node specimens submitted for evaluation of metastatic disease. *Am J Surg Pathol* **25**, 961–3.

161. Gershenwald J.E., Thompson W., Mansfield P.F., Lee J.E., Colome M.I., Tseng C.H., Lee J.J., Balch C.M., Reintgen D.S., Ross M.I. (1999). Multi-institutional melanoma lymphatic mapping experience: the prognostic value of sentinel lymph node status in 612 stage I or II melanoma patients. *J Clin Oncol* **17**, 976–83.

162. Bautista N.C., Cohen S., Anders K.H. (1994). Benign melanocytic nevus cells in axillary lymph nodes. A prospective incidence and immunohistochemical study with literature review. *Am J Clin Pathol* **102**, 102–8.

163. Urso C., Borgognoni L., Saieva C., Ferrara G., Tinacci G., Begliomini B., Reali U. (2006). Sentinel lymph node biopsy in patients with "atypical Spitz tumors": a report on 12 cases. *Hum Pathol* **37**, 816–23.

164. Thompson J., Shaw H. (2007). Sentinel node mapping for melanoma: results of trials and current applications. *Surg Oncol Clin N Am* **16**, 35–54.

165. Morton D., Thompson J., Cochran A., Mozzillo N., Elashoff R., Essner R., Niewig O., Roses D., Hoekstra H., Karakousis C., Reintgen D., Coventry B., Glass E., Wang H., MSLT Group. (2006). Sentinel-node biopsy or nodal observation in melanoma. *N Engl J Med* **355**, 1307–17.

166. Weiss S.W., Gnepp D.R., Bratthauer G.L. (1989). Palisaded myofibroblastoma. A benign mesenchymal tumor of lymph node. *Am J Surg Pathol* **13**, 341–6.

167. Hisaoka M., Hashiomoto H., Daimaru Y. (1998). Intranodal palisaded myofibroblastoma with so-called amianthoid fibers: a report of two cases with a review of the literature. *Pathol Int* **48**, 307–12.

168. Rossi A., Bulgarini A., Rondanelli E., Incensati R. (1995). Intranodal palisaded myofibroblastoma: report of three new cases. *Tumori* **81**, 464–8.

169. Chan J.K., Tsang W.Y., Pau M.Y., Tang M.C., Pang S.W., Fletcher C.D. (1993). Lymphangiomyomatosis and angiomyolipoma: closely related entities characterized by hamartomatous proliferation of HMB-45-positive smooth muscle. *Histopathology* **22**, 445–55.

170. Chan J.K., Frizzera G., Fletcher C.D., Rosai J. (1992). Primary vascular tumors of lymph nodes other than Kaposi's sarcoma: analysis of 39 cases and delineation of two new entities. *Am J Surg Pathol* **16**, 335–50.

171. Lin O., Frizzera G. (1997). Angiomyoid and follicular dendritic cell proliferative lesions in Castleman's disease of hyaline-vascular type: a study of 10 cases. *Am J Surg Pathol* **21**, 1295–1306.

172. Cho N.H., Yang W.I., Lee W.J. (1997). Spindle and epithelioid haemangioendothelioma of the inguinal lymph nodes. *Histopathology* **30**, 595–8.

173. Finkbeiner W.E., Egbert B.M., Groundwater J.R., Sagebiel R.W. (1982). Kaposi's sarcoma in young homosexual men: a histopathologic study with particular reference to lymph node involvement. *Arch Pathol Lab Med* **106**, 261–4.

174. Fraga M., Forteza J. (2007). Diagnosis of Hodgkin's disease: an update on histopathological and immunophenotypical features. *Histol Histopathol* **22**, 923–35.

175. Colby T.V., Hoppe R.T., Warnke R.A. (1982). Hodgkin's disease: a clinicopathologic study of 659 cases. *Cancer* **49**, 1848–58.

176. Colby T.V., Warnke R.A. (1980). The histology of the initial relapse of Hodgkin's disease. *Cancer* **45**, 289–92.

177. Strum S.B., Park J.K., Rappaport H. (1970). Observation of cells resembling Sternberg-Reed cells in conditions other than Hodgkin's disease. *Cancer* **26**, 176–90.

178. Dolginow D., Colby T.V. (1981). Recurrent Hodgkin's disease in treated sites. *Cancer* **48**, 1124–6.

179. Colby T.V., Hoppe R.T., Warnke R.A. (1981). Hodgkin's disease at autopsy: 1972–1977. *Cancer* **47**, 1852–62.

180. Re D., Kuppers R., Diehl V. (2005). Molecular pathogenesis of Hodgkin's lymphoma. *J Clin Oncol* **23**, 6379–86.

181. Thomas R., Re D., Zander T., Wolf J., Diehl V. (2002). Epidemiology and etiology of Hodgkin's lymphoma. *Ann Oncol* **13** (suppl 4), 147–52.

182. Pileri S., Ascani S., Leoncini L., Sabattini E., Zinzani P., Piccaluga P., Pileri A., Giunti M., Falini B., Balis G., Stein H. (2002). Hodgkin's lymphoma: the pathologist's viewpoint. *J Clin Pathol* **55**, 162–76.

183. MacLennan K.A., Bennett M.H., Vaughan H.B., Vaughan H.G. (1992). Diagnosis and grading of nodular sclerosing Hodgkin's disease: a study of 2190 patients. *Int Rev Exp Pathol* **33**, 27–51.

184. Strickler J.G., Michie S.A., Warnke R.A., Dorfman R.F. (1986). The "syncytial variant" of nodular sclerosing Hodgkin's disease. *Am J Surg Pathol* **10**, 470–7.

185. MacLennan K.A., Bennett M.H., Tu A., Hudson B.V., Easterling J., Hudson G.V., Jelliffe A.M. (1989). Relationship of histopathologic features to survival and relapse in nodular sclerosing Hodgkin's disease: a study of 1,659 patients. *Cancer* **64**, 1686–93.

186. Kuppers R., Schmitz R., Distler V., Renne C., Brauninger A., Hansmann M. (2005). Pathogenesis of Hodgkin's lymphoma. *Eur J Haematol* Suppl **66**, 26–33.

187. Ashton-Key M., Thorpe P.A., Allen J.P., Isaacson P.G. (1995). Follicular Hodgkin's disease. *Am J Surg Pathol* **19**, 1294–9.

188. Browne P., Petrosyan K., Hernandez A., Chan J. (2003). The B-cell transcription factors BSAP, Oct2, and BOB1 and the pan-B-cell markers CD20, CD22, and CD79a are useful in the differential diagnosis of classic Hodgkin lymphoma. *Am J Clin Pathol* **120**, 767–77.

189. Buettner M., Greiner A., Avramidou A., Jack H.-M., Niedobitek G. (2005). Evidence of abortive plasma cell differentiation in Hodgkin and Reed-Sternberg cells of classical Hodgkin lymphoma. *Hematol Oncol* **23**, 127–32.

190. Diehl V., Sextro M., Fanklin J., Hansmann M.L., Harris N., Jaffe E., Poppema S., Harris M., Franssila K., van Krieken J., Marafioti T., Anagnostopoulos I., Stein H. (1999). Clinical presentation, course, and prognostic factors in lymphocyte-predominant Hodgkin's disease and lymphocyte-rich classical Hodgkin's disease: report from the European Task Force on Lymphoma Project on Lymphocyte-Predominant Hodgkin's Disease. *J Clin Oncol* **17**, 776–83.

191. Kuppers R., Klein U., Hansmann M., Rajewsky K. (1999). Cellular origin of human B-cell lymphomas. *N Engl J Med* **341**, 1520–9.

192. Lukes R.J., Butler J.J. (1966). The pathology and nomenclature of Hodgkin's disease. *Cancer Res* **26**, 1063–83.

193. Rudiger T., Ott G., Ott M., Muller-Hermelink H. (1998). Differential diagnosis between classic Hodgkin's lymphoma, T-cell-rich B-cell lymphoma and paragranuloma by paraffin immunohistochemistry. *Am J Surg Pathol* **22**, 1184–91.

194. Tzankov A., Zimpfer A., Pehrs A., Lugli A., Went P., Maurer R., Pileri S., Dirhofer S. (2003). Expression of B-cell markers in classical Hodgkin lymphoma: a tissue microarray analysis of 330 cases. *Mod Pathol* **16**, 1141–7.

195. van Spronsen D., Vrints L., Hofstra G., Crommelin M., Coebergh J., Breed W. (1997). Disappearance of prognostic significance of histopathological grading of nodular sclerosing Hodgkin's disease for unselected patients, 1972–92. *Br J Haematol* **96**, 322–7.

196. Weiss L.M., Chen Y.-Y., Liu X.-F., Shibata D. (1991). Epstein-Barr virus and Hodgkin's disease: a correlative in situ hybridization and polymerase chain reaction study. *Am J Pathol* **139**, 1259–65.

197. Lister T.A., Crowther D., Sutcliffe S.B., et al (1989). Report of a committee convened to discuss the evaluation and staging of patients with Hodgkin's disease: Cotswolds meeting. *J Clin Oncol* **7**, 1630–6.

198. Kamel O.W., Gelb A.B., Shibuya R.B., Warnke R.A. (1993). Leu7 (CD57) reactivity distinguishes nodular lymphocyte predominance Hodgkin's disease, T cell rich B cell lymphoma and follicular lymphoma. *Am J Pathol* **142**, 541–6.

199. Mason D.Y., Banks P.M., Chan J., Cleary M.L., Delsol G., De Wolf-Peeters C., Falini B., Gatter K., Grogan T.M., Harris N.L., Isaacson P.G., Jaffe E.S., Knowles D.M., Muller-Hermelink H., Pileri S., Piris M., Stein H., Ralfkiaer E., Warnke R. (1994). Nodular lymphocyte predominance Hodgkin's disease: a distinct clinicopathological entity. *Am J Surg Pathol* **18**, 528–30.

200. Fan Z., Natkunam Y., Bair E., Tibshirani R., Warnke R. (2003). Characterization of variant patterns of nodular lymphocyte predominant Hodgkin's lymphoma with immunohistologic and clinical correlation. *Am J Surg Pathol* **27**, 1346–56.

201. Boudova L., Torlakovic E., Delabie J., Reimer P., Pfistner B., Wiedenmann S., Diehl V., Muller-Hermelink H., Rudiger T. (2003). Nodular lymphocyte-predominant Hodgkin lymphoma with nodules resembling T-cell/histiocyte-rich B-cell lymphoma: differential diagnosis between nodular lymphocyte-predominant Hodgkin lymphoma and T-cell/histiocyte-rich B-cell lymphoma. *Blood* **102**, 3753–8.

202. Algara P., Martinez P., Sanchez L., Villuendas R., Orradre J.L., Oliva H., Piris M.A. (1991). Lymphocyte predominance Hodgkin's disease (nodular paragranuloma) – a bcl-2 negative germinal centre lymphoma. *Histopathology* **19**, 69–75.

203. Anagnostopoulos I., Hansmann M.L., Franssila K., Harris M., Harris N.L., Jaffe E.S., van Krieken J.H.J.M., Poppema S., Marafioti T., Franklin J., Sextro M., Diehl V., Stein H. (2000). European Task Force on Lymphoma project on lymphocyte predominance Hodgkin's disease: histologic and immunohistological analysis of submitted cases reveals 2 types of Hodgkin disease with a nodular growth and abundant lymphocytes. *Blood* **96**, 1889–99.

204. Chittal S.M., Alard C., Rossi J.F., Al Saati T., Le Tourneau A., Diebold J., Delsol G. (1990). Further phenotypic evidence that nodular, lymphocyte-predominant Hodgkin's disease is a large B-cell lymphoma in evolution. *Am J Surg Pathol* **14**, 1024–35.

205. Hansmann M.L., Stein H., Fellbaum C., Hui P.K., Parwaresch M.R., Lennert K. (1989). Nodular paragranuloma can transform into high-grade malignant lymphoma of B type. *Hum Pathol* **20**, 1169–75.

206. Hansmann M.L., Stein H., Dallenbach F., Fellbaum C. (1991). Diffuse lymphocyte-predominant Hodgkin's disease (diffuse paragranuloma): a variant of the B-cell-derived nodular type. *Am J Pathol* **138**, 29–36.

207. Marafioti T., Hummel M., Anagnostopoulos I., Foss H.D., Falini B., Delsol G., Isaacson P.G., Pileri S., Stein H. (1997). Origin of nodular lymphocyte-predominant Hodgkin's disease from a clonal expansion of highly mutated germinal-center B cells. *N Engl J Med* **337**, 453–8.

208. Marafioti T., Hummel M., Foss H., Laumen H., Korbjuhn P., Anagnostopoulos I., Lammert H., Demel G., Theil J., Wirth T., Stein H. (2000). Leukocyte-specific phosphoprotein-1 and PU.1: two useful markers for distinguishing T-cell-rich lymphoma from lymphocyte-predominant Hodgkin's disease. *Haematologica* **89**, 957–64.

209. Ohno T., Striblem J.A., Wu G., Hinrichs S.H., Weisenburger D.D., Chan W.C. (1997). Clonality in nodular lymphocyte-predominant Hodgkin's disease. *N Engl J Med* **337**, 459–65.

210. Regula D.P., Hoppe R.T., Weiss L.M. (1988). Nodular and diffuse types of lymphocyte predominance Hodgkin's disease. *N Engl J Med* **318**, 214–9.

211. von Wasielewski R., Werner M., Fischer R., Hansmann M., Hubner K., Hasencleaver D., Franklin J., Sextro M., Diehl V., Georgii A. (1997). Lymphocyte-predominant Hodgkin's disease. An immunohistochemical analysis of 208 reviewed Hodgkin's disease cases from the German Hodgkin Study Group. *Am J Pathol* **150**, 793–803.

212. Wickert R.S., Weisenburger D.D., Tierens A., Greiner T.C., Chan W.C. (1995). Clonal relationship between lymphocyte predominance Hodgkin's disease and concurrent or subsequent large-cell lymphoma of B lineage. *Blood* **86**, 2312–20.

213. Jaffe E., Harris N., Stein H., Vardiman J. (2001). *Pathology and Genetics of Tumours of Haematopoietic and Lymphoid Tissues.* Lyon, France: IARC Press.

214. The International Non-Hodgkin Lymphoma Prognostic Factors Project (1993). A predictive model for aggressive non-Hodgkin lymphoma. *N Engl J Med* **329**, 987–94.

215. Anderson J.R., Armitage J.O., Weisenburger D.D. (1998). Epidemiology of the non-Hodgkin's lymphomas: distributions of the major subtypes differ by geographic locations. Non-Hodgkin's Lymphoma Classification Project. *Ann Oncol* **9**, 717–20.

216. Turner N., Dusheiko G., Jones A. (2003). Hepatitis C and B-cell lymphoma. *Ann Oncol* **14**, 1341–5.

217. The Non-Hodgkin's Lymphoma Pathologic Classification Project (1982). National Cancer Institute sponsored study of classifications of non-Hodgkin lymphomas: summary and description of a working formulation for clinical usage. *Cancer* **49**, 2112–35.

218. The Non-Hodgkin's Lymphoma Classification Project (1993). A clinical evaluation of the International Lymphoma Study Group classification of non-Hodgkin lymphoma. *Blood* **89**, 3909–18.

219. Harris N.L., Jaffe E.S., Stein H., Banks P.M., Chan J.K.C., Cleary M.L., Delsol G., De Wolf-Peeters C., Falini B., Gatter K.C., Grogan T.M., Isaacson P.G., Knowles D.M., Mason D.Y., Muller-Hermelink H.-K., Pileri S.A., Piris M.A., Ralfkiaer E., Warnke R.A. (1994). A revised European-American classification of lymphoid neoplasms. A proposal from the International Lymphoma Study Group. *Blood* **84**, 1361–92.

220. Momose H., Jaffe E.S., Shin S.S., Chen Y.Y., Weiss L.M. (1992). Chronic lymphocytic leukemia/small lymphocytic lymphoma with Reed-Sternberg-like cells and possible transformation to Hodgkin's disease. Mediation by Epstein-Barr virus. *Am J Surg Pathol* **16**, 859–67.

221. Cheson B.D., Bennett J.M., Rai K.R., Grever M.R., Kay N.E., Schiffer C.A., Oken M.M., Keating M.J., Boldt D.H., Kempin S.J. (1988). Guidelines for clinical protocols for chronic lymphocytic leukemia: recommendations of the National Cancer Institute-sponsored working group. *Am J Hematol* **29**, 152–63.

222. Ben-Ezra J., Burke J.S., Swartz W.G., Brownell M.D., Brynes R.K., Hill L.R., Nathwani B.N., Oken M.M., Wolf B.C., Woodruff R. (1989). Small lymphocytic lymphoma: aclinicopathologic analysis of 268 cases. *Blood* **73**, 579–87.

223. Dick F.R., Maca R.D. (1978). The lymph node in chronic lymphocytic leukemia. *Cancer* **41**, 283–292.

224. Pugh W.C., Manning J.T., Butler J.J. (1988). Paraimmunoblastic variant of small lymphocytic lymphoma/leukemia. *Am J Surg Pathol* **12**, 907–17.

225. DiGiuseppe J.A., Borowitz M.J. (1998). Clinical utility of flow cytometry in the chronic lymphoid leukemias. *Semin Oncol* **25**, 6–10.

226. Zukerberg L.R., Medeiros L.J., Ferry J.A., Harris N.L. (1993). Diffuse low-grade B-cell lymphomas: four clinically distinct subtypes defined by a combination of morphologic and immunophenotypic features. *Am J Clin Pathol* **100**, 373–85.

227. Rai K., Sawitsky A., Cronkite E., Chanana A., Levy R., Pasternack B. (1975). Clinical staging of chronic lymphocytic leukemia. *Blood* **46**, 219.

228. Binet J. (1999). Prognostic factors in chronic lymphocytic leukaemia. *Haematologica* **84**, 96–7.

229. O'Brien A., del Giglio A., Keating M. (1995). Advances in the biology and treatment of B-cell chronic lymphocytic leukemia. *Blood* **85**, 307–18.

230. Rassenti L., Huynh L., Toy T., Chen L., Keating M., Gribben J., Neuberg D., Flinn I., Rai K., Byrd J., Kay N., Greaves A., Weiss A., Kipps T. (2004). ZAP-70 compared with immunoglobulin heavy-chain gene mutation status as a predictor of disease progression in chronic lymphocytic leukemia. *N Engl J Med* **351**, 893–901.

231. Juliusson G., Merup M. (1998). Cytogenetics in chronic lymphocytic leukemia. *Semin Oncol* **25**, 19–26.

232. Chiorazzi N., Rai K., Ferrarini M. (2005). Chronic lymphocytic leukemia. *N Engl J Med* **352**, 804–15.

233. Wiestner A., Rosenwald A., Barry T., Wright G., Davis R., Henrickson S., Zhao H., Ibbotson R., Orchard J., Davis Z., Stetler-Stevenson M., Raffeld M., Arthur D., Marti G., Wilson W., Hamblin T., Oscier D., Staudt L. (2003). ZAP-70 expression identifies a chronic lymphocytic leukemia subtype with unmutated immunoglobulin genes, inferior clinical outcome, and distinct gene expression profile. *Blood* **101**, 4944–51.

234. Dohner H., Stilgenbauer S., Dohner K., Bentz M., Lichter P. (1999). Chromosome aberrations in B-cell chronic lymphocytic leukemia: reassessment based on molecular cytogenetic analysis. *J Mol Med* **77**, 266–81.

235. Pangalis G.A., Angelopoulou M.K., Vassilakopoulos T.P., Siakantaris M.P., Kittas C. (1999). B-chronic lymphocytic leukemia, small lymphocytic lymphoma, and lymphoplasmacytic lymphoma, including Waldenstrom's macroglobulinemia: a clinical, morphologic, and biologic spectrum of similar disorders. *Semin Hematol* **36**, 104–14.

236. Lin P., Medeiros L. (2005). Lymphoplasmacytic lymphoma/Waldenstrom macroglobulinemia. An evolving concept. *Adv Anat Pathol* **12**, 246–55.

237. Schop R.F., Fonseca R. (2003). Genetics and cytogenetics of Waldenstrom's macroglobulinemia. *Semin Oncol* **39**, 142–5.

238. Owen R., Treon S., Al-Katib A., Fonseca R., Greipp P., McMaster M., Morra E., Pangalis G., San Miguel J., Branagan A., Dimopoulos M. (2003). Clinicopathological definition of Waldenstrom's macroglobulinemia: consensus panel recommendations from the Second International Workshop on Waldenstrom's Macroglobulinemia. *Semin Oncol* **30**, 110–15.

239. Lin B.T., Weiss L.M. (1997). Primary plasmacytoma of lymph nodes. *Hum Pathol* **28**, 1083–90.

240. Addis B., Isaacson P., Billings J. (1980). Plasmacytoma of lymph nodes. *Cancer* **46**, 340–6.

241. Bergsagel P., Kuehl W. (2005). Molecular pathogenesis and a consequent classification of multiple myeloma. *J Clin Oncol* **23**, 6333–8.

242. Liebisch P., Dohner H. (2006). Cytogenetics and molecular cytogenetics in multiple myeloma. *Eur J Cancer* **42**, 1520–9.

243. Chang K.L., Stroup R., Weiss L.M. (1992). Hairy cell leukemia. Current status. *Am J Clin Pathol* **97**, 719–38.

244. Mercieca J., Puga M., Matutes E., Moskovic E., Salim S., Catovsky D. (1994). Incidence and significance of abdominal lymphadenopathy in hairy cell leukemia. *Leuk Lymphoma* **14**, 79–83.

245. Hakimian D., Tallman M., Hogan D., Rademaker A., Rose E., Nemcek A. (1994). Prospective evaluation of internal adenopathy in a cohort of 43 patients with hairy cell leukemia. *J Clin Oncol* **12**, 268–72.

246. Nathwani B.N., Drachenberg M.R., Hernandez A.M., Levine A.M., Sheibani K. (1999). Nodal monocytoid B-cell lymphoma (nodal marginal-zone B-cell lymphoma). *Semin Hematol* **36**, 128–38.

247. Arcaini L., Paulli M., Boveri E., Magrini U., Lazzarino M. (2003). Marginal zone-related neoplasms of splenic and nodal origin. *Haematologica* **88**, 80–93.

248. Traverse-Glehen A., Felman P., Callet-Bauchu E., Gazzo S., Baseggio L., Bryon P., Thieblemont C., Coiffier B., Salles G., Berger F. (2006). A clinicopathological study of nodal marginal zone B-cell lymphoma. A report on 21 cases. *Histopathology* **48**, 162–73.

249. Ngan B.Y., Warnke R.A., Wilson M., Takagi K., Cleary M.L., Dorfman R.F. (1991). Monocytoid B-cell lymphoma: a study of 36 cases. *Hum Pathol* **22**, 409–21.

250. Nathwani B.N., Mohrmann R.S., Brynes R.K., Taylor C.R., Hansmann M.L., Sheibani K. (1992). Monocytoid B-cell lymphomas: an assessment of diagnostic criteria and a perspective on histogenesis. *Hum Pathol* **23**, 1061–71.

251. Fisher R.I., Dahlberg S., Nathwani B.N., Banks P.M., Miller T.P., Grogan T.M. (1995). A clinical analysis of two indolent lymphoma entities: mantle cell lymphoma and marginal zone lymphoma (including the mucosa-associated lymphoid tissue and monocytoid B-cell categories): a Southwest Oncology Group study. *Blood* **85**, 1075–82.

252. Arcaini L., Paulli M., Burcheri S., Rossi A., Spina M., Passamonti F., Lucioni M., Motta T., Canzonieri V., Montanari M., Bonoldi E., Gallamini A., Uziel L., Crugnola M., Ramponi A., Montanari F., Pascutto C., Morra E., Lazzarino M., Intergruppo Italiano Linfomi. (2007). Primary nodal marginal zone B-cell lymphoma: clinical features and prognostic assessment of a rare disease. *Br J Haematol* **136**, 301–4.

253. Maes B., De Wolfe-Peeters C. (2002). Marginal zone cell lymphoma – an update on recent advances. *Histopathology* **40**, 117–26.

254. Nathwani B., Drachenberg M., Hernandez A. (2000). Primary nodal marginal zone lymphomas of splenic and MALT type. *Am J Surg Pathol* **24**, 317–19.

255. Campo E., Miquel R., Krenacs L., Sorbara L., Raffeld M., Jaffe E.S. (1999). Primary nodal marginal zone lymphomas of splenic and MALT type. *Am J Surg Pathol* **23**, 59–68.

256. Shin S.S., Sheibani K., Fishleder A., Ben-Ezra J., Bailey A., Koo C.H., Burke J.S., Tubbs R., Rappaport H. (1991). Monocytoid B-cell lymphoma in patients with Sjogren's syndrome: a clinicopathologic study of 13 patients. *Hum Pathol* **22**, 422–30.

257. Royer B., Cazals-Hatem D., Sibilia J., Agbalika F., Cayuela J.M., Soussi T., Maloisel F., Clauvel J.P., Brouet J.C., Mariette X. (1997). Lymphomas in patients with Sjogren's syndrome are marginal zone B-cell neoplasms, arise in diverse extranodal and nodal sites, and are not associated with viruses. *Blood* **90**, 766–75.

258. Nizze H., Cogliatti S.B., von Schilling C., Feller A.C., Lennert K. (1991). Monocytoid B-cell lymphoma: morphological variants and relationship to low-grade B-cell lymphoma of the mucosa-associated lymphoid tissue. *Histopathology* **18**, 403–14.

259. Isaacson P. (2005). Update on MALT lymphomas. *Best Pract Res Clin Haematol* **18**, 57–8.

260. Isaacson P., Du M. (2004). MALT lymphoma: from morphology to molecules. *Nat Rev Cancer* **4**, 644–53.

261. Farinha P., Gascoyne R. (2005). Molecular pathogenesis of mucosa-associated lymphoid tissue lymphoma. *J Clin Oncol* **23**, 6370–8.

262. Streubel B., Vinatzer U., Lamprecht A., Raderer M., Chott A. (2005). t(3;14)(p14.1;q32) involving IGH and FOXP1 is a novel recurrent chromosomal aberration in MALT lymphoma. *Leukemia* **19**, 652–8.

263. Mollejo M., Lloret E., Marguez J., Piris M.A., Isaacson P.G. (1997). Lymph node involvement by splenic marginal zone lymphoma: morphological and immunohistochemical features. *Am J Surg Pathol* **21**, 772–80.

264. Gine E., Montoto S., Bosch F., Arenillas L., Mercadal S., Villamor N., Martinez A., Colomo L., Campo E., Montserrat E., Lopez-Guillermo A. (2006). The follicular lymphoma international prognostic index (FLIPI) and the histological subtype are the most important factors to predict histological transformation in follicular lymphoma. *Ann Oncol* **17**, 1539–45.

265. Nathwani B.N., Anderson J.R., Armitage J.O., Cavalli F., Diebold J., Drachenberg M.R., Harris N.L., MacLennan K.A., Muller-Hermelink H.K., Ullrich R.A., Weisenburger D.D. (1999). Clinical significance of follicular lymphoma with monocytoid B cells. *Hum Pathol* **30**, 263–8.

266. Pinto A., Hutchison R.E., Grant L.H., Trevenen C.L., Berard C.W. (1990). Follicular lymphomas in pediatric patients. *Mod Pathol* **3**, 308–13.

267. Isaacson P. (1996). Malignant lymphomas with a follicular growth pattern. *Histopathology* **28**, 487–95.

268. Goates J.J., Kamel O.W., LeBrun D.P., Benharroch D., Dorfman R.F. (1994). Floral variant of follicular lymphoma. Immunological and molecular studies support a neoplastic process. *Am J Surg Pathol* **18**, 37–47.

269. Mann R.B., Berard C.W. (1982). Criteria for the cytologic subclassification of follicular lymphomas: a proposed alternative method. *Hematol Oncol* **1**, 187–92.

270. Ott G., Katzenberger T., Lohr A., Kindelberger S., Rudiger T., Wilhelm M., Kalla J., Rosenwald A., Muller J., Ott M., Muller-Hermelink H. (2002). Cytomorphologic, immunohistochemical, and cytogenetic profiles of follicular lymphoma: 2 types of follicular lymphoma grade 3. *Blood* **99**, 3806–12.

271. Lorsbach R.B., Shay-Seymore D., Moore J., Banks P.M., Hasserjian R.P., Sandlund J.T., Behm F.G. (2002). Clinicopathologic analysis of follicular lymphoma occurring in children. *Blood* **99**, 1959–64.

272. Bartlett N.L., Rizeq M., Dorfman R.F., Halpern J., Horning S.J. (1994). Follicular large-cell lymphoma: intermediate or low grade? *J Clin Oncol* **12**, 1349–57.

273. Davies A. (2006). Clinical and molecular prognostic factors in follicular lymphoma. *Curr Oncol Rep* **8**, 359–367.

274. Goodlad J., Batstone P., Hamilton D., Kernohan N., Levison D., White J. (2006). BCL2 gene abnormalities define distinct clinical subsets of follicular lymphoma. *Histopathology* **49**, 229–41.

275. Solal-Celigny P. (2006). Follicular lymphoma international prognostic index. *Curr Treat Options Oncol* **7**, 270–5.

276. Metter G.E., Nathwani B.N., Burke J.S., Winberg C.D., Mann R.B., Barcos M., Kjeldsberg C.R., Whitcomb C.C., Dixon D.O., Miller T.P., Jones S.E. (1985).

Morphological subclassification of follicular lymphoma: variability of diagnosis among hematopathologists, a collaborative study between the Repository Center and Pathology Panel for Lymphoma Clinical Studies. *J Clin Oncol* **3**, 25–38.

277. Nathwani B.N., Metter G.E., Miller T.P., Burke J.S., Mann R.B., Barcos M., Kjeldsberg C.R., Dixon D.O., Winberg C.D., Whitcomb C.C. (1986). What should be the morphologic criteria for the subdivision of follicular lymphomas? *Blood* **68**, 837–45.

278. Hans C.P., Weisenburger D.D., Vose J.M., Hock L.M., Lynch J.C., Aoun P., Greiner T.C., Chan W.C., Bociek R.G., Bierman P.J., Armitage J.O. (2003). A significant diffuse component predicts for inferior survival in grade 3 follicular lymphoma, but cytologic subtypes do not predict survival. *Blood* **101**, 2363–7.

279. Warnke R.A., Weiss L.M., Chan J.K.C., Cleary M.L., Dorfman R.F. (1995). *Tumors of the Lymph Nodes and Spleen.* (3rd ed.). Washington, D.C.: Armed Forces Institute of Pathology.

280. Kojima M., Yamanaka S., Yoshida T., Shimizu K., Murayama K., Ohno Y., Itoh H., Motoori T., Masawa N., Nakamura S. (2006). Histological variety of floral variant of follicular lymphoma. *APMIS* **114**, 626–32.

281. Du M., Diss T.C., Liu H., Ye H., Hamoudi R., Cebecadas J., Dong H., Harris N., Chan J., Rees J., Dogan A., Isaacson P. (2002). KSHV- and EBV-associated germinotropic lymphoproliferative disorder. *Blood* **100**, 3415–18.

282. Yatabe Y., Suzuki R., Matsuno Y., Tobinai K., Ichinohazama R., Tamaru J., Mizoguchi Y., Hashimoto Y., Kojima M., Uike N., Okamoto M., Isoda K., Ichimura K., Morishima Y., Seto M., Suchi T., Nakamura S. (2001). Morphological spectrum of cyclin D1-positive mantle cell lymphoma: study of 168 cases. *Pathol Int* **51**, 747–61.

283. Kurtin P.J. (1998). Mantle cell lymphoma. *Adv Anat Pathol* **5**, 376–98.

284. Campo E., Raffeld M., Jaffe E.S. (1999). Mantle-cell lymphoma. *Semin Hematol* **36**, 115–27.

285. Banks P.M., Chan J., Cleary M.L., Delsol G., DeWolf-Peeters C., Gatter K., Grogan T.M., Harris N.L., Isaacson P.G., Jaffe E.S. (1992). Mantle cell lymphoma. A proposal for unification of morphologic, immunologic, and molecular data. *Am J Surg Pathol* **16**, 637–40.

286. Argatoff L.H., Connors J.M., Klasa R.J., Horsman D.E., Gascoyne R.D. (1997). Mantle cell lymphoma: a clinicopathologic study of 80 cases. *Blood* **89**, 2067–78.

287. Samaha H., Dumontet C., Ketterer N., Moullet I., Thieblemont C., Bouafia F., Callet-Bauchu E., Felman P., Berger F., Salles G., Coiffier B. (1998). Mantle cell lymphoma: a retrospective study of 121 cases. *Leukemia* **12**, 1281–7.

288. Bertoni F., Rinaldi A., Zucca E., Cavalli F. (2006). Update on the molecular biology of mantle cell lymphoma. *Hematol Oncol* **24**, 22–7.

289. Rosenwald A., Wright G., Wiestner A., Chan W., et al (2003). The proliferation gene expression signature is a quantitative integrator of oncogenic events that predicts survival in mantle cell lymphoma. *Cancer Cell* **3**, 185–97.

290. Ott G., Kalla J., Ott M., Schryen B., et al (1997). Blastoid variants of mantle cell lymphoma: frequent bcl-1 rearrangements at the major translocation cluster region and tetraploid chromosome clones. *Blood* **89**, 1421–9.

291. Zoldan M., Inghirami G., Masuda Y., Vandekerckhove F., et al (1996). Large-cell variants of mantle cell lymphoma: cytologic characteristics and p53 anomalies may predict poor outcome. *Br J Haematol* **93**, 475–86.

292. Martinez N., Camacho R., Algara P., Rodriguez A., Dopazo A., Ruiz-Ballesteros E., Martin P., Martinez-Climent J., Solano F., Mollejo M., Piris M. (2003). The

molecular signature of mantle cell lymphoma reveals multiple signals favoring cell survival. *Cancer Res* **63**, 8226–32.

293. Fu K., Weisenburger D., Greiner T., Dave S., Wright G., Rosenwald A., Chiorazzi M., Iqbal J., Gesk S., Siebert R., de Jong D., Jaffe E., Wilson W., Delabie J., Ott G., Dave B., Sanger W., Smith L., Rimsza L., Braziel R., Muller-Hermelink H., Campo E., Gascoyne R., Staudt L., Chan W. (2005). Cyclin D1-negative mantle cell lymphoma: a clinicopathologic study based on gene expression profiling. *Blood* **106**, 4315–21.

294. Hans C., Weisenberger D., Greiner T., Gascoyne R., Delabie J., Ott G., Muller-Hermelink H., Campo E., Braziel R., Jaffe E., Pan Z., Farinha P., Smith L., Falini B., Banham A., Rosenwald A., Staudt L., Connors J., Armitage J., Chan W. (2004). Confirmation of the molecular classification of diffuse large B-cell lymphoma by immunohistochemistry using a tissue microarray. *Blood* **103**, 275–82.

295. Kwak L.W., Wilson M., Weiss L.M., Horning S.J., Warnke R.A., Dorfman R.F. (1991). Clinical significance of morphologic subdivision in diffuse large cell lymphoma. *Cancer* **68**, 1988–93.

296. Alizadeh A.A., Eisen M.B., Davis R.E., Ma C., Lossos I.S., Rosenwald A., Boldrick J.C., Sabet H., Tran T., Yu X., Powell J.I., Yang L., Marti G.E., Moore T., Hudson J., Lu L., Lewis D.B., Tibshirani R., Sherlock G., Chann W.C., Greiner T.C., Weisenburger D.D., Armitage J.O., Warnke R., Levy R., Wilson W., Grever M.R., Byrd J.C., Botstein D., Brown P.O., Staudt L.M. (2000). Distinct types of diffuse large B-cell lymphoma identified by gene expression profiling. *Nature* **403**, 503–11.

297. Rosenwald A., Wright G., Chan W., Connors J., Campo E., Fisher R., Gascoyne R., Muller-Hermelink H., Smeland E., Giltnane J., Hurt E., Zhao H., Averett L., Yang L., Wilson W., Jaffe E., Simon R., Klausner R., Powell J., Duffey P., Longo D., Greiner T., Weisenburger D., Sanger W., Dave B., Lynch J., Vose J., Armitage J., Montserrat E., Lopez-Guillermo A., Grogan T., Miller T., LeBlanc M., Ott G., Kvaloy S., Delabie J., Holte H., Krajci P., Stokke T., Staudt L., Lymphoma/Leukemia Molecular Profiling Project. (2002). The use of molecular profiling to predict survival after chemotherapy for diffuse large-B-cell lymphoma. *N Engl J Med* **346**, 1937–47.

298. Muris J., Meijer C., Vos W., van Kriken J., Jiwa N., Ossenkoppele G., Oudejans J. (2006). Immunohistochemical profiling based on Bcl-2, CD10 and MUM1 expression improves risk stratification in patients with primary nodal diffuse large B cell lymphoma. *J Pathol* **208**, 714–23.

299. Winter J., Weller E., Horning S., Krajewska M., Variakoojis D., Habermann T., Fisher R., Kurtin P., Macon W., Chhanabhai M., Felgar R., Hsi E., Medeiros L., Weick J., Reed J., Gascoyne R. (2006). Prognostic significance of Bcl-6 protein expression in DLBCL treated with CHOP or R-CHOP: a prospective correlative study. *Blood* **107**, 4207–13.

300. Shivakumar L., Armitage J. (2006). Bcl-2 gene expression as a predictor of outcome in diffuse large B-cell lymphoma. *Clin Lymphoma Myeloma* **6**, 455–7.

301. Abramson J., Shipp M. (2005). Advances in the biology and therapy of diffuse large B-cell lymphoma: moving toward a molecularly targeted approach. *Blood* **106**, 1164–74.

302. Berglund M., Thunberg U., Amini R., Book M., Roos G., Erlanson M., Linderoth J., Dictor M., Jerkeman M., Cavallin-Stahl E., Sundstrom C., Rehn-Eriksson S., Backlin C., Hagberg H., Rosenquist R., Enblad G. (2005). Evaluation of immunophenotype in diffuse large B-cell lymphoma and its impact on prognosis. *Mod Pathol* **18**, 1113–20.

303. Lossos I., Czerwinski D., Alizadeh A., Wechser M., Tibshirani R., Botstein D., Levy R. (2004). Prediction of survival in diffuse large-B-cell lymphoma based on the expression of six genes. *N Engl J Med* **350**, 1828–37.

304. Lossos I., Morgensztern D. (2006). Prognostic biomarkers in diffuse large B-cell lymphoma. *J Clin Oncol* **24**, 995–1007.

305. Tsang W.Y., Chan J.K., Tang S.K., Tse C.C., Cheung M.M. (1992). Large cell lymphoma with fibrillary matrix. *Histopathology* **20**, 80–2.

306. Tse C.C., Chan J.K., Yuen R.W., Ng C.S. (1991). Malignant lymphoma with myxoid stroma: a new pattern in need of recognition. *Histopathology* **18**, 31–5.

307. Kinney M.C., Glick A.D., Stein H., Collins R.D. (1990). Comparison of anaplastic large cell Ki-1 lymphomas and microvillous lymphomas in their immunologic and ultrastructural features. *Am J Surg Pathol* **14**, 1047–60.

308. Ripp J., Loiue D., Chan W., Nawaz H., Portlock C. (2002). T-cell rich B-cell lymphoma: clinical distinctiveness and response to treatment in 45 patients. *Leuk Lymphoma* **43**, 1573–80.

309. Delabie J., Vandenberghe E., Kennes C., Verhoef G., Foschini M.P., Stul M., Cassiman J.J., Wolf-Peeters C.D. (1992). Histiocyte-rich B-cell lymphoma. A distinct clinicopathologic entity possibly related to lymphocyte predominant Hodgkin's disease, paragranuloma subtype. *Am J Surg Pathol* **16**, 37–48.

310. Khalidi H.S., Brynes R.K., Browne P., Koo C.H., Battifora H., Medeiroa L.J. (1998). Intravascular large B-cell lymphoma: the CD5 antigen is expressed by a subset of cases. *Mod Pathol* **11**, 983–8.

311. Delecluse H.J., Anagnostopoulos I., Dallenbach F., Hummel M., Marafioti T., Schneider U., Huhn D., Schmidt-Westhausen A., Reichart P.A., Gross U., Stein H. (1997). Plasmablastic lymphomas of the oral cavity: a new entity associated with the human immunodeficiency virus infection. *Blood* **89**, 1413–20.

312. Carbone A., Gaidano G., Gloghini A., Ferlito A., Rinaldo A., Stein H. (1999). AIDS-related plasmablastic lymphomas of the oral cavity and jaws: a diagnostic dilemma. *Ann Otol Rhinol Laryngol* **108**, 95–9.

313. Ansari M.Q., Dawson D.B., Nador R., Rutherford C., Schneider N.R., Latimer M.J., Picker L., Knowles D.M., McKenna R.W. (1996). Primary body cavity-based AIDS-related lymphomas. *Am J Clin Pathol* **105**, 221–9.

314. DiGiuseppe J., Nelson W., Seifter E., Boitnott J., Mann R. (1994). Intravascular lymphomatosis: a clinicopathologic study of 10 cases and assessment of response to chemotherapy. *J Clin Pathol* **12**, 2573–9.

315. Perrone T., Frizzera G., Rosai J. (1986). Mediastinal diffuse large-cell lymphoma with sclerosis: a clinicopathologic study of 60 cases. *Am J Surg Pathol* **10**, 176–91.

316. Davis R.E., Dorfman R.F., Warnke R.A. (1990). Primary large cell lymphoma of the thymus: a diffuse B-cell neoplasm presenting as primary mediastinal lymphoma. *Hum Pathol* **21**, 1262–8.

317. Abou-Elella A.A., Weisenburger D.D., Vose J.M., Kollath J.P., Lynch J.C., Bast M.A., Bierman P.J., Greiner T.C., Chan W.C., Armitage J.O. (1999). Primary mediastinal large B-cell lymphoma: a clinicopathologic study of 43 patients from the Nebraska Lymphoma Study Group. *J Clin Oncol* **17**, 784–90.

318. Paulli M., Strater J., Gianelli U., Rousset M.T., Gambacorta M., Orlandi E., Klersy C., Lavabre-Bertrand T., Morra E., Manegold C., Lazzarino M., Magrini U., Moller P. (1999). Mediastinal B-cell lymphoma: a study of its histomorphologic spectrum based on 109 cases. *Hum Pathol* **30**, 178–87.

319. Rosenwald A., Wright G., Leroy K., Yu X., Gaulard P., Gascoyne R., Chan W., Zhao T., Haioun C., Greiner T., Weisenburger D., Lynch J., Vose J., Armitage J., Smeland E., Kvaloy S., Holte H., Delabie J., Campo E., Montserrat E.,

Lopez-Guillermo A., Ott G., Muller-Hermelink H., Connors J., Braziel R., Grogan T., Fisher R., Miller T., LeBlanc M., Chiorazzi M., Zhao H., Yang L., Powell J., Wilson W., Jaffe E., Simon R., Klausner R., Staudt L. (2003). Molecular diagnosis of primary mediastinal B cell lymphoma identifies a clinically favorable subgroup of diffuse large B cell lymphoma related to Hodgkin lymphoma. *J Exp Med* **198**, 851–62.

320. Savage K., Monti S., Kutok J., Cattoretti G., Neuberg D., DeLeval L., Kurtin P., Dal Cin P., Ladd C., Feuerhake F., Aguiar R., Li S., Salles G., Berger F., Jing W., Pinkus G., Habermann T., Dalla-Favera R., Harris N., Aster J., Golub T., Shipp M. (2003). The molecular signature of mediastinal large B-cell lymphoma differs from that of other diffuse large B-cell lymphomas and shares features with classical Hodgkin lymphoma. *Blood* **102**, 3871–9.

321. Rodig S., Savage K., LaCasce A., Weng A., Harris N., Shipp M., Hsi E., Gascoyne R., Kutok J. (2007). Expression of TRAF1 and nuclear c-Rel distinguishes primary mediastinal large cell lymphoma from other types of diffuse large B-cell lymphoma. *Am J Surg Pathol* **31**, 106–12.

322. Magrath I. (1990). The pathogenesis of Burkitt's lymphoma. *Adv Cancer Res* **53**, 133–270.

323. Yano T., van Krieken J.H.J.M., Magrath I., Longo D.L., Jaffe E.S., Raffeld M. (1992). Histogenetic correlations between subcategories of small noncleaved cell lymphomas. *Blood* **79**, 1282–90.

324. Hutchison R.E., Murphy S., Fairclough D.L., Shuster J.J., Sullivan M.P., Link M.P., Donaldson S.S., Berard C.W. (1989). Diffuse small noncleaved cell lymphoma in children, Burkitt's versus non-Burkitt's types. *Cancer* **64**, 23–38.

325. Dave S., Fu K., Wright G., Lam L., Kluin P., Boerma E., Greiner T., Weisenburger D., Rosenwald A., Ott G., Muller-Hermelink H., Gascoyne R., Delabie J., Rimsza L., Braziel R., Grogan T., Campo E., Jaffe E., Dave B., Sanger W., Bast M., Vose J., Armitage J., Connors J., Smeland E., Kvaloy S., Holte H., Fisher R., Miller T., Montserrat E., Wilson W., Bahl M., Zhao H., Yank L., Powell J., Simon R., Chan W., Staudt L. (2006). Molecular diagnosis of Burkitt's lymphoma. *N Engl J Med* **354**, 2431–42.

326. Hummel M., Bentink S., Berger H., Klapper W., Wessendorf S., Barth T., Bernd H., Cogliatti S., Dierlamm J., Feller A., Hansmann M., Haralambieva E., Harder L., Hasenclever D., Kuhn M., Lenze D., Lichter P., Martin-Subero J., Moller P., Muller-Hermelink H., Ott G., Parwaresch R., Pott C., Rosenwald A., Rosolowski M., Schwaenen C., Sturzenhofecker B., Szczepanowski M., Trautmann H., Wacker H., Spang R., Loeffler M., Trumper L., Stein H., Siebert R. (2006). A biologic definition of Burkitt's lymphoma from transcriptional and genomic profiling. *N Engl J Med* **354**, 2419–30.

327. Braziel R., Arber D., Slovak M., Gulley M., Spier C., Kjeldsberg C., Unger J., Miller T., Tubbs R., Leith C., Fisher R., Grogan T. (2001). The Burkitt-like lymphomas: a Southwest Oncology Group study delineating phenotypic, genotypic, and clinical features. *Blood* **97**, 3713–20.

328. Murphy S., Fairclough D., Hutchinson R., Berard C. (1989). Non-Hodgkin's lymphomas of childhood: an analysis of the histology, staging, and response to treatment of 338 cases at a single institution. *J Clin Oncol* **7**, 186–93.

329. Lin P., Jones D., Dorfman D., Medeiros J. (2000). Precursor B-cell lymphoblastic lymphoma. *Am J Surg Pathol* **24**, 1480–90.

330. Nathwani B.N., Diamond L.W., Winberg C.D., Kim H., Bearman R.M., Glick J., Jones S.E., Gams R.A., Nissen N.I., Rappaport H. (1981). Lymphoblastic lymphoma: a clinicopathologic study of 95 patients. *Cancer* **48**, 2347–57.

331. Griffith R.C., Kelly D.R., Nathwani B.N., Shuster J.J., Murphy S.B., Hvizdala E., Sullivan M.P., Berard C.W. (1987). A morphologic study of childhood lymphoma of the lymphoblastic type. The Pediatric Oncology Group experience. *Cancer* **59**, 1126–31.

332. Weiss L.M., Bindl J.M., Picozzi V.J., Link M.P., Warnke R.A. (1986). Lymphoblastic lymphoma: an immunophenotype study of 26 cases with comparison to T cell acute lymphoblastic leukemia. *Blood* **67**, 474–8.

333. Soslow R.A., Bhargava V., Warnke R.A. (1997). MIC2, TdT, bcl-2, and CD34 expression in paraffin-embedded high grade lymphoma/acute lymphoblastic leukemia distinguishes between distinct clinicopathologic entities. *Hum Pathol* **28**, 1158–65.

334. Inhorn R.C., Aster J.C., Roach S.A., Slapak C.A., Soiffer R., Tantravahi R., Stone R.M. (1995). A syndrome of lymphoblastic lymphoma, eosinophilia, and myeloid hyperplasia/malignancy associated with t(8;13)(p11;q11): description of a distinctive clinicopathologic entity. *Blood* **85**, 1887.

335. Bagg A. (2004). Role of molecular studies in the classification of lymphoma. *Expert Rev Mol Diagn* **4**, 83–97.

336. Savage K., Chhanabhai M., Gascoyne R., Connors J. (2004). Characterization of peripheral T-cell lymphomas in a single North American institution by the WHO classification. *Ann Oncol* **15**, 1467–75.

337. Kikuchi M., Mitsui T., Takeshita M., Okamura H., Naitoh H., Eimoto T. (1986). Virus associated adult T-cell leukemia (ATL) in Japan: clinical, histological and immunological studies. *Hematol Oncol* **4**, 81.

338. Kagami Y., Suzuki R., Yaji H., Yatabe Y., Takeuchi T., Maeda S., Kondo E., Kojima M., Motoori T., Mizoguchi Y., Okamoto M., Ohnishi K., Yamabe H., Seto M., Ogura M., Koshikawa T., Takahashi T., Kurita S., Morishima.Y., Suchi T., Nakamura S. (1999). Nodal cytotoxic lymphoma spectrum: a clinicopathologic study of 66 patients. *Am J Surg Pathol* **23**, 1184–200.

339. Lones M.A., Lopez-Terrada D., Weiss L.M., Shintaku I.P., Nichols W.S., Said J.W. (1997). Donor origin of posttransplant lymphoproliferative disorder localized in a liver allograft. Demonstration by flourescence in situ hybridization. *Arch Pathol Lab Med* **121**, 701–6.

340. Attygalle A., Chuang S., Diss T., Du M., Isaacson P., Dogan A. (2007). Distinguishing angioimmunoblastic T-cell lymphoma from peripheral T-cell lymphoma, unspecified, using morphology, immunophenotype, and molecular genetics. *Histopathology* **50**, 498–508.

341. Dupuis J., Boye K., Martin N., Copie-Bergman C., Plonquet A., Fabiani B., Baglin A.-C., Haioun C., Delfau-Larue M.-H., Gaulard P. (2006). Expression of CXCL13 by neoplastic cells in angioimmunoblastic T-cell lymphoma (AITL): a new diagnostic marker providing evidence that AITL derives from follicular helper T cells. *Am J Surg Pathol* **30**, 490–4.

342. Weiss L.M., Jaffe E.S., Liu X., Chen Y., Shibata D., Medeiros L.J. (1992). Detection and localization of Epstein-Barr viral genomes in angioimmunoblastic lymphadenopathy and angioimmunoblastic lymphadenopathy-like lymphomas. *Blood* **79**, 1789–95.

343. Ree H.J., Kadin M.E., Kikuchi M., Ko Y.H., Go J.H., Suzumiya J., Kim D.S. (1998). Angioimmunoblastic lymphoma (AILD-type T-cell lymphoma) with hyperplastic germinal centers. *Am J Surg Pathol* **22**, 643–55.

344. Grogg K., Attygalle A., Macon W., Remstein E., Kurtin P., Dogan A. (2005). Angioimmunoblastic T-cell lymphoma: a neoplasm of germinal-center T-helper cells? *Blood* **106**, 1501–2.

345. Rudinger T., Ichinohasama R., Ott M.M., Muller-Deubert S., Miura I., Ott G., ller-Hermelink H.K. (2000). Peripheral T-cell lymphoma with distinct perifollicular growth pattern: a distinct subtype of T-cell lymphoma? *Am J Surg Pathol* **24**, 117–22.

346. Patsouris E., Noel H., Lennert K. (1988). Histological and immunohistological findings in lymphoepithelioid cell lymphoma (Lennert's lymphoma). *Am J Surg Pathol* **12**, 341–50.

347. Horning S.J., Weiss L.M., Crabtree G.S., Warnke R.A. (1986). Clinical and phenotypic diversity of T cell lymphomas. *Blood* **67**, 1578–82.

348. Chott A., Augustin I., Wra F., Hanak H., Ohlinger W., Radaszkiewicz T. (1990). Peripheral T-cell lymphomas – a clinicopathologic study of 75 cases. *Hum Pathol* **21**, 1117–25.

349. de Bruin P.C., Kummer J.A., van der Valk P., van Heerde P., Kluin P.M., Willemze R. (1994). Granzyme B-expressing peripheral T-cell lymphomas: neoplastic equivalents of activated cytotoxic T cells with preference for mucosa-associated lymphoid tissue localization. *Blood* **84**, 3785–91.

350. Berge R., Oudejans J., Ossenkoppele G., Meijer C. (2003). ALK-negative systemic anaplastic large cell lymphoma: differential diagnostic and prognostic aspects – a review. *J Pathol* **200**, 4–15.

351. Chan J.K.C. (1998). Anaplastic large cell lymphoma: redefining its morphologic spectrum and importance of recognition of the ALK-positive subset. *Adv Anat Pathol* **5**, 281–313.

352. Kinney M.C., Kadin M.E. (1999). The pathologic and clinical spectrum of anaplastic large cell lymphoma and correlation with ALK gene dysregulation. *Am J Clin Pathol* **111**, S56–67.

353. Chan J.K.C., Ng C.S., Hui P.K., et al (1989). Anaplastic large cell Ki-1 lymphoma. Delineation of two morphological types. *Histopathology* **15**, 11–34.

354. Jaffe E. (2001). Anaplastic large cell lymphoma: the shifting sands of diagnostic hematopathology. *Mod Pathol* **14**, 219–28.

355. Vassallo J., Lamant L., Brugieres L., Gaillard F., Campo E., Brousset P., Delsol G. (2006). ALK-positive anaplastic large cell lymphoma mimicking nodular sclerosis Hodgkin's lymphoma: report of 10 cases. *Am J Surg Pathol* **30**, 223–9.

356. Benharroch D., Meguerian-Bedoyan Z., Lamant L., Amin C., Brugieres L., Terrier-Lacombe M.J., et al (1998). ALK-positive lymphoma: a single disease with a broad spectrum of morphology. *Blood* **91**, 2076–84.

357. deBruin P.C., Beljaards R.C., VanHeerde P., van der Valk P., Noorduyn L.A., van Krieken J.H., Kluin-Nelemans J.C., Willemze R., Meijer C.J.L.M., Van J.M. (1993). Differences in clinical behaviour and immunophenotype between primary cutaneous and primary nodal anaplastic large cell lymphoma of T-cell or null cell phenotype. *Histopathology* **23**, 127–35.

358. Hodges K.B., Collins R.D., Greer J.P., Kadin M.E., Kinney M.C. (1999). Transformation of the small cell variant Ki-1+ lymphoma to anaplastic large cell lymphoma: pathologic and clinical features. *Am J Surg Pathol* **23**, 49–58.

359. Chan J.K.C., Buchanan R., Fletcher C.D.M. (1991). Sarcomatoid variant of anaplastic large cell Ki-1 anaplastic large-cell lymphoma. *J Clin Oncol* **9**, 539–47.

360. Falini B., Pileri S., Zinzani P.L., Carbone A., Zagonel V., Wolf-Peeters C., Verhoef G., Menestrina F., Todeschini G., Paulli M., Lazzarino M., Giardini R., Aiello A., Foss H.D., Araujo I., Fizzotti M., Pelicci P.G., Flenghi L., Martelli M.F., Santucci A. (1999). ALK+ lymphoma: clinico-pathological findings and outcome. *Blood* **93**, 2697–706.

361. Colby T., Burke J., Hoppe R.T. (1981). Lymph node biopsy in mycosis fungoides. *Cancer* **47**, 351–9.

362. Izban K.F., Hsi E.D., Alkan S. (1998). Immunohistochemical analysis of mycosis fungoides on paraffin-embedded tissue sections. *Mod Pathol* **11**, 978–82.

363. Weiss L.M., Hu E., Wood G.S., Moulds C., Cleary M., Warnke R., Sklar J. (1985). Clonal rearrangements of the T cell receptor gene in mycosis fungoides and dermatopathic lymphadenopathy. *N Engl J Med* **313**, 539–44.

364. Kern D., Kidd P., Moe R., Hanke D., Olerud J. (1998). Analysis of T-cell receptor gene rearrangement in lymph nodes of patients with mycosis fungoides. Prognostic implications. *Arch Dermatol* **134**, 158–64.

365. Scheffer E., Meijer C., van Vloten W. (1980). Dermatopathic lymphadenopathy and lymph node involvement in mycosis fungoides. *Cancer* **45**, 137–48.

366. Olsen E., Vonderheid E., Pimpinelli N., Wilemze R., Kim Y., Knobler R., Zackheim H., Duvic M., Estrach T., Lamberg S., Wood G., Dummer R., Ranki A., Burg G., Heald P., Pittelkow M., Bernengo M., Sterry W., Laroche L., Trautinger F., Whittaker S. (2007). Revisions to the staging and classification of mycosis fungoides and Sezary syndrome: a proposal of the International Society for Cutaneous Lymphomas (ISCL) and the Cutaneous Lymphoma Task Force of the European Organization of Research and Treatment of Cancer (EORTC). In press.

367. Jaffe E.S., Clark J., Steis R., et al (1985). Lymph node pathology of HTLV and HTLV-associated neoplasms. *Cancer Res* **45**, 4662s–4s.

368. Jaffe E.S., Blattner W.A., Blayney D.W. (1984). The pathologic spectrum of adult T-cell leukemia/lymphoma in the United States. Human T-cell leukemia/lymphoma virus-associated lymphoid malignancies. *Am J Surg Pathol* **8**, 263–75.

369. Matutes E., Brito-Babapulle V., Swansbury J., Ellis J., Morilla R., Dearden C., Sempere A., Catovsky D. (1991). Clinical and laboratory features of 78 cases of T-prolymphocytic leukemia. *Blood* **78**, 3269–74.

370. Matutes E., Garcia T., O'Brien M., Catovsky D. (1986). The morphological spectrum of T-prolymphocytic leukaemia. *Br J Haematol* **64**, 111–24.

371. Semenzato G., Zambello R., Starkebaum G., Oshimi K., Loughran T. (1997). The lymphoproliferative disease of granular lymphocytes: update criteria for diagnosis. *Blood* **89**, 256–60.

372. DiGiuseppe J.A., Louie D.C., Williams J.E., Miller D.T., Griffin C.A., Mann R.B., Borowitz M.J. (1997). Blastic natural killer cell leukemia/lymphoma: a clinicopathologic study. *Am J Surg Pathol* **21**, 1223–30.

373. Hasserjian R., Harris N. (2007). NK-cell lymphomas and leukemias: a spectrum of tumors with variable manifestations and immunophenotype. *Am J Clin Pathol* **127**, 860–8.

374. Barrionuevo C., Zaharia M., Martinez M., Taxa L., Misad O., Moscol A., Sarria G., Guerrero I., Casanova L., Flores C., Zevallos-Giampietri E.A. (2007). Extranodal NK/T-cell lymphoma, nasal type: study of clinicopathologic and prognosis factors in a series of 78 cases from Peru. *Appl Immunohistochem Mol Morphol* **15**, 38–44.

375. Weiss L.M., Arber D.A., Strickler J.G. (1994). Nasal T cell lymphoma. *Ann Oncol* **5**, 39–42.

376. Chan J.K., Sin V.C., Wong K.F., Ng C.S., Tsang W.Y., Chan C.H., Cheung M.M., Lau W.H. (1997). Nonnasal lymphoma expressing the natural killer cell marker CD56: a clinicopathologic study of 49 cases of an uncommon aggressive neoplasm. *Blood* **89**, 4501–13.

377. Wright D. (1997). Enteropathy associated T cell lymphoma. *Cancer Surv* **30**, 249–61.

378. Chott A., Haedicke W., Mosberger I., Fodinger M., Winkler K., Mannhalter C., Muller-Hermelink H. (1998). Most CD56+ intestinal lymphomas are CD8+ CD5−T-cell lymphomas of monomorphic small to medium size histology. *Am J Pathol* **153**, 1483–90.

379. Chott A., Vesely M., Simonitsch I., Mosberger I., Hanak H. (1999). Classification of intestinal T-cell neoplasms and their differential diagnosis. *Am J Clin Pathol* **111**, S68–74.

380. Sallah S., Smith S.V., Lony L.C., Woodard P., Schmitz J.L., Folds J.D. (1997). Gamma/delta T-cell hepatosplenic lymphoma: review of the literature, diagnosis by flow cytometry and concomitant autoimmune hemolytic anemia. *Ann Hematol* **74**, 139–42.

381. Salhany K.E., Macon W.R., Choi J.K., Elenitsas R., Lessin S.R., Felgar R.E., Wilson D.M., Przyblski G.K., Lister J., Wasik M.A., Swerdlow S.H. (1998). Subcutaneous panniculitis-like T-cell lymphoma: clinicopathologic, immunophenotypic, and genotypic analysis of alpha/beta and gamma/delta subtypes. *Am J Surg Pathol* **22**, 881–93.

382. Dargent J.L., Roufosse C., Delville J.P., Kentos A., Delplace J., Kornreich A., Cochauz P., Hilbert P., Pradier O., Feremans W. (1998). Subcutaneous panniculitis-like T-cell lymphoma: further evidence for a distinct neoplasm originating from large granular lymphocytes of T/NK phenotype. *J Cutan Pathol* **25**, 394–400.

383. Macon W.R., Levy N.B., Kurtin P.J., Salhany K.E., Elkhalifa M.Y., Casey T.T., Craig F.E., Vnencak-Jones C.L., Gulley M.L., Park J.P., Cousar J.B. (2001). Hepatosplenic alpha beta T-cell lymphomas – a report of 14 cases and comparison with hepatosplenic gamma delta T-cell lymphomas. *Am J Surg Pathol* **25**, 285–96.

384. Cooke C.B., Krenacs L., Stetler-Stevenson M., et al (1996). Hepatosplenic T-cell lymphoma: a distinct clinicopathologic entity of cytotoxic gd T-cell origin. *Blood* **88**, 4265–74.

385. Kumar S., Krenacs L., Medeiros J., Elenitoba-Johnson K., Greiner T., Sorbara L., Kingma D., Raffeld M., Jaffe E. (1998). Subcutaneous panniculitic T-cell lymphoma is a tumor of cytotoxic T-lymphocytes. *Hum Pathol* **29**, 397–403.

386. Gonzalez C.L., Medeiros L.J., Jaffe E.S. (1991). Composite lymphoma. A clinicopathologic analysis of nine patients with Hodgkin's disease and B-cell non-Hodgkin's lymphoma. *Am J Clin Pathol* **96**, 81–9.

387. Zarate-Osorno A., Medeiros L.J., Longo D.L., Jaffe E.S. (1992). Non-Hodgkin's lymphomas arising in patients successfully treated for Hodgkin's disease. A clinical, histologic, and immunophenotypic study of 14 cases. *Am J Surg Pathol* **16**, 885–95.

388. Zarate-Osorno A., Medeiros L.J., Kingma D.W., Longo D.L., Jaffe E.S. (1993). Hodgkin's disease following non-Hodgkin's lymphoma. A clinicopathologic and immunophenotypic study of nine cases. *Am J Surg Pathol* **17**, 123–32.

389. Traverse-Glehen A., Pittaluga S., Gaulard P., Sorbara L., Alonso M., Raffeld M., Jaffe E. (2005). Mediastinal gray zone lymphoma: the missing link between classic Hodgkin's lymphoma and mediastinal large B-cell lymphoma. *Am J Surg Pathol* **29**, 1411–21.

390. Huang K., Weinstock M., Clarke C., McMillan A., Hoppe R., Kim Y. (2007). Second lymphomas and other malignant neoplasms in patients with mycosis fungoides and Sezary syndrome: evidence from population-based and clinical cohorts. *Arch Dermatol* **143**, 45–50.

391. Knowles D.M. (1999). Immunodeficiency-associated lymphoproliferative disorders. *Mod Pathol* **12**, 200–17.

392. Elenitoba-Johnson K.S., Jaffe E.S. (1997). Lymphoproliferative disorders associated with congenital immunodeficiencies. *Semin Diagn Pathol* **14**, 35–47.

393. Lim M., Straus S., Dale J., Fleisher T., Stetler-Stevenson M., Strober W., Sneller M.C., Puck J., Lenardo M., Elenitoba-Johnson K., Lin A., Raffeld M., Jaffe E. (1998). Pathological findings in human autoimmune lymphoproliferative syndrome. *Am J Pathol* **153**, 1541–50.

394. Maia D.M., Garwacki C.P. (1999). X-linked lymphoproliferative disease: pathology and diagnosis. *Pediatr Dev Pathol* **2**, 72–7.

395. Davi F., Delecluse H.J., Guiet P., Gabarre J., Fayon A., Gentilhomme O., Felman P., Bayle C., Audouin J., Bryon P.A., Diebold J., Raphael M. (1998). Burkitt-like lymphomas in AIDS patients: characterization within a series of 103 human immunodeficiency virus-associated non-Hodgkin's lymphomas. *J Clin Oncol* **16**, 3788–95.

396. Nador R.G., Cesarman E., Chadburn A., Dawson D.B., Ansari M.Q., J.S., Knowles D.M. (1996). Primary effusion lymphoma: a distinct clinicopathologic entity associated with the Kaposi's sarcoma-associated herpes virus. *Blood* **88**, 645–56.

397. Swerdlow S. (1997). Classification of the posttransplant lymphoproliferative disorders: from the past to the present. *Semin Diagn Pathol* **14**, 2–7.

398. Chadburn A., Cesarman E., Knowles D. (1997). Molecular pathology of post-transplantation lymphoproliferative disorders. *Semin Diagn Pathol* **14**, 15–26.

399. Pitman S., Huang Q., Zuppan C., Rowsell E., Cao J., Berdeja J., Weiss L., Wang J. (2006). Hodgkin lymphoma-like posttransplant lymphoproliferative disorder (HL-like PTLD) simulates monomorphic B-cell PTLD both clinically and pathologically. *Am J Surg Pathol* **30**, 470–6.

400. Chadburn A. (1997). Molecular pathology of the post-transplantation lymphoproliferative disorders. *Semin Diagn Pathol* **14**, 15–26.

401. Kamel O.W. (1997). Iatrogenic lymphoproliferative disorders in nontransplantation settings. *Semin Diagn Pathol* **14**, 27–34.

402. Kamel O.W., van de Rijn M., LeBrun D.P., Weiss L.M., Warnke R.A., Dorfman R.F. (1994). Lymphoproliferative lesions in patients with rheumatoid arthritis and dermatomyositis: frequency of Epstein-Barr virus and other features associated with immunosuppression. *Hum Pathol* **25**, 638–43.

403. Kamel O.W., Weiss L.M., van de R.M., Colby T.V., Kingma D.W., Jaffe E.S. (1996). Hodgkin's disease and lymphoproliferations resembling Hodgkin's disease in patients receiving long-term low-dose methotrexate therapy. *Am J Surg Pathol* **20**, 1279–87.

404. Abruzzo L., Rosales C., Medeiros L., Vega F., Luthra R., Manning J., Keating M., Jones D. Epstein-Barr virus-positive B-cell lymphoproliferative disorders arising in immunodeficient patients previously treated with fludarabine for low-grade B-cell neoplasms. *Am J Surg Pathol* **26**, 630–6.

405. Shimoyama Y., Oyama T., Asano N., Oshiro A., Suzuki R., Kagami Y., Morishima Y., Nakamura S. (2006). Senile Epstein-Barr virus-associated B-cell lymphoproliferative disorders: a mini review. *J Clin Exp Hematopathol* **46**, 1–4.

406. Oyama T., Ichimura K., Suzuki R., Suzumiya J., Ohshima K., Yatabe Y., Yokoi T., Kojima M., Kamiya Y., Tajo H., Kagami Y., Ogura M., Saito H., Morishima Y., Nakamura S. (2003). Senile EBV + B-cell lymphoproliferative disorders: a clinicopathologic study of 22 patients. *Am J Surg Pathol* **27**, 16–26.

407. Favara B.E., Feller A.C., Paulli M., Jaffe E., Weiss L.M., Arico M., Bucsky P., Egeler M., Elinder G., Gadner H., Gresik M., Henter J.-I., Imashuku S., Janka-Schaub G., Jaffe R., Ladisch S., Nezelof C. (1997). A contemporary classification

of histiocytic disorders. The WHO Committee on Histiocytic/Reticulum Cell Proliferations. Reclassification Working Group of the Histiocyte Society. *Med Pediatr Oncol* **29**, 157–66.

408. Kamel O.W., Gocke C.D., Kell D.L., Cleary M.L., Warnke R.A. (1995). True histiocytic lymphoma: a study of 12 cases based on current definition. *Leuk Lymphoma* **18**, 81–6.

409. Copie-Bergman C., Wotherspoon A.C., Norton A.J., Diss T.C., Isaacson P.G. (1998). True histiocytic lymphoma. A morphologic, immunohistochemical and molecular genetic study of 13 cases. *Am J Surg Pathol* **22**, 1386–92.

410. Bloomfield C.D., Arthur D.C., Frizzera G., Levine E.G., Peterson B.A., Gajl-Peczalska K.J. (1983). Nonrandom chromosome abnormalities in lymphoma. *Cancer Res* **43**, 2975–84.

411. Hanson C.A., Jaszcz W., Kersey J.H., Astorga M.G., Peterson B.A., Gajl-Peczalska K.J., Frizzera G. (1989). True histiocytic lymphoma: histopathologic, immuno-phenotypic and genotypic analysis. *Br J Haematol* **73**, 187–98.

412. Ralfkiaer E., Delsol G., O'Connor N.T.J., Brandktzaeg P., Brousset P., Vejlsgaard G.L., Mason D.Y. (1990). Malignant lymphomas of true histiocytic origin. A clinical, histological, immunophenotypic and genotypic study. *J Pathol* **160**, 9–17.

413. Vos J., Abbondanzo S.L., Barekman C., et al (2005). Histiocytic sarcoma: a study of five cases including the histiocyte marker CD163. *Mod Pathol* **18**, 693–704.

414. Nichols C.R., Roth B.J., Heerema N., Griep J., Tricot G. (1990). Hematologic neoplasia associated with primary mediastinal germ-cell tumors. *N Engl J Med* **322**, 1425–9.

415. Soria C., Orradre J.L., Garcia-Almagro D., Martinez B., Algara P., Piris M.A. (1992). True histiocytic lymphoma (monocytic sarcoma). *Am J Dermatol* **14**, 511–17.

416. Lieberman P.H., Jones C.R., Steinman R.M., Erlandson R.A., Smith J., Gee T., Huvos A., Garin-Chesa P., Filippa D.A., Urmacher C., Gangi M.D., Sperber M. (1996). Langerhans cell (eosinophilic) granulomatosis: a clinicopathologic study encompassing 50 years. *Am J Surg Pathol* **20**, 519–52.

417. The French Langerhans' Cell Histiocytosis Group (1996). A multicentre retro-spective survey of Langerhans' cell histiocytosis: 348 cases observed between 1983 and 1993. *Arch Dis Child* **75**, 17–24.

418. Howarth D.M., Gilchrist G.S., Mullan B.P., Wiseman G.A., Edmonson J.H., Schomberg P.J. (1999). Langerhans cell histiocytosis: diagnosis, natural history, management, and outcome. *Cancer* **85**, 2278–90.

419. Motoi M., Helbron D., Kaiserling E., Lennert K. (1980). Eosinophilic granuloma of lymph nodes: a variant of histiocytosis X. *Histopathology* **4**, 585–606.

420. Burns B.F., Colby T.V., Dorfman R.F. (1983). Langerhans' cell granulomatosis (histiocytosis X) associated with malignant lymphomas. *Am J Surg Pathol* **7**, 529–33.

421. Favara B.E., Steele A. (1997). Langerhans cell histiocytosis of lymph nodes: a morphological assessment of 43 biopsies. *Pediatr Pathol Lab Med* **17**, 769–87.

422. Willman C.L., Busque L., Griffith B.B., Favara B.E., McClain K.L., Duncan M.H., Gilliland D.G. (1994). Langerhans'-cell histiocytosis (histiocytosis X) – a clonal proliferative disease. *N Engl J Med* **331**, 154–60.

423. Geissmann F., Lepelletier Y., Fraitag S., Valladeau J., Bodemer C., Debre M., Leborgne M., Saeland S., Brousse N. (2001). Differentiation of Langerhans cells in Langerhans cell histiocytosis. *Blood* **97**, 1241–8.

424. Coppes-Zantinga A., Egeler R.M. (2002). The Langerhans cell histiocytosis X files revealed. *Br J Haematol* **116**, 3–9.

425. Favara B.E., Jaffe R. (1987). Pathology of Langerhans cell histiocytosis. *Hematol Oncol Clin North Am* **1**, 75–97.

426. Hage C., Willman C.L., Favara B.E., Isaacson P.G. (1993). Langerhans' cell histiocytosis (histiocytosis X): immunophenotype and growth fraction. *Hum Pathol* **24**, 840–5.

427. Egeler R.M., Favara B.E., van Meurs M., Laman J.D., Claassen E. (1999). Differential in situ cytokine profiles of Langerhans-like cells and T cells in Langerhans cell histiocytosis: abundant expression of cytokines relevant to disease and treatment. *Blood* **94**, 4195–201.

428. Pileri S.A., Grogan T.M., Banks P., Harris N., Campo E., Chan J.K., Favera R.D., Delsol G., De Wolf-Peeters C., Falini B., Gascoyne R., Gaulard P., Gatter K.C., Isaacson P.G., Jaffe E.S., Kluin P., Knowles D.M., Mason D.Y., Mori S., Muller-Hermelink H.K., Piris M.A., Ralfkiaer E., Stein H., Su I.J., Warnke R.A., Weiss L.M. (2002). Tumours of histiocytes and accessory dendritic cells: an immunohistochemical approach to classification from the International Lymphoma Study Group based on 61 cases. *Histopathology* **41**, 1–29.

429. Ben-Ezra J., Bailey A., Azumi N., Delsol G., Stroup R., Sheibani K., Rappaport H. (1991). Malignant histiocytosis X. A distinct clinicopathologic entity. *Cancer* **68**, 1050–60.

430. Wood C., Wood G.S., Deneau D.G., Oseroff A., Beckstead J.H., Malin J. (1984). Malignant histiocytosis X. Report of rapidly fatal case in an elderly man. *Cancer* **54**, 347–52.

431. Weiss L.M., Berry G.J., Dorfman R.F., Banks P., Kaiserling E., Curtis J., Rosai J., Warnke R.A. (1990). Spindle cell neoplasms of lymph nodes of probable reticulum cell lineage. True reticulum cell sarcoma? *Am J Surg Pathol* **14**, 405–14.

432. Pillay K., Solomon R., Daubenton J.D., Sinclair-Smith C.C. (2004). Interdigitating dendritic cell sarcoma: a report of four paediatric cases and review of the literature. *Histopathology* **44**, 283–91.

433. Vasef M.A., Zaatari G.S., Chan W.C., Sun N.C., Weiss L.M., Brynes R.K. (1995). Dendritic cell tumors associated with low-grade B-cell malignancies. Report of three cases. *Am J Clin Pathol* **104**, 696–701.

434. Chan J.K., Fletcher C.D., Nayler S.J., Cooper K. (1997). Follicular dendritic cell sarcoma. Clinicopathologic analysis of 17 cases suggesting a malignant potential higher than currently recognized. *Cancer* **79**, 294–313.

435. Becroft D.M.O., Dix M.R., Gillman J.C., MacGregor B.J.L., Shaw R.L. (1973). Benign sinus histiocytosis with massive lymphadenopathy: transient immunological defects in a child with mediastinal involvement. *J Clin Pathol* **26**, 463–9.

436. Monda L., Warnke R., Rosai J. (1986). A primary lymph node malignancy with features suggestive of dendritic reticulum cell differentiation. A report of 4 cases. *Am J Surg Pathol* **122**, 562–72.

437. Perez-Ordonez B., Erlandson R.A., Rosai J. (1996). Follicular dendritic cell tumor: report of 13 additional cases of a distinctive entity. *Am J Surg Pathol* **20**, 944–55.

438. Perez-Ordonez B., Rosai J. (1998). Follicular dendritic cell tumor: review of the entity. *Semin Diagn Pathol* **15**, 144–54.

439. Chan J.K.C., Fletcher C.D.M., Nayler S., Cooper K. (1997). Follicular dendritic cell sarcoma. Clinicopathologic analysis of 17 cases suggesting a malignant potential higher than currently recognized. *Cancer* **79**, 294–313.

440. Andriko J.W., Kaldjian E.P., Tsokos M., Abbondanzo S.L., Jaffe E.S. (1998). Reticulum cell neoplasms of lymph nodes: a clinicopathologic study of 11 cases with recognition of a new subtype derived from fibroblastic reticular cells. *Am J Surg Pathol* **22**, 1048–58.

441. Bastain B., Ott G., Muller-Deubert S. (1998). Primary cutaneous natural killer/ T-cell lymphoma. *Arch Dermatol* **134**, 109–11.

442. Matano S., Nakamura S., Annen Y., Hattori N., Kobayashi K., Kyoda K., Sugimoto T. (1999). Monomorphic agranular natural killer cell lymphoma/leukemia with no Epstein-Barr virus association. *Acta Haematol* **101**, 206–8.

443. Petrella T., Dalac S., Maynadie M., et al (1999). CD4+ CD56+ cutaneous neoplasms: a distinct hematological entity? Groupe Francais d'Etude des Lymphomes Cutanes (GFELC). *Am J Surg Pathol* **23**, 137–46.

444. Petrella T., Comeau M.R., Maynadie M., Couillault G., de Muret A., Maliszewski C.R., Dalac S., Durlach A., Galibert L. (2002). 'Agranular CD4+ CD56+ hematodermic neoplasm' (blastic NK-cell lymphoma) originates from a population of CD56+ precursor cells related to plasmacytoid monocytes. *Am J Surg Pathol* **26**, 852–62.

445. Urosevic M., Conrad C., Kamarashev J., et al (2005). CD4+CD56+ hematodermic neoplasms bear a plasmacytoid dendritic cell phenotype. *Hum Pathol* **36**, 1020–4.

446. O'Malley D. (2007). Benign extramedullary myeloid proliferations. *Mod Pathol* **20**, 405–15.

447. Neiman R.S., Barcos M., Berard C., Bonner H., Mann R., Rydell R.E., Bennett J.M. (1981). Granulocytic sarcoma: a clinicopathologic study of 61 biopsied cases. *Cancer* **48**, 1426–37.

448. Traweek S.T., Arber D.A., Rappaport H., Brynes R.K. (1993). Extramedullary myeloid cell tumors. An immunohistochemical and morphologic study of 28 cases. *Am J Surg Pathol* **17**, 1011–19.

449. Travis W.D., Li C.Y. (1988). Pathology of the lymph node and spleen in systemic mast cell disease. *Mod Pathol* **1**, 4–14.

INDEX

acute infectious mononucleosis, 39–42,
45, 115, 199, 222
differential diagnosis, 41
EBV association, 39, 173
gene rearrangement studies, 42
Age-Adjusted International Prognostic
Index, 169
aggressive NK-cell leukemia, 210,
211–212
ALPS. *see* autoimmune
lymphoproliferative syndrome
(ALPS)
anaplastic large-cell lymphoma
ALK-negative type, 197–200
differential diagnosis, 199–200
immunophenotype 197
ALK-positive type, 200–205
differential diagnosis, 203–205
non-Hodgkin association, 237
angiofollicular hyperplasia w/
eosinophilia, 20
angioimmunoblastic T-cell lymphoma,
187–190
differential diagnosis, 189–190
gene rearrangement studies, 188, 190
immunohistochemical studies, 188
angiomyolipoma, 91
angiomyomatous hamartoma, 93–95
angiosarcoma
high-grade, 100
low-grade (hemangioendothelioma),
97–98
lymph node metastases, 89
Association of the Directors of Anatomic
and Surgical Pathology (ADASP)
lymph node specimen
recommendations, 2
ataxia telangiectasia, 128, 220, 222
atypical mycobacterial infection, 67–68,
69
autoimmune lymphoproliferative
syndrome (ALPS), 223–224

bacillary angiomatosis, 78–79
Bartonella henselae, 71, 73, 78
B-cell lymphomas. *see also* diffuse
large-B-cell lymphoma
B-cell non-Hodgkin
classical Hodgkin, composite,
216–217
sequential Hodgkin, 217

extranodal marginal B-cell lymphoma,
142
histiocyte-rich-B-cell lymphoma, 174
benign epithelial inclusions, 82–84
benign lymphadenopathies. *see*
lymphadenopathies, benign
benign mammary epithelial inclusions,
83
biopsies, types of, 1
blastic NK-cell lymphoma, 248
blood vessels, of lymph nodes, 5
breast carcinoma, 88
breast inclusions, 82–84
British National Lymphoma
Investigation, 107
Burkitt lymphoma, 175–181
cytologic variants, 177–179
differential diagnosis, 180
endemic form, 176
genetic hallmark, 179–180
and HIV infection, 224–225
immunophenotype, 179
sporadic form, 176
prognostic factors, 180
transitional form, 176

carcinoma, 84–86
breast carcinoma, 88
lymphoepithelioma-like carcinomas,
111
metastasis/micrometastasis/isolated
tumor cells, 86
metastatic lobular carcinoma, 138
metastatic thyroid carcinoma, 83
nasopharyngeal, undifferentiated,
111
noncaseating granuloma association, 67
primary neuroendocrine carcinomas,
84
spindled metastatic carcinoma, 89, 246
squamous carcinoma, 83
Castleman disease, 25–32
hyaline-vascular cell type, 25, 26
multicentric Castleman disease, 25, 30,
31
multicentric plasma cell type, 25
symptoms of, 29, 30
treatments for, 30
vascular lesion with, 95–97
cat scratch lymphadenitis, 71–73 *see also*
Bartonella henselae

vs. Kikuchi histiocytic necrotizing
lymphadenitis, 73
chemotherapy. *see also* treatment
for anaplastic large-cell lymphoma/
ALK-positive type, 200
for Burkitt lymphoma, 180
for Castleman disease, 30
for extranodal NK/T-cell lymphoma,
nasal type, 212
for histiocytic sarcoma, 234
for mantle cell lymphoma, 156
for nodal marginal zone B-cell
lymphoma, 138
for posttransplantation
lymphoproliferative disorders,
228
for precursor B-lymphoblastic
lymphoma/leukemia, 181
for precursor T-lymphoblastic
lymphoma/leukemia, 183
Chlamydia trachomatis, 73
chronic lymphocytic leukemia/small
lymphocytic lymphoma, 125–130
classical Hodgkin lymphoma, 101–115
B-cell non-Hodgkin composite,
216–217
diagnosis, 102–111
histologic appearance, 105–108
HIV-associated malignant lymphoma,
225
immunohistochemical studies,
110–111
molecular studies/differential diagnosis,
111–115
pathoetiologies of, 101
subtypes, 105–110
symptoms, 102
treatment, 102
clear cell sarcoma, 89
composite lymphomas, 216–219
classical Hodgkin
B-cell non-Hodgkin, 216–217
T-cell lymphoma, 219
definition of, 216
gray-zone lymphoma, 217–218
sequential Hodgkin/B-cell lymphoma,
217
cortex, of lymph nodes, primary/
secondary follicles, 5
Crow-Fukase disease (POEMS
syndrome), 30

cytomegalovirus (CMV) lymphadenitis, 40, 42–43
cytophagocytosis/hemophagocytosis, in histiocytic sarcoma, 236

dermatopathic lymphadenitis, 45–48, 206, 207
differential diagnosis
    of acute infectious mononucleosis, 41
    of aging-related immunosuppression, 233
    of anaplastic large-cell lymphoma
        ALK-negative type, 199–200
        ALK-positive type, 203–205
    of angioimmunoblastic T-cell lymphoma, 189–190
    of bacillary angiomatosis, 79
    of Burkitt lymphoma, 180
    of carcinoma/melanoma, 57
    of cat scratch lymphadenitis, 73
    of chronic lymphocytic leukemia/small lymphocytic lymphoma, 129
    of classical Hodgkin lymphoma, 111–115
    of CMV lymphadenitis, 43
    of dermatopathic lymphadenitis, 47
    of diffuse large-B-cell lymphoma, 172–173
    of fibroblastic reticulum cell neoplasm, 249
    of follicular dendritic cell sarcoma, 246
    of follicular lymphoma, 154
    of hairy cell leukemia, 137
    of histiocytic sarcoma, 234–237
    of HIV-associated florid follicular hyperplasia, 33
    of HIV-related benign lymphadenopathy, 33
    of immunoglobulin deposition lymphadenopathy, 80
    of interdigitating dendritic cell sarcoma, 243–244
    of Kikuchi histiocytic necrotizing lymphadenitis, 63
    of Kikuchi necrotizing histiocytic lymphadenitis, 63
    of Langerhans cell histiocytosis, 240–241
    of Langerhans cell sarcoma, 241
    of lymphoplasmacytic lymphoma, 132
    of mantle cell lymphoma, 161
    of mast cell neoplasia, 256
    of monocytoid B-cell hyperplasia, 48
    of multicentric Castleman disease, 31
    of myeloid sarcoma, 253
    of myofibroblastoma, 90
    of nodular lymphocyte-predominant Hodgkin lymphoma, 119–120
    of non-Hodgkin lymphoma, 63
    of peripheral T-cell lymphoma, 208
        unspecified, 194
    of plasmacytoma, 135
    of precursor B-lymphoblastic lymphoma/leukemia, 182–183
    of precursor T-lymphoblastic lymphoma/leukemia, 186–187
    of proteinaceous lymphadenopathy, 80
    of reactive paracortical hyperplasia, 38
    of Rosai-Dorfman disease, 56
    of splenic marginal zone lymphoma, involving lymph nodes and primary nodal marginal zone lymphoma, splenic type, 145
    of T-cell/histiocyte-rich-B-cell lymphoma, 174
    of Whipple lymphadenopathy, 51
diffuse large-B-cell lymphoma, 161–175, 169
    age range/gender dominance, 162
    associated HIV lymphomas, 225
    differential diagnosis, 172–173
    immunohistochemical studies, 168, 172
    pathogenesis, 162
    prognostic factors, 169
    T-cell/histiocyte-rich B-cell variant, 165
    vs. mantle cell lymphoma variants, 174
    vs. reactive paracortical hyperplasia, 173

effusion lymphoma, primary, 226–227
endometriosis, 82
enteropathy-associated T-cell lymphoma, 213
epithelial lesions, 82–86
    benign epithelial inclusions, 82–84
    carcinoma, 84–86
epithelioid hemangioma, 95
    vs. Kimura disease, 95
epithelioid sarcoma, 89
Epstein Barr Virus (EBV), 39–42
    associations
        acute infectious mononucleosis, 39, 173
        aggressive NK-cell leukemia, 211
        aging-related immunosuppression, 233
        angioimmunoblastic T-cell lymphoma, 187
        B-cell lymphoproliferative disorders, 231
        Burkitt lymphoma, 175
        classical Hodgkin lymphoma, 101, 108, 111
        CMV lymphadenitis, 42–43
        diffuse large B-cell lymphoma, 161
        extranodal NK/T-cell lymphoma, nasal type, 212
        germinotropic lymphoproliferative disorder, 156
        hemophagocytic lymphohistiocytosis, 58
        HIV malignant lymphoma, 225
        methotrexate-associated lymphoproliferative disorders, 231
        monocytoid B-cell hyperplasia, 48
        non-Hodgkin lymphoma, 123
        NK/T-cell lymphoma, 59
        posttransplantation lymphoproliferative disorders, 228
excisional lymph node biopsies, 1
extramedullary hematopoiesis, 250–251
extranodal marginal B-cell lymphoma of mucosa-associated lymphoid tissue (MALT) involving lymph nodes, 142
extranodal NK/T-cell lymphoma, nasal type, 212

familial hemophagocytic lymphohistiocytosis, 58
fibroblastic reticulum cell neoplasm, 247–249
fibroblastic reticulum cells, 5
fine-needle aspiration biopsies, 1
florid follicular hyperplasia, 33
flow cytometry, 1
    interpretation pitfalls, 2
    supplemental to immunohistochemical analysis, 2
fludarabine-associated lymphoproliferative disorders, 231
fluorescence in situ hybridization (FISH) studies, 1
    of Burkitt lymphoma, 179, 180
    of chronic lymphocytic leukemia/small lymphocytic lymphoma, 127
    of mantle cell lymphoma, 161
    of nodular lymphocyte-predominant Hodgkin lymphoma, 119
    of plasmacytoma, 134
follicles
    primary/secondary follicles, 5
follicular dendritic cell sarcoma, 244–246
follicular lymphoma, 145–156
    vs. reactive follicular hyperplasia, 15, 173
        gene rearrangement studies, 17
        immunohistological studies, 15
fungal lymphadenitis, 70

gene rearrangement studies
    for acute infectious mononucleosis, 42
    for angioimmunoblastic T-cell lymphoma, 189, 190
    for diffuse large-B-cell lymphoma, 174
    for peripheral T-cell lymphoma, unspecified, 194
    reactive vs. neoplastic follicular proliferations, 17
germinal centers
    progressive transformation of, 36–37

vascularization of, in Kimura disease, 20
glandular inclusions, 82
glomeruloid hemangioma, 31
granulotomatous necrotizing lymphadenitis, 64
gray-zone lymphoma, 217–218

hairy cell leukemia, 135–137
Hand-Schüller-Christian disease (multifocal unisystem disease), 238
hemangioendothelioma (low-grade angiosarcoma), 97–98
hematodermic neoplasm, 248
hemophagocytic lymphohistiocytosis, 58–59
  symptoms, 58
hemophagocytosis, in histiocytic sarcoma, 236
hepatosplenic T-cell lymphoma, 213–215
herpes simplex lymphadenitis, 43–44
high-grade angiosarcoma, 100
highly-active antiretroviral therapy (HAART)
  for Castleman disease, 30
histiocytic/dendritic cell neoplasms, 234–249
  fibroblastic reticulum cell neoplasm, 247–249
  follicular dendritic cell sarcoma, 244–246
  histiocytic sarcoma, 234–237
  interdigitating dendritic cell sarcoma, 241–244
  Langerhans cell histiocytosis, 237–241
  Langerhans cell sarcoma, 241
histiocytosis, nonspecific sinus, 48
histiocytosis X. see Langerhans cell histiocytosis
Hodgkin lymphoma, 31, 41, 101–121
  classical, 101–115
    B-cell non-Hodgkin composite, 216–217
    diagnosis, 102–111
    histologic appearance, 105–108
    HIV-associated malignant lymphoma, 225
    identical vs. dizygotic twins, concordance rate, 101
    immunohistochemical studies, 110–111
    molecular studies/differential diagnosis, 111–115
    pathoetiologies of, 101
    presentation, 102
    subtypes, 105–110
    treatment, 102
  nodular-lymphocyte-predominant, 115–121

association with progressive transformation of germinal centers, 36
    complications of, 121
    differential diagnosis, 119–120
    hallmarks, 117
    immunohistochemical studies, 117–119
    molecular biologic studies, 116
  sequential
    composite with B-cell lymphoma, 217
    vs. progressive transformation of germinal centers, 37
    vs. reactive paracortical hyperplasia, 38
    vs. T-cell/histiocyte-rich B-cell lymphoma, 175
human immunodeficiency virus (HIV), 22
  associated malignant lymphomas, 224–230
    Burkitt lymphoma, 224–225
    classical Hodgkin lymphoma, 225
    diffuse large B-cell lymphoma, 225
    EBV, 225
    plasmablastic lymphoma, 226
    primary effusion lymphoma, 226–227
  and Castleman disease, 30
  HIV-related benign lymphadenopathy, 32–35
  and Kaposi sarcoma, 98
  and lymphoepithelial cysts, 83
  risk factors of, 32–33
hyaline-vascular type Castleman disease, 25, 26
hyper-IgM syndrome, 222–223
hyperplasias
  drug-induced reactive paracortical hyperplasia, 38–39
  florid follicular hyperplasia, 33
  monocytoid B-cell hyperplasia, 48–51
  nonspecific reactive hyperplasia, 230
  postvaccinal reactive paracortical hyperplasia, 44
  reactive follicular hyperplasia, 15–17
  reactive paracortical hyperplasia, 38–39
  reactive plasmacytic hyperplasia, 228–229
  sinus hyperplasia, 48

immunodeficiency-associated lymphoproliferative disorders, 220–233
  association with aging, 231–233
  immunosuppression associated treatment of other diseases, 231–233
    fludarabine-associated lymphoproliferative disorders, 231

methotrexate-associated lymphoproliferative disorders, 231
  primary immunodeficiency syndromes, 220–224
    ALPS, 223–224
    ataxia telangiectasia, 222
    HIV-associated malignant lymphomas, 224–230
    hyper-IgM syndrome, 222–223
    posttransplantation lymphoproliferative disorders, 228–230
    Wiskott-Aldrich syndrome, 221–222
    X-linked lymphoproliferative disorder, 222
immunoglobulin deposition lymphadenopathy, 80–81
  differential diagnosis, 80
immunophenotypic studies
  of aggressive NK-cell leukemia, 212
  of angioimmunoblastic T-cell lymphoma, 189
  of classical Hodgkin lymphoma, 110–111
  of cytospin preparations, 1
  of dermatopathic lymphadenitis, 47
  of diffuse large B-cell lymphoma, 168, 172
  of enteropathy-associated T-cell lymphoma, 213
  of extranodal NK/T-cell lymphoma, nasal type, 212
  of hairy cell leukemia, 136
  of histiocytic sarcoma, 236
  of mast cell neoplasia, 255
  of mycosis fungoides, 206
  of myeloid sarcoma, 253
  of nodal marginal zone B-cell lymphoma, 140
  of nodular lymphocyte-predominant Hodgkin lymphoma, 117–119
  of peripheral T-cell lymphoma, unspecified, 196
  of plasmacytoma, 133
  of precursor B-lymphoblastic lymphoma/leukemia, 181–182
  of precursor T-lymphoblastic lymphoma/leukemia, 183–185
  of splenic marginal zone lymphoma involving lymph nodes/primary nodal marginal zone lymphoma of splenic type, 145
  of subcutaneous panniculitis-like T-cell lymphoma, 215
  of T-cell prolymphocytic leukemia, 209
immunosuppression associated treatment of other diseases, 231–233

fludarabine-associated
lymphoproliferative disorders,
231
methotrexate-associated
lymphoproliferative disorders,
231
immunosuppression associated with
aging, 231–233
inclusions
benign epithelial inclusions, 82–84
benign mammary epithelial inclusions,
82–83
benign thyroid inclusions, 83
breast inclusions, 82
endometrial stroma association, 82
glandular inclusions, 82
herpetic, with herpetic simplex
lymphadenitis, 43
intracytoplasmic (Russell bodies), 133
intranuclear eosinophilic, 44
intranuclear PAS-positive inclusions,
131
Mullerian inclusions, 82
nuclear pseudoinclusions, 247
salivary gland inclusions, 82
thyroid inclusions, 82
viral, with cytomegaly, 43
inflammatory pseudotumor, 75–76
differential diagnosis, 76
inguinal lymphadenopathy, 22, 143
interdigitating dendritic cell sarcoma,
241–244
International Prognostic Index, 169
intestinal lipodystrophy (Whipple
lymphadenopathy), 51
intranodal hemorrhagic spindle-cell
tumor, w/amianthoid fibers, 90

Kaposi sarcoma, 31, 35, 98–100
associations
HIV infection, 98
multicentric Castleman disease, 98
and bacillary angiomatosis, 79
and inflammatory pseudotumors, 76
vs. vascular transformation of lymph
node sinuses, 77
Kawasaki disease, 65–66
symptoms of, 65
treatment of, 65
Kikuchi histiocytic necrotizing
lymphadenitis, 61–64
differential diagnosis, 63
symptoms, 61
vs. cat scratch lymphadenitis, 73
Kimura disease, 19–21
treatment of, 20
vs. angiofollicular hyperplasia w/
eosinophilia, 20
vs. epithelioid hemangioma, 95

Langerhans cell histiocytosis, 237–241

Langerhans cell sarcoma, 241
leiomyosarcoma, 89
lepromatous lymphadenitis, 69
Letterer-Siwe disease (multifocal,
multisystem disease), 238
leukemias
adult T-cell leukemia, 208–209
aggressive NK-cell leukemia, 211–212
chronic lymphocytic leukemia, 125–130
hairy cell leukemia, 135–137
precursor B-lymphoblastic lymphoma/
leukemia, 181–183
precursor T-lymphoblastic lymphoma/
leukemia, 183–187
T-cell large granular lymphocytic
leukemia, 211
T-cell prolymphocytic leukemia,
209–210
lipomatosis, 89
lymphadenitis
cat scratch, 71–73
CMV, 42–43
dermatopathic, 45–48
lymphadenopathies, benign, 13–81
autoimmune disease, 18–19
bacillary angiomatosis, 78–79
Castleman disease, 25–32
due to connective tissue alteration, 73
due to endogenous material deposition,
53
due to exogenous material deposition,
51–52
germinal centers, progressive
transformation of, 36–37
hemophagocytic lymphohistiocytosis,
58–59
HIV-related, 32–35
immunoglobulin deposition
lymphadenopathy, 80–81
w/infectious primary granulomatous
pattern, 67–73
atypical mycobacterial infection, 69
cat scratch lymphadenitis, 71–73
fungal lymphadenitis, 70
lepromatous lymphadenitis, 69
lymphogranuloma venereum, 73
tuberculosis, 69
yersinial lymphadenitis, 73
inflammatory pseudotumors, 75–76
interstitial substance deposition, 79
Kawasaki disease, 65–66
Kikuchi histiocytic necrotizing
lymphadenitis, 61–64
Kimura disease, 19–21
lymphadenitis
CMV, 42–43
dermatopathic, 45–48
herpes simplex, 43–44
monocytoid B-cell hyperplasia, 48–51
mononucleosis, acute infectious, 39–42
with necrosis

complete, 59–61
extensive, 59
w/noninfectious primary
granulomatous pattern, 66–73
granulomatous inflammation in
malignant neoplasms, 67
sarcoidosis, 67–69
nonspecific sinus histiocytosis, 48
paracortical hyperplasia, reactive, 38–39
drug-induced, 44–45
postvaccinal, 44
pneumocytis lymphadenitis, 81
proteinaceous lymphadenopathy, 79–80
reactive follicular hyperplasia, 15–17
Rosai-Dorfman disease, 53–57
sinuses
sinus hyperplasia, 48
vascular transformation of, 76–78
syphilis, 22
systemic lupus erythematosus, 64–65
toxoplasmosis, 22–23
Whipple lymphadenopathy, 51
lymphangiomyomatosis, 91
lymph node dissections, 1
lymph nodes (normal)
structure/cells, 5–12
B-cells, 11–12
blood vessels, 5
cortex: primary/secondary follicles, 5
fibroblastic reticulum cells, 5
mantle zone, 5
paracortical zone, 7–10
sinuses, 10
T-cells, 11–12
Warthin-Finkeldey cells, 7
trafficking/immune response, 10–12
tumorlike lesions of, 89–100
lymph node specimens, ADASP
recommendations for, 2
lymphocyte-predominant Hodgkin
lymphoma, 36, 37, 175
lymphoepithelial cysts, 83
lymphoepithelioma-like carcinomas, 111
lymphogranuloma venereum, 73 see also
Chlamydia trachomatis
lymphoplasmacytic lymphoma, 130–133

mantle cell lymphoma, 156–161, 174
mantle zone, of lymph nodes, 5
mast cell neoplasia, 253–256
Merkel cells, with primary
neuroendocrine carcinoma, 84
metastatic lobular carcinoma, 137
metastatic neoplasm
assessment/treatment, 1
metastatic thyroid carcinoma, 83
methotrexate-associated
lymphoproliferative disorders, 231
monocytoid B-cell hyperplasia, 48–51, 71
mononucleosis, acute infectious, 39–42
Mullerian inclusions, 82

multicentric Castleman disease, 25, 30
  differential diagnosis of, 31
  and Kaposi sarcoma, 98
  risk factors of, 31
multifocal, multisystem disease
        (Letterer-Siwe disease), 238
multifocal unisystem disease (Hand-
        Schüller-Christian disease), 238
mycobacterial infection, atypical, 69
Mycobacterium avium, 51
mycosis fungoides/Sezary syndrome,
        205–208
myeloid/mast cell neoplasms, 250–256
        extramedullary hematopoiesis,
              250–251
        mast cell neoplasia, 253–256
        myeloid sarcoma, 251–253
myofibroblastoma, palisaded, 90

nasopharyngeal carcinoma,
        undifferentiated, 111
needle core biopsies, 1
neuroendocrine carcinoma (primary),
        with Merkel cells, 84
nevomelanocytic lesions, 86–88
NK-cell leukemia, aggressive, 211–212
NK/T-cell lymphoma, 59
NK/T-cell lymphoma, extranodal/nasal
        type, 212
nodal angiomatosis, 79
nodular-lymphocyte-predominant
        Hodgkin lymphoma, 115–121
  complications of, 121
  FISH studies of, 119
  hallmarks, 117
  immunohistochemical studies,
        117–119
  molecular biologic studies, 116
non-Hodgkin lymphoma, 31, 41
  definition, 123
  differential diagnosis, 63
  presentation, 123
non-Hodgkin lymphoma, types, 123–215
  adult T-cell leukemia/lymphoma,
        208–209
  aggressive NK-cell leukemia, 211–212
  anaplastic large-cell
        ALK-negative type, 197–200
        ALK-positive type, 200–205
  angioimmunoblastic T-cell lymphoma,
        187–190
  Burkitt lymphoma, 175–181
  chronic lymphocytic leukemia/small
        lymphocytic lymphoma, 125–130
  diffuse large B-cell lymphoma, 161–175
  enteropathy-associated T-cell
        lymphoma, 213
  extranodal marginal B-cell lymphoma
        of mucosa-associated lymphoid
        tissue involving lymph nodes,
        142

extranodal NK/T-cell lymphoma, nasal
        type, 212
  follicular lymphoma, 145–156
  hairy cell leukemia, 135–137
  hepatosplenic T-cell lymphoma, 213–
        215
  lymphoplasmacytic lymphoma, 130–
        133
  mantle cell lymphoma, 156–161
  mature T-cell/NK-cell neoplasms, 187
  mycosis fungoides/Sezary syndrome,
        205–208
  other mature T-/NK-cell-neoplasms,
        210
  peripheral T-cell lymphoma,
        unspecified, 190–196
  plasmacytoma, 133–135
  precursor B-lymphoblastic lymphoma/
        leukemia, 181–183
  precursor T-lymphoblastic lymphoma/
        leukemia, 183–187
  splenic marginal zone, involving lymph
        nodes and primary nodal
        marginal zone lymphoma,
        splenic type, 143–145
  subcutaneous panniculitis-like T-cell
        lymphoma, 215
  T-cell large granular lymphocytic
        leukemia, 211
  T-cell prolymphocytic leukemia,
        209–210
nonspecific reactive hyperplasia, 230
nonspecific sinus histiocytosis, 48

occult primary tumors, 84
oculocutaneous telangiectasia, 222

palisaded myofibroblastoma, 90
paracortical hyperplasia
        and ALPS, 223
        postvaccinal reactive, 44
        reactive, 38, 38–39, 173
paracortical zone, of lymph nodes,
        7–10
        and B-cell response, 11–12
perilymphadenitis, 22
peripheral T-cell lymphoma, 27, 174
peripheral T-cell lymphoma, unspecified,
        190–196
        differential diagnosis, 194
        histologic variants, 192–193
plasmablastic lymphoma, 226
plasmacytic hyperplasia, reactive,
        228–229, 230
plasmacytoma, 31, 133–135
Pneumocytis carinii, 81
POEMS syndrome (Crow-Fukase
        disease)
  and Castleman disease, 30
polymerase chain reaction (PCR)
        studies, 2

polymorphic posttransplantation
        lymphoproliferative disorders,
        229–230
posttransplantation lymphoproliferative
        disorders, 228–230
postvaccinal reactive paracortical
        hyperplasia, 44
precursor B-lymphoblastic lymphoma/
        leukemia, 181–183
        differential diagnosis, 182–183
        immunophenotyping studies, 181–182
precursor plasmacytoid dendritic cell
        neoplasm, 248
precursor T-lymphoblastic lymphoma/
        leukemia, 183–187
        differential diagnosis, 186–187
        immunophenotyping studies, 184–186
        prognostic factors, adverse, 186
primary follicles, 5
prognostic factors
        of Burkitt lymphoma, 180
        of diffuse large-B-cell lymphoma, 169
        of Langerhans cell histiocytosis, 240
        of precursor T-lymphoblastic
              lymphoma/leukemia, 186
proteinaceous lymphadenopathy, 79–80
        differential diagnosis, 80
        symptoms of, 79
pseudotumor, inflammatory, 69, 75–76,
        78

reactive follicular hyperplasia, 15–17
        and autoimmune disease, 18
        and Kimura disease, 20
        vs. follicular lymphoma, 15, 173
              gene rearrangement studies, 17
              immunohistological studies, 15
reactive lymphadenopathies. *see*
        lymphadenopathies, reactive
reactive paracortical hyperplasia, 38–39
        differential diagnosis of, 38
        vs. diffuse large-B-cell lymphoma, 173
        vs. Hodgkin lymphoma, 38
reactive plasmacytic hyperplasia,
        228–229, 230
rhabdomyosarcoma, 89
risk factors
        of HIV infection, 32–33
        for multicentric Castleman disease, 31
Rosai-Dorfman disease, 56, 53–57, 237,
        241

salivary gland inclusions, 82
sarcoidosis, 67–69
schwannoma, benign, 90
secondary follicles, 5
senile EBV-positive
        lymphoproliferations, 231
sentinel lymph node biopsies, 1
        for malignant lymphoma, 88
sequential Hodgkin lymphoma

composite with B-cell lymphoma, 217
Sezary syndrome, 205–208
sinuses, of lymph nodes, 10
    vs. Kaposi sarcoma, 78
sinus histiocytosis, nonspecific, 48
sinus hyperplasia, 48
Sjögren syndrome, 19, 83
small lymphocytic lymphoma, 125–130
smooth muscle neoplasms, 90–93
solitary eosinophilic disease (solitary
    eosinophilic granuloma), 238
Southern blot studies, 2
specimens/studies, 1–3
spindle-cell carcinoma, 89, 246
Spitz nevi, 87
splenectomy
    for Castleman disease, 30
splenic marginal zone lymphoma,
    involving lymph nodes and
    primary nodal marginal zone
    lymphoma, splenic type,
    143–145
squamous carcinoma, 83
stroma, endometrial, 82
stromal tumors/tumorlike lesions,
    89–100
    angiomyomatous hamartoma, 93–95
    angiosarcoma (high-grade), 100
    epithelioid hemangioma, 95
    hemangioendothelioma, 97–98
    lipomatosis, 89
    palisaded myofibroblastoma, 90
    smooth muscle neoplasms, 90–93
    vascular lesion w/Castleman disease,
    95–97
    vascular tumors/tumorlike lesions, 93
symptoms
    of Castleman disease, 29, 30
    of classical Hodgkin lymphoma, 102
    of hemophagocytic
    lymphohistiocytosis, 58
    of Kawasaki disease, 65
    of Kikuchi histiocytic necrotizing
    lymphadenitis, 61
    of proteinaceous lymphadenopathy, 79

of Whipple lymphadenopathy, 51
synovial sarcoma, 89
syphilis, 22
systemic lupus erythematosus, 64, 64–65

T-cell lymphomas
    angioimmunoblastic T-cell lymphoma,
    187–190
    enteropathy-associated T-cell
    lymphoma, 213
    extranodal NK/T-cell lymphoma, nasal
    type, 212
    peripheral T-cell lymphoma, 174
    peripheral T-cell lymphoma,
    unspecified, 190–196
    subcutaneous panniculitis-like T-cell
    lymphoma, 215
    T-cell large granular lymphocytic
    leukemia, 211
    T-cell/NK-cell neoplasms, 187
    T-cell prolymphocytic leukemia,
    209–210
T-cell/histiocyte-rich-B-cell lymphoma,
    174
thyroid inclusions, 82
Toxoplasma gondii parasite, 22
toxoplasmosis, 22–23
treatment. *see also* chemotherapy
    of B-cell lymphoma, 218
    of Castleman disease, 30
    of chronic lymphocytic leukemia/small
    lymphocytic lymphoma, 125
    of classical Hodgkin lymphoma, 102
    of extramedullary hematopoiesis, 250
    of follicular dendritic cell sarcoma, 244
    of Kawasaki disease, 65
    of Kimura disease, 20
    of metastatic neoplasm, 1
    of peripheral T-cell lymphoma,
    unspecified, 190
    of posttransplantation
    lymphoproliferative disorders,
    228
    of smooth muscle neoplasm, 91–92
    of Whipple lymphadenopathy, 51

tuberculosis, 69

unifocal disease (solitary eosinophilic
    granuloma), 238

vascular lesions
    and angiomyomatous hamartoma, 93
    in lymph nodes, 93
    and primary stromal tumors, 89
    w/Castleman disease, 95–97
VDRL/RPR screening tests, for syphilis,
    22

Warthin-Finkeldey cells, 7, 44
Warthin tumors, 83
Whipple lymphadenopathy (intestinal
    lipodystrophy), 51
    differential diagnosis, 51
    symptoms, 51
    treatment, 51
Wiskott-Aldrich syndrome, 221–222
World Health Organization (WHO),
    classifications
    chronic lymphocytic leukemia/small
    lymphocytic lymphoma, 125
    diffuse large B-cell lymphoma, 169
    follicular lymphoma, 145, 148
    Hodgkin lymphoma, 101, 105–110
    of mast cell neoplasia, 253
    mature T-cell/NK-cell neoplasms,
    187
    non-Hodgkin lymphoma, 123
    other mature T-cell/NK-cell neoplasms,
    210
    peripheral T-cell lymphoma,
    unspecified, 190, 192–193
    posttransplant lymphoproliferative
    disorders, 228

X-linked lymphoproliferative disorder,
    222

Yersinia enterocolitica, 73
yersinial lymphadenitis, 73
Yersinia pseudotuberculosis, 73